SLOW SEX

"Like everything else in this fast-forward world, our sex lives have been infected by the virus of hurry. *Slow Sex* is the perfect antidote. With warmth and wisdom, Diana Richardson shows how slowing down in the bedroom can bring us better sex, better relationships, and a better world. What are you waiting for? The time has come to unleash your inner tortoise in the bedroom!"

CARL HONORÉ, AUTHOR OF *IN PRAISE OF SLOWNESS*

"How rare it is for a book to appear about sex and sensuality with a truly fresh and innovative approach. Diana Richardson has crafted a masterpiece that is warm, evocative, timely, and accessible to everyone. Her wise and inviting style will welcome you into a fascinating new world where your experience of sexuality will be forever changed. If you've wanted just one book that could give you the most simple and powerful access into the ancient, beautiful world of Tantra, here it is . . ."

MARC DAVID, AUTHOR OF *THE SLOW DOWN DIET* AND FOUNDER OF THE INSTITUTE FOR THE PSYCHOLOGY OF EATING

SLOW SEX

THE PATH TO FULFILLING AND SUSTAINABLE SEXUALITY

DIANA RICHARDSON

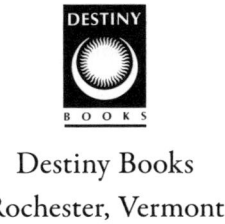

Destiny Books
Rochester, Vermont

Destiny Books
One Park Street
Rochester, Vermont 05767
www.DestinyBooks.com

Destiny Books is a division of Inner Traditions International

Copyright © 2011 by Diana Richardson
Art in chapters 4 and 5 copyright © 2004, 2010, 2011 by Diana Richardson
Art in chapter 10 copyright © 2011 by Gabriel Tempesta

All rights reserved. No part of this book may be reproduced or utilized in any form or by any means, electronic or mechanical, including photocopying, recording, or by any information storage and retrieval system, without permission in writing from the publisher.

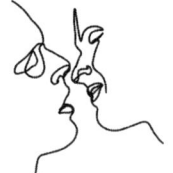

Volume III
of
Tantric Sex for Lovers
Boxed Set

Slow Sex

Printed and bound in India by Replika Press Pvt. Ltd.

10　9　8　7　6　5　4　3　2　1

Text design and layout by Virginia Scott Bowman
This book was typeset in Garamond Premier Pro with Perpetua, Avant Garde,
　　Posterama Text, and Swiss used as display typefaces
Artwork in chapters 4 and 5 prepared by Alfredo Hernando, Madrid, Spain.
Artwork in chapter 10 (with the exception of fig. 10.3) prepared by Gabriel
　　Tempesta, Wolcott, Vermont, **www.tempestart.homestead.com**

To send correspondence to the author of this book, mail a first-class letter to the author c/o Inner Traditions • Bear & Company, One Park Street, Rochester, VT 05767, and we will forward the communication or contact the author directly at **www.livinglove.com** or **info@livinglove.com**.

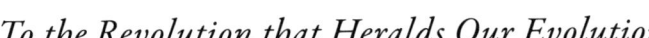

To the Revolution that Heralds Our Evolution

Recently, I invited my longest-standing erotic partner to read Diana's book on conscious sex. Our "love connection" had been dead for more than twenty years. No ecstatic experience left, dead, dead, dead.

We naturally, effortlessly started following the instructions in the book, inspired and transported by something in it, something new and loving, some energy and wisdom emanating from its pages. Lo and behold, we spent the next two weeks in five- to nine-hour sessions, reaching a state so beautiful I wanted to stay there forever.

I had never understood why people called sex "making love" and here we were making, within ourselves and between us, a tangible love energy. My intelligent penis "knew" when my partner's vagina was open. It knew to stay cool, in that receptive state where *it* was guiding me, *it* knew when to penetrate and how. My heart was in joy, my whole body felt touched by her vagina. We remained for hours in this glow, losing all sense of time. A few times I felt her heart touching my penis from very deep in the vagina. She had not self-lubricated in decades; she had lost contact with the vagina, now *it* became alive. At one point she said, glowing in deep appreciation and love: "I feel like a woman for the first time in my life."

CONTENTS

	Acknowledgments	viii
	Introduction: Curing the Speed Disease	1
1	Slow Sex: A Physical and Spiritual Revolution	5
2	The Sexual Power of Relaxation	11
3	The Sexual Power of Awareness	22
4	The Sexual Power of Quality	33
5	The Sexual Power of Rhythm	54
6	The Sexual Power of Pleasure	65
7	The Sexual Power of Thought	71
8	The Sexual Power of the Sacred	78
9	The Sexual Power of the Story	95
10	Your Personal Slow Sex Practice	99
	Appendix: True Male and Female Qualities versus Conditioned Distortions	163
	Books and Resources	166

ACKNOWLEDGMENTS

My heartfelt thanks to Marc David, whose book *The Slow Down Diet* arrived in my life as if by divine hand to become an inspiration far beyond anything I had ever anticipated. I am very grateful for his generosity in allowing me to use his words, which appear as short extracts throughout this book.

I also wish to extend my deepest gratitude to the couples I have met in my workshops over the years for their trust, and for giving me endless inspiration and encouragement by being living and loving endorsements that man and woman thrive and flourish on slow sex.

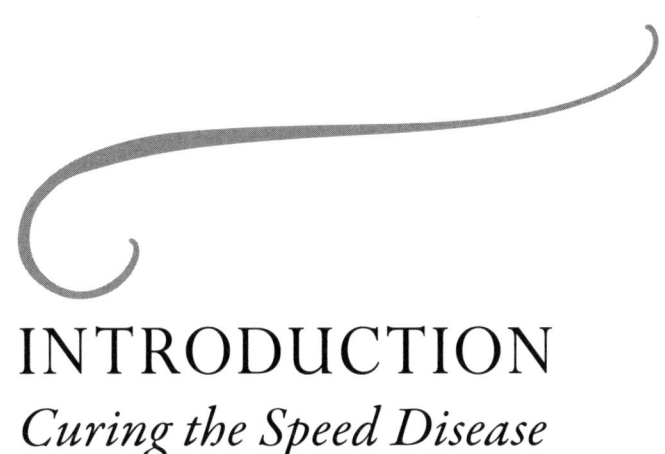

INTRODUCTION
Curing the Speed Disease

In keeping with the emerging Slow Food movement, I was delighted when my publisher suggested that I write a book entitled *Slow Sex*. This is a subject that is dear to my heart. My partner, Michael, and I have been facilitating weeklong "Making Love" retreats for couples since 1993. During these retreats we teach couples to take a fresh approach toward sex—to slow down and be fully present to each moment while having sex together, rather than practice more active sex that strives so intensely toward orgasm that it misses the subtler nuances of union along the way.

In short, we teach couples how to cultivate a slow sex practice. It is crystal clear to both of us that when couples engage in sex at a more leisurely pace, in which each moment is slowly savored and relished with awareness, they experience more sensitivity, sensuality, and satisfaction. Afterward they feel deeply nourished by love, empowered as a couple, and significantly, equally empowered as individuals too.

Recently a friend suggested I read *The Slow Down Diet: Eating for Pleasure, Energy, and Weight Loss* by Marc David. This book turned out to be an exceptional source of information, insight, and inspiration—not just in relation to food, but also in relation to sex. Marc David is a professional nutritionist with a master's degree in the psychology of eating. Through his own personal experiences in the practice of yoga, he became acquainted with the existence of eight universal metabolic enhancers that are *transubstantial,* meaning "above and beyond the realm of matter." Two examples of these universal metabolic forces are relaxation and awareness. When applied directly to eating, they are the greatest enhancers of digestion, nutrition, and maintenance of appropriate body weight. That is, when we slow down enough to be fully aware of the food we are eating—taste it, savor it, and make time for relaxation at the dining table—the food nourishes us in ways that no food can when it is wolfed down or gobbled on the run.

Every cell in my body resonated deeply with David's words. I realized that the transubstantial metabolic enhancers he recommends for health, nutrition, and maintenance of optimum weight are undeniably similar to the suggestions I offer couples seeking more satisfying sexual experiences and more loving relationships. These universal metabolic forces and their powerful effects on human sexuality hold absolutely true in my own personal experience. Just as we allow our food to nourish our bodies by eating more slowly, by practicing slow sex we allow our sexual relationships to nourish our bodies, hearts, and souls.

The first step is to change our minds about sex. A shift in perspective opens new doors of experience for the body, giving it space to express itself. Usually our *ideas* about sex are forced onto the body, pushing it to cooperate and fulfill the many expectations and desires we associate with sex. Such pressures have made sex a hurried and single-minded act, whereas the body is inwardly thrilled with a slow, languid, expansive sexual exchange. Rather than *do* so much in sex, the body prefers to *be* in sex. This requires an acute awareness of the present moment. In slow sex, instead of getting involved in building to a climax, you take a step back and witness yourself. You are not so hot; instead you become more cool. Slowness takes the heat out of sex, which is a good thing, because bliss and ecstasy plant their delicate roots in a cool environment, not a hot one.

For the same reason, sexual arousal is not a prerequisite. You don't need to heat up with excitement. Instead, you discover how to fall back into your body, to be more aware and relaxed, with a sense of not really going anywhere special. It doesn't require lots of energy to engage in, or sustain, slow sex. And herein lies one of the main blessings of a slow sex practice—it is a sustainable practice particularly well suited to long-term committed couples. Over a period of many years it is natural for a couple to experience a certain amount of cooling down in sex, because it's simply not possible to stay hot and excited about each other forever. There has to be some maturing, some settling, some turning inward toward resources that lie within yourself, rather than outside of yourself. The nature of heat is that it has to cool down eventually. Coolness is sustainable and it has an eternal quality. This makes slow sex a practice that can grow, deepen, and develop over time. It is a practice that generates love and harmony, creating balance within each person and between two lovers.

This book presents slow sex as a practice for contemporary couples, but it has ancient roots in Eastern spiritual traditions—such as Tantra from India and Taoism from China—that have found expression in a number of current Western sexual movements. Certain Tantric lineages embraced sexual practice to bring about an expansion of consciousness, and as a doorway to the Divine. Taoist inner alchemy practices cultivate sexual energy in order to empower the body and boost health.

"There are very long and rich traditions of sexual mysticism that can be traced back before the origins of Christianity in the West," writes Arthur Versluis in his book *The Secret History of Western Sexual Mysticism,* "and for all the efforts of the 'orthodox' to extirpate it, erotic mysticism still recurs time and again, perpetually renewed, like the phoenix." Versluis believes that sexual mysticism is particularly attractive in the present day and age because it resonates with a deep human need for connection—with another individual, but also to nature and to the Divine. Fulfillment of these needs has eroded in modern Western culture, where disconnection and isolation tend to prevail. I can say with certainty that slow sex is a practice of sexual mysticism that gently heals and restores our isolating severed connections. Sex has a higher potential—sex is able to carry us beyond duality into a spiritual unity that brings us closer to ourselves, the other, nature, and God.

Among the early proponents of contemporary spiritual sexuality was Alice Bunker Stockham, one of the first women to graduate from medical school in the United States, who published a book called *Karezza: Ethics of Marriage* in 1903. Stockham's text states that there is deeper purpose and meaning to the reproductive faculties and functions than is generally understood and taught. She writes about a physical union that can include a joyful soul communion that promotes soul growth and development. So although spirituality in sex may be new to many of us, we can see that sex has been used for higher purposes over and over again in different ways and in very different cultures from ancient times to the present.

Slow sex as a practice leads to a form of spiritual marriage that meets deep human needs for connection and generates a positive rejuvenating energy in a couple, which then spills over into the community. Slow sex represents the only viable way forward for us—as man and woman together—to create a loving and sustainable humanity. It is a powerful way to create peace for ourselves and for the world.

1

SLOW SEX
A Physical and Spiritual Revolution

Slow sex provides a simple and effective antidote to the ever-accelerating pace of modern life, allowing lovers to rest in a still point at the center of a turning world. Through the workshops we offer to couples, my partner and I have been able to see the profound effect that just one week of relaxing slow sex can have on a couple's relationship. We are true believers in the power of taking it slow, but sometimes it appears as if the whole world is bent on spinning faster and faster around us.

That is why it was so thrilling for me to read *The Slow Down Diet* by Marc David. David writes about slowing down in relation to food and I am concerned with slowing down while having sex, but we are really talking about the same thing—the ability to be fully present and aware in the current moment so that we can actually experience life on an inner cellular level, rather than racing through it so quickly that everything flies by in a blur.

David says that for food to be truly nourishing, the invisible "atmospheric" factors—*how* we eat—are even more important than the physical substances we actually consume. I have already mentioned two of the eight universal metabolic enhancers that he defines—relaxation and awareness. The other six are quality, rhythm, pleasure, thought, the sacred, and the story.

In essence, and in my own way, my teaching conveys the need to incorporate these great universal metabolic enhancers into the sexual act, organically elevating the physical exchange into something spiritual and fulfilling. I have also observed that the satisfaction of slow sex acts as a nutrient that boosts the immune system, with rejuvenating effects that increase vitality, creativity, and love. At the same time, slow sex naturally reduces the emphasis on food and eating because we find nourishment and fulfillment elsewhere. It naturally supports weight loss and brings balance into the system, not through vigorous calorie-burning sex, but through extended, deeply satisfying, sensitive sex.

I suggest, for instance, that couples incorporate relaxation and awareness into the sexual act. These two simple "Love Keys" (as I call these universal metabolic enhancers) can greatly transform the sexual experience from a perhaps short-lived and repetitive event into a captivating, extended, and inspiring one. When a couple embraces the universal metabolic enhancers, doing so creates a rarified atmosphere that strengthens and amplifies the field of love surrounding them. In an environment such as this, an inner radiance and vitality will remain as an afterglow.

Such expanded dimensions can even open up when only one person introduces metabolic enhancers into the atmosphere. Just as a sensitive person in the presence of a genuinely spiritual individual may experience a type of transmitted phenomenon that ignites feelings of being more open, alive, expanded, and present, when one person slows down in sex, the second person is naturally drawn into the expanded energy field and will tune in to and link up with the universal metabolizers. The slower we can learn to be, the more we can relax and hold awareness of the present moment; gradually the practice of slowness will begin to positively impact every aspect of living.

The conventional definition of metabolism implies it is a purely physical function, "the sum total of all the chemical reactions in the body." Marc David's understanding goes beyond that, defining metabolism as "the sum total of all the chemical reactions in the body, plus the sum total of all our thoughts, feelings, beliefs, and experiences" (*The Slow Down Diet,* page 8).

David believes that these metabolizers have been in existence for a long time but have been completely overlooked because:

> First, we've been moving too fast to notice them, since their chemical power is activated only when the requisite level of "slowness" has been met. Second, we've believed that a metabolic enhancer must be exclusively of the order of a food, a pill, or a push-up, yet the eight universal metabolizers are of a different category. (*The Slow Down Diet,* page 9)

As a professional nutritionist and expert in the psychology of eating, Marc David has applied these universal metabolic insights to people who seek his guidance for nutritional and weight issues. He observed their responses to his unusual dietary suggestions and noted the undeniably positive impact on the entire system. He writes:

> The bottom line was this: These folks achieved more by doing less. The people I'm speaking of stopped fighting food and started embracing it. . . . They ceased being victimized by food, by their bodies, and by anyone else's standards and instead took responsibility for making simple but profound changes that created an empowered metabolic state. They slowed down and trusted life. (*The Slow Down Diet,* page 11)

I can say exactly the same thing about the couples who have attended our slow sex workshops. When couples learn to relax into the present moment while having sex, their entire experience is transformed into something deeply touching and nourishing for body and being. The entire metabolism is profoundly influenced and empowered. Because the eight universal metabolic enhancers defined by David apply just as directly to our sexuality as they do to our physical nutrition, I have decided to organize the book around them, just as he has done in *The Slow Down Diet*.

As a way of approaching slow sex, each of the eight universal metabolic enhancers will appear as the focus of a separate chapter. Each chapter will act as an umbrella covering relevant information and guidelines. At times it will be necessary to repeat some information as the sexual themes intertwine and form a bigger picture.

> Chapter 2, "The Sexual Power of Relaxation," focuses on relaxing away from *doing* and into simply *being* while having sex—away from goal-oriented sex that strives toward the climax of orgasm, and toward sex that allows things to evolve of their own accord.
>
> Chapter 3, "The Sexual Power of Awareness," focuses on awareness as the missing link to expressing our higher sexual potential. Through awareness we awaken to the body on an inner level and tune in to our intrinsic sexual vitality.
>
> Chapter 4, "The Sexual Power of Quality," focuses on the sexual intelligence lying within our human bodies. It recognizes the fact that our genitals have an innate wisdom about how to connect when we give them the chance and space to communicate in their own language.
>
> Chapter 5, "The Sexual Power of Rhythm," focuses primarily on the difference between male and female rhythms. These polarity differences are understood as complementary forces that can be embraced to bring sex to a higher level of expression.
>
> Chapter 6, "The Sexual Power of Pleasure," focuses on the need for a shift from sensation to sensitivity. Slowness increases sensitivity and trust in the body, and activates the metabolic power of pleasure.
>
> Chapter 7, "The Sexual Power of Thought," focuses on the capacity to think and fantasize, and how these can act as distractions. However, thought can also be used in positive ways that will stimulate the sexual metabolism.

Chapter 8, "The Sexual Power of the Sacred," focuses on sensitivity and coolness as the bridge to divine ecstatic experiences. It explains the healing and purifying power of the genitals.

Chapter 9, "The Sexual Power of the Story," focuses on the inherent human aspects of sex and the historical personal aspects, as well as evaluating slow sex as a step in human evolution.

Each of these is a key to transforming your sex life, often in ways that feel surprisingly easy and natural. As you read each chapter, any insights or curiosities that are stimulated in you as a consequence can be put immediately into practice when you are next with your partner. You need to bear in mind that it's not *what* you do, but *how* you do it, so in that sense it's easy to make subtle changes with little effort. Naturally it's impossible to incorporate all the different aspects at once and expect to get it right the very first time you try slow sex. Sometimes people take to the new way very easily, as if it were second nature, but this tends to be more the exception than the rule.

In a more sensitive society, the opposite would be true—slow sex would be the rule, not the exception. However, we have fundamental misconceptions about sex that act as a barrier to a simple, innocent, and spiritual sexual experience. Because sex has been practiced and presented in a certain way, generation upon generation, it is helpful to have an awareness of our collective conditioning, along with patience and compassion for yourself and your partner. Don't expect instant results! It's more of an unfolding based on exploration and discovery. You become a pioneer of your inner world. You simply start from where you are today—misunderstandings included. To an extent you undergo a process of unlearning what we've all inherited and rediscovering what is real and true. Each time you and your partner get together you will continue to make small exploratory steps, experimenting, incorporating what you discovered (or learned) the previous time, and gradually developing a new sexual language together.

At the end of some chapters, sensitivity and awareness exercises are suggested as a way to tune in to, support, and enhance the cellular perception of the body. The final chapter, chapter 10, "Your Personal Slow Sex Practice," will pull together all of the previous information, offering basic suggestions on how to get started with your own personal practice.

This book is not a technical manual in the sense of being focused on *what you do;* rather, the approach is one of exploring *how you do it.* Much information on "how to proceed" and how to create the atmosphere necessary for an uplifting experience is embedded in the chapters ahead. As you read, you may perhaps begin to notice a subtle shift in the way you view and understand sex. And as I see it, this is the way to go—first and foremost, a change of mind is required. We need a new vision of sex that brings about a change or revolution in our ideas. When there is a change in the mind, the body will easily and willingly respond.

Whenever I get into the details of sex I will often begin by apologizing, because I tend to talk in generalizations that have the effect of bringing us all onto much the same level. As if we are all afloat in the same sexual boat. However, each one of us has an individual personal experience and sexual history, so it is likely that *not* everything I say will hold true for each person. If something does not ring true for you, it means only that it is not true for you as an individual, not that what is said is false; because *generally* speaking, what is said about sex is true. As an overall invitation, please feel free to discard anything that does not ring true for you. And at the same time, be open to something you may have *thought* is not true for you, as well as being interested in what is true for others.

Whether we like it or not, our sexuality affects our total being. Each of us feels the impact of sex from the moment of arrival on Earth in a human body, even if our adult lives may ultimately include rare or no sexual interactions with another person. The conventional and accepted speedy way we have sex circumscribes and reduces our experience of living in our extraordinarily beautiful human bodies. Slow sex enables us to physically and consciously create love and happiness, nourishing us on extremely profound and life-changing levels.

2

THE SEXUAL POWER OF RELAXATION

Many of us are under the mistaken impression that relaxation is some kind of floppy, collapsed, and more-or-less dead state. This is definitely not true. Deep relaxation brings about a state of inner aliveness and vitality. The real by-product of relaxation is a sense of regeneration, of feeling refreshed and uplifted.

THE BREVITY OF THE SEX ACT

Humans are living not only longer, but faster. We seem to be speeding up by the day and by the decade. The stress levels that accompany all this speed are acute and cumulative, and penetrate deeply into many aspects of our lives, including our sex lives. Generally speaking, sex often is, and has always been, a speedy and short-lived event. If what we see in the movies and what we know from our own sexual experiences is anything to go by, then sex is mostly comprised of fleeting encounters of the "wham, bam, thank you, ma'am!" variety.

At present the universal average time of a sexual encounter is estimated to be anywhere from two to three minutes—a time span of 120 to 180 seconds out of a day in which we live through 86,400 seconds.

These "quickies" seem to serve one main purpose, and that is (for the man especially) to have an orgasm as quickly as possible.

Reaching orgasm means that sex is usually finished shortly after it starts. The perhaps much longed-for, or much fantasized, event is compressed into an astoundingly brief period of time. As humans we seem to mimic the animals around us, who are very efficient in their reproduction. They get the job over and done at high speed, because there is usually only one chance, and it's now. But as humans we are granted the privilege of choice. We can engage in sex at any time of the day, week, or year, because we are not restricted to hormonally dictated mating seasons. So why do humans tend to want to get sex over with so quickly, particularly when we have more options in the matter than our animal friends? And then, even with the privilege of choice, strangely enough it often happens that we continually have the urge for the same thing, over and over. It's as if we are caught in a cycle of unfulfilled sexual desire—longing for it, getting it, but only as a temporary measure. Soon the urge or desire will arise again, but satisfying it doesn't seem to leave us in a state of peace and contentment.

Seldom does one hear about a sexual engagement that is consciously extended, hour upon hour. My first really long lovemaking experience was thirteen hours nonstop, from dusk to dawn. At that point I had been more accustomed to five or six hours at a time. And then, at some time further on in my exploration, my new lover and I were in bed for a solid twenty-one days, apart from the minimum of time required to care for bodily needs. We ate only occasionally, finding ourselves satiated by something other than food. We were "in" love, constantly fused in an ecstatic state of timelessness and rapture, suspended in a miraculous web of the unfolding moment. We did not sleep, as we had no need of it. Night merged with day, day with night, in one continuum of sexual presence, passion, and spontaneity, literally tapped into an awesome, abundant source of life.

Some people experience similar remarkable exchanges and interactions of a higher frequency, but invariably these connections happen spontaneously, and are likely to be relatively isolated. Usually a person is unable to consciously create similar experiences on a sustained basis as a style of sexual expression.

The Tedium of Repetition

Even though there is certainly pleasure to be had in sexual quickies, the experience is essentially brief and there is simply not enough time for anything exotic or extraordinary to happen between two bodies. Bodies are similar to musical instruments, and usually need to first be tuned individually. Then they need time to warm up and attune to each other. Only then is it possible for the sounds to dance together in the creation of a musically engaging piece. But usually, where the musical creativity of sex is concerned, many people will admit that the experience can be repetitive and a little bit boring (unless we change partners to spice things up). The repetition is not inherent to sex itself, but occurs because we are sticking to certain sexual habits and patterns. In some cases it's even an addiction—doing more or less the same thing, year in and year out. We don't really know how to bring variety and creativity into our sexual encounters. The full spectrum of human sexual experience allows us to consciously choose to make a fundamental shift in our sexual ways. When we are able to transcend our habits and patterns, we are easily able to generate and make love in the way we were designed by the Divine. Through engaging in a more informed style of sexual interaction we are able to create love, joy, and sustenance for ourselves.

RELAXATION IS VITAL FOR THE SEXUAL METABOLISM

The way forward for us as humans is to engage in sex with increasing ease, leisure, and relaxation. In taking speed and stress out of the sexual act, we remove the performance pressure that comes with filling expectations and achieving goals. We allow time and space for the experience, in the sense of being able to extend the meeting as a matter of choice. A slow approach in sex acts like a "medicine" that is easily able to resolve and heal many long-term sexual problems and wounds that cause unhappiness, separation, and insecurity. The majority of our problems can be reduced to our sexual problems, so it is obvious that we need to make some changes.

Being, Rather than Doing

Relaxation is generally something we afford ourselves only when most of our daily tasks are done. Trying to fit everything into our busy schedules frequently creates time-management stress, and we give little value to the benefits of sheer relaxation and the joy of doing nothing. When the endless list is more or less complete, only then do we grant ourselves permission to take a break. Often by this stage we fall into an exhausted sleep or drift off into a doze. Perhaps we read a book or watch television. These moments definitely represent time off, but they don't amount to true relaxation, which is highly refreshing in its effects.

Many of us afford ourselves very little in the way of relaxation because we believe that to be "doing" something has intrinsic value. In fact, we sometimes feel that we are doing something wrong or feel guilty if we are doing, literally, nothing. Simply relaxing into a space of being, or non-doing, is judged by ourselves, and perhaps by others, as laziness or a lack of ambition and goals. We don't approve of that in our speed- and goal-driven culture.

THE GOAL OF ORGASM INTERFERES WITH RELAXATION

Relaxation becomes a challenge when we have survival stress and anxiety compounded by many different goals to achieve, and dreams and expectations to fulfill. Sex, likewise, is filled to the brim with goals and expectations. We enter sex with an agenda, with a clear sense of knowing exactly what we want or expect. Then we set about engineering these desired results with intention and tension. We base our approach on previous experiences, which are, in turn, rooted in conventional ideas about sex that we unconsciously inherit from our society.

In sex it is not common to simply relax and enjoy what is happening in the moment, waiting to see where our bodies want to take us, allowing things to evolve of their own accord. Our desire to have an orgasm, or "come," is often why most of us want sex in the first place. Having the goal of orgasm causes stress about performance and satisfaction, so we rush toward the finish to make sure we get there. We get ahead of the body and use the body, pushing it, forcing it to obey and follow the mind's instructions. However, the pressure and tension we bring into the situation has the ultimate and actual effect of making us less sensitive. The sheer speed of it all deadens us to the vitality and inner aliveness streaming through our human flesh. Being distracted by an anticipated orgasm and working toward building to a climax literally prevents us from being rooted in the body, from being in the here and now, connected to the actual moment-by-moment experience of the body.

Having orgasm as a goal causes a kind of absence because the focus lies slightly ahead of where we actually are. It make us always more interested in the *next* penetration, and not particularly interested in *this* one, because the next one will bring us closer to the desired goal, to the climax. In being one step ahead of ourselves, we miss the pure joy of devoting total attention to each glorious penetration, man giving and woman receiving in perfect communion. When we can be more still in mind and body, we can listen to our inner wisdom and and honor the natural ways of the body. Slowing down and relaxing away from goals will open up a new window of sexual experience to explore. Finding full value in sex, pursuing its human aspects and its great potential, lies beyond the boundaries of the common quickie.

Premature Ejaculation

Man has an easier time than woman in the quickie approach, in that sex is usually over when the man ejaculates. Often the man will finish well before the woman has sufficiently warmed up to the experience.

For the majority of women, reaching an orgasm within a few minutes of penetration is not so easy. Ten, fifteen, or twenty minutes are not necessarily enough either. Women will often require additional stimulation of the clitoris in order to reach a climax. Yet the majority of men are not really able to hold back their ejaculation in order to intentionally extend lovemaking. Ejaculation will usually be experienced as an overwhelming wave, impossible to stop or sidestep. It takes control of the body, somewhat like a sneeze that suddenly emerges from nowhere and takes you over. To intentionally refrain from ejaculation, a man must from time to time relax back into his body and take several deep breaths. These pauses take the focus off increasing the excitement and help to bring more attention to the body in the present moment. As soon as orgasm as the goal of sex is dropped, relaxation into the present follows naturally.

The underlying reason for a man's premature ejaculation is too much stress and tension, particularly in the form of sexual stimulation and excitement, which (as we will explore in later chapters) has little to do with pure pleasure and ecstasy. There are also many psychological stresses that create tension and contraction in the system, such as performance pressure and wanting to be successful, fear of not being good enough, fear of coming too soon, wanting to satisfy and please, ego desire to be this particular woman's best lover ever, and so on. With relaxation, ejaculation can easily be postponed. The effort and stimulation necessary to achieve orgasm falls away, with the result that the whole system relaxes and the body is then able to be more present. If you want to avoid premature ejaculation, then drop the idea that orgasm is central to sex. Slowing down movements will automatically reduce the level of excitement, which is a good thing; it's what we want. Even if a man has suffered from untimely ejaculation all his life, miracles are definitely possible when a relaxed sexual attitude is adopted. One man shared during a couples retreat several years ago that he had been able to overcome a thirty-year premature ejaculation problem *overnight,* simply by monitoring and reducing his level of excitement.

The suggestion to reduce the level of excitement holds true for women, too. If a woman wishes to make love for longer periods of time, she should reduce movements that cause stimulation and excitement, instead holding still at times, poised and present. One particularly good reason for a woman to avoid high levels of stimulation is that her excitement is frequently the trigger for a man's early ejaculation. Fortunately, it is well within a woman's power to relax back into herself and thereby postpone her partner's ejaculation. Instead of going for an orgasm, she creates a situation that is inviting and welcoming, without being exciting. Remaining in the cooler zone of sexual experience will naturally keep a man's ejaculation at bay.

The Containment of Semen Empowers Man
One tablespoon of semen is incredibly powerful stuff, almost atomic in its potency. In addition to sperm cells, seminal fluid contains an immense amount of protein, vitamins, minerals, and amino acids, as well as vital energies. Semen contained within the male body represents tremendous individual potential and creative power. It should really be viewed as a type of liquid gold, and not taken so lightly. Dispersed semen represents a loss of personal energy resources, particularly when a man's climax involves the buildup of much tension and stress that leave behind traces in the body, brain chemistry, and psyche. The vast majority of men will admit that after an orgasm they feel depleted, low in energy, disconnected, or withdrawn. Containment of semen will empower a man because the vital substances nourish his intelligence and creativity; he becomes more centered and master of himself.

Relaxation happens easily when we change the idea that orgasm has to happen as a necessary part of sex. When we take away the goal or intention of orgasm, there is no need for a push toward the finish line. With nowhere to go there is no hurry, so everything can unfold in a unique organic way. There is no need to force the body along a certain direction because the body's innate intelligence has other plans in store for us.

DEEP SLOW BREATHING INVITES RELAXATION

Relaxation is supported through deep slow breathing, because breath brings an infusion of vitality to the system. Deep slow breathing causes an increase in the release of endorphins—neurochemicals produced by the body that act like opiates—into the system, which helps to produce relaxation and a sense of well-being. When we neglect to pay attention to our breath, it often remains only in the chest and shoulders. It's beneficial to invite the breath downward through the diaphragm and into the belly, allowing the belly to rise and fall with the in-breaths and out-breaths. And if you wish you can imagine, or with practice perhaps even feel, that the breath is able to internally caress the genital area.

Conscious breathing in the direction of the genitals during sex increases the oxygen intake and enhances the whole metabolism, providing you with sexual vitality and aliveness. Throughout lovemaking, simply paying acute attention to the process of the in-breaths and the out-breaths can shift you to another realm of experience. Normally breathing is involuntary and happens whether we're thinking about it or not, which makes it extremely easy to slip out of conscious connection with the breath. It is a function of the autonomic nervous system, meaning that its function is independent of the conscious mind. We are not able to consciously affect most processes of our autonomic nervous system, but we can take an active part in our breathing process. The extent to which you relax and deepen the breath as you make love will definitely pay off with the rewards of greater presence, enhanced cellular sensitivity, and inner expansion.

Some people like to make a little ritual of taking several deep slow breaths before actually doing anything. For instance, before you start the ignition of your car, stop, take a couple of breaths as you relax your shoulders. Or, when practicing slow sex, take a couple of conscious breaths and become centered in your body for a few moments before you hug your partner. And again, take several breaths before you bring your lips together in a sealed kiss, repeatedly using breath to relax and prepare you for any meeting and exchange. The same thing can be done when a man poises with his penis at the entrance to the vagina, immediately prior to actual penetration. And then once inside, stopping frequently for a couple of deep breaths along the way. The penis can travel breath by breath and fraction by fraction into the vagina, and this journey into woman's body can last for many pleasurable minutes. Once fully inside, a man can remain within the depths, alert and breathing consciously for an extended period of time.

When you touch your partner's body, hold your hands still and give your partner your full inner attention as you take a few breaths into your belly or genitals. Or breathe deeply and consciously as you slowly caress your partner's body with a feather-light touch. Avoid any kind of stimulation that will trigger the desire for orgasm, which can easily leave us a bit breathless. Or at least take a few breathing breaks between bouts of excitement. A little excitement, then relax and breathe; then a little more excitement, and again relax. Whenever you find yourself focusing on the next penetration and eventual orgasm, if you stop all movement and be still for a while, taking a few deep breaths, it will help you to cool down and relax into the here and now.

LINING UP THE BONES

I have found that the depth of relaxation depends substantially on the physical body position; literally, how the bones line up as a skeleton. Relaxation requires a certain physical poise, which means physical alignment, and alignment brings presence to a body and grace to movement. A certain tension level is required to hold most upright sitting positions, and tension is part of our physical integrity, but any extra or habitual tension can be consciously released. The body will usually respond to this conscious letting go and relaxation of tensions with a spontaneous deep breath in gratitude.

CREATE TIME FOR SEX

It is much easier to be relaxed about sex when you grant yourself adequate space and time for the sexual exchange. To support relaxation you can actually make an appointment with your partner for sex, in the same way that you make time for meals, work, the gym, friends, and children. Set aside enough time and space to allow yourselves to warm up and physically attune to each other. Decide together on the time and place for the experience.

Exercises: Daily Observation and Conscious Relaxation Practices

◉ Scanning from Head to Toe for Tension

You can do this simple practice at any time of the day and in almost any place. The body gets tense and a bit contracted without our realizing it, and this type of tension has a compressing effect on your body energy during daily life, which also carries over into sex. The body carries many subtle and not-so-subtle tensions. As you make love (or sit, walk, drive, and so on), repeatedly scan your body from head to toe, or toe to head, and deliberately and consciously relax any areas of tension that you encounter. The following are some classic places where we hold tension without realizing it:

- Around the mouth
- In the joints of the jaw (the temporomandibular joint, or TMJ)
- In the neck and shoulders
- In the solar plexus (the soft spot below the upside-down V formed by the rib cage)
- In the belly
- In the feet

◉ Relaxing the Pelvic Floor

Another central and significant place to consciously relax is the pelvic floor, which means the web of muscles and tissues that surround the anus and genitals. Invariably this muscular floor will be slightly contracted and pulled upward, without our being aware of this tension. Let go of any tightness you discover there, and do so a hundred times during the day or whenever you happen to remember. Intentionally relaxing and releasing any subtle holding and tension in the muscles will allow the pelvic floor to widen and drop slightly.

- For a woman, relaxing the pelvic floor means taking the attention to the vagina and relaxing any tightness or holding discovered there.
- For a man it means consciously relaxing and letting go of the anus and the muscles of the buttocks.

To feel the difference between tension and then relaxation, you can first exaggerate the tension, and then release it. Tighten genitals and anus, pulling upward and inward, hold for a few seconds, and then release slowly.

☉ Make Conscious Relaxation an Everyday Practice

Invariably, as soon as our attention has moved away from the part we have consciously relaxed, the tension gradually begins to return and assert itself. So scanning the body from head to toe and relaxing tensions can be done intermittently. We will probably never completely rid ourselves of these subtle tensions, and that is really not the aim or goal. The aim is to remember that you are first and foremost a body—and to notice when and where you are tense, and then to intentionally relax these tense parts. Let go, take a deep breath, and feel your body. This little process is something to be done billions of times, not just once or twice. Relaxation of different body parts creates inner space and expansion and is usually followed by a wave of sensitivity on a delicate cellular level.

There are myriad small, insignificant daily actions in which we can practice conscious relaxation: brushing our teeth, washing dishes, preparing food, driving, opening and closing doors, sitting at the computer, and standing in line at the bank or checkout, to name but a few. Paying attention to your level of relaxation during the day will support your experience in bed, and vice versa.

3

THE SEXUAL POWER OF AWARENESS

If you have tried scanning your body and relaxing any tense areas that you notice, that in itself was an act of awareness. So if you are not sure what awareness means, and you managed to relax your jaw, shoulders, and belly, you are already using that particular witnessing power or aptitude. Awareness is not far away from us, and indeed, we would not be able to survive without a certain level of awareness. At the same time, we know remarkably little about the power of awareness and how it can change our every moment.

AWARENESS IS THE MISSING LINK

For human beings, awareness during sex is the missing link to expressing and living our higher sexual potential. This uniquely human capacity to observe ourselves as if from a distance has a tremendously powerful impact on metabolism and sexual responsiveness. Awareness acts as a highly potent aphrodisiac. Through awareness we awaken to the body on an inner level and tune in to our intrinsic, God-given sexual vitality. Awareness is the capacity to observe and witness oneself—as a body and as a mind filled with the thoughts that distance us from the body—in any given moment of any given day, including, of course, while we are having sex. As Marc David notes:

> One of the most unusual scientific revelations of the last century is the mathematical proof that the act of observing any phenomenon in the universe—be it the flight of a bird or the rotation of a planet—has a direct influence upon that phenomenon. According to the laws of physics, we have no choice but to alter the bird's course or the planet's speed simply by focusing our awareness on it. So if we have the power to tweak the orbit of a heavenly body, it should come as no surprise that vitamin A—awareness—also has a profound impact on the human body. (*The Slow Down Diet,* page 62)

Awareness is the driving force behind slow sex. As we become intensely aware of each and every breath, touch, movement, or shift of the body, the sexual experience unfolds and flows easily and effortlessly moment by moment. And if we so wish, the exchange can continue for hours on end according to, and being guided by, what wants to happen between the bodies themselves. For extended lovemaking there needs to be no agenda, no goal, just an appreciation of the here-and-now experience. So to some extent you are faced with dropping the ego and the sexual personality with its demands, likes and dislikes, habits and addictions. Slowness is basic to a shift in sexual experience—slowing down in all you do, giving yourself the space to tune in to yourself. Be slow in your approach to the other person as well, and above all be slow, easy, and relaxed as you join your bodies and become one.

Relaxation and awareness actually go hand in hand, because you have to become more aware of your physical body in order to release any tension, clenching, tightness, or holding. Awareness, therefore, precedes relaxation, and relaxation in turn deepens the awareness. When you consciously relax you will usually feel an inner wave of vitality, light, or aliveness expanding through the body. The delight of these inner sensations in turn engages the awareness, enabling you to fall into even deeper relaxation.

Once we find our way into the intangible present through awareness, we develop the qualities and radiance of true "presence." Awareness is the capacity to be alert to what *is*. It's the ability to be in touch with what is happening inside you and around you this very moment. When we build awareness into our sexual expression, it is the most powerful metabolic force.

IT'S NOT WHAT YOU DO BUT HOW YOU DO IT

As we explore further we will discover that it is well-nigh impossible to make rules about how to be slow. Creating a shift in our sexual experience is definitely not about following a set of rules; it's more of an inquiry. It's an ongoing effort to feel yourself and be self-observant during sex. It is examining not only what you are doing, but more importantly, how you are doing it. We simply do whatever we do as consciously as possible, with all the alertness we can muster in any given moment.

We usually say in our workshops that when you are making love, everything and anything goes, because it's not what you do, but how you do it. Any act done with awareness is changed by that awareness itself, so the "what" can be transformed through the "how." In this way being slow can never be a special sexual technique. It is not something you can do as such, because slowness is actually an outcome or by-product of what happens when an action is carried out with awareness.

You may already have discovered how difficult it is to *do* slow, especially when accustomed to a faster approach. Most of us have had the experience of driving along in a car, totally engaged in the movement and momentum, when all of a sudden a road sign saying "Slow" or "Stop" appears. At such a point, being forced to go slowly is a disturbance that can lead to irritation and frustration. Imagine, then, during sex when you are in full swing and then unexpectedly you remember the suggestion to go slow. Or you have it fixed in your mind that you have to be slow because you have been instructed to be slow. With this kind of rule-oriented attitude, the exploration of slowness will be tedious, not easy. In fact being slow will probably be the last thing you feel like doing when in the throes of a sexual encounter. The mind likes to do things right and stick with the rules, but this lack of flexibility closes the door to exploration. An inquiry requires curiosity, alertness, and a willingness to step into the unknown.

BEING CONSCIOUS
INSTEAD OF MECHANICAL

The bottom-line truth is that most of the time we humans are not fully present in, or aware in, our beautifully sensitive fleshy bodies. We are not really connected to them on an inner level. We habitually use them in mechanical ways and do not really pay attention during most of our activities, except when physical pain is experienced. We remember the spine when we unexpectedly have a backache or the knee only when it hurts every time we bend it. Over time, especially as our bodies begin to show signs of wear and tear, our associations with the body can become negative and draining, not positive, nourishing, and uplifting.

Seldom do we focus ourselves sufficiently to consciously experience the actual "how" of what we are doing. Because we do the same things again and again, there is a mechanization in the way we conduct our daily activities—walk, sit, stand, lie down, drive, cook, clean, shower, shave, shampoo, or whatever. We don't use our awareness. How are you sitting right now, as you are reading, for instance? Where is your body and how is your spine, your head, your neck? Collapsed forward or in one connected line? Shoulders up or down? Jaw clenched or relaxed? Breathing? When did you last consciously feel your breath? Are you holding your breath or is it shallow? Enjoy a deep breath right now!

As we get busy dealing with the demands of the day, our focus is, for the most part, outside of the body. Our attention is on achievement, getting something done, but not on the physical process involved in getting there. We lack a certain presence in all of our activities, including, of course, sex. We all have personal goals and doggedly set off each time in a mechanical, driven way in an attempt to reach a pleasing end. And as mentioned before, satisfying our immediate desires causes us to be absent, marginally present to the moment, ourselves, the other.

USE AWARENESS TO REMAIN IN THE NOW

As your level of awareness grows, everything becomes slower and more deliberate, creating an opportunity to feel and follow the wisdom and intelligence residing within the human body. A change in sexual experience becomes possible with the insight that the goal or habit of orgasm acts as a temptation in the future (see previous chapter), seducing us away from an awareness of the simple, authentic here and now.

Imagine for a moment that you have been used to spinning happily along in an automatic car and then unexpectedly you have to adjust to a less familiar manual shift. With a manual shift, gears are changed by hand in a more sequenced step-by-step way, coordinating with the clutch and engine speed. More awareness is needed, naturally, especially in the beginning when it is quite easy to stall the car. You are required to pay attention to the engine, tune in to its sounds, listen to the engine revolutions until they reach the right pitch, then do some speedy fancy footwork to release the gas, press the clutch, shift the gear with your hand, then release the clutch, and reapply pressure to the accelerator, all in one flowing move. These shifts are repeated again and again depending on traffic density or the road's curves, shifting gears down and up again. At first this kind of deliberate driving is bound to feel awkward and unfamiliar, and to get it right takes practice, but before long it becomes an integral part of driving. Eventually the moves will flow smoothly, but maintaining attention to the sound of the engine is an ongoing process.

We can change our patterns of lovemaking in much the same way. Instead of accelerating immediately to top gear, we can consciously cause a change in the course of events by choosing to become more aware of each shift in the situation. And the transition begins with *not* running after something, which makes it simpler. We do not fast-forward directly toward orgasm. Deliberately and with intention we stay here, remaining present. We already have some kind of awareness of the components required to pull an orgasm together, so to create the opposite and not dash forward must be an option as well. When we withdraw from fantasy or stimulation or anything that puts pressure on or inflames the situation, we forestall the urge that so easily becomes a compulsion. We no longer feel forced to give in to the pressing urgency to climax and release.

Open Eyes Increase Awareness

Our eyes are tools that put us in direct contact with our immediate surroundings in the present. Often sex takes place with closed eyes and in the dark, and usually sexual fantasy involves closed eyes, but during slow sex you can begin to experiment with keeping them open and receptive. You can begin to make a practice of receiving with your eyes when you are looking at nature, imagining that nature is looking back at you. You reverse the perspective of vision. You are not looking out, but are being looked into by the other. This can be done with a tree, a flower, a bird, a beautiful sunset, the moon, stars, snowcapped peaks, a waterfall, the sunrise, or any lovely creation of nature, including another human being. The eyes can just be open, receiving, and inviting. (See the soft vision exercise at the end of this chapter.)

With the eyes open, staying in awareness, we naturally slow down to the extent that the usual triggers for climax are minimized. Sounds like contrary sexual advice, doesn't it? Usually the recommendation would be to maximize whatever brings us to a peak, but here we are placing attention on a critical point. We want to gently simmer and not boil over. We are monitoring ourselves—noticing what we are doing and how we are doing it—by engaging our awareness.

ENERGY FOLLOWS ATTENTION

Direct your awareness to your own body during lovemaking. You take the focus away from your partner's body and direct it inwardly toward yourself. As you relax and remain present to what is, you become better able to actually feel what is happening in your own body. Instead of attention being focused on orgasm or the other, you have the opportunity and space to turn inward and connect to your inner world at the outset.

The physical body ought to be given primary place in your field of awareness. When you focus on being rather than on doing, you can now bring attention, using your inner eye, to a flesh and bone level. And here you uncover new realms, a cosmos of cellular aliveness and vitality that is the domain of the invisible inner body. Uniting with the inner world makes a world of difference to your experience of sex, because you enter the domain of your awe-inspiring senses.

Allowing your awareness to penetrate the body tissues brings you alive to your embodied self. Love is made with and between bodies, and the body acts as an anchor to the present—a simple bridge to the inner qualities of sensitivity, being, and love.

Shifting focus from outer stimuli to the sensitivity of the inner body requires some practice, which means it may take time to get the knack of feeling yourself from another perspective. It's no big deal, really; instead of the more familiar "up and out," where the attention is focused outside yourself, you draw back and pull your attention into your own body. Simple. Your attention becomes free to move inward, and you will observe that if you put your attention on any pleasing inner experience, that sensitivity, energy, vitality, aliveness, chi, prana, or life force (call it what you will) actually increases. That's the power of awareness. Any sensations of streaming, tingling, vibrating, or warmth, for instance, will respond to the awareness and amplify, expanding deliciously into other parts of the body.

In *The Slow Down Diet* I found confirmation of this thrilling inner phenomenon:

In the yoga tradition there's a saying that has helped practitioners reach for greater levels of mastery in working with the body: "Where attention goes, energy flows." Decades of research in biofeedback have certainly proved this axiom, for when we focus on most any area of the body we can increase blood flow, alter bioelectric potential, and influence the secretion of numerous biochemicals. (*The Slow Down Diet*, page 75)

In other words, all these physiological responses to awareness create pleasurable, engaging, sensitive subtle sensations within the body. These experiences are touching and fulfilling; they make you feel better about yourself, improving your sense of self-worth and dignity. With awareness you can set out on a journey into the abundant delights and thrills of relaxation. As you become more aware, you relax more. And the more you relax, the more your awareness increases. With more awareness, relaxation can deepen even further. And so it goes, ad infinitum. The forces of the universal metabolic enhancers complement and weave together in a magical, mysterious, consciousness-enhancing way.

COME HOME TO YOURSELF

The fundamental step to developing awareness is to come back to yourself. In order to shift your attention "in and down," rather than "up and out," begin by making the effort of being more aware of your body, noticing how it feels and where it feels. As suggested earlier, sometimes it's easier to become more aware of tensions if you first tighten and deliberately exaggerate the level of tension. Contract and tighten your upper body for a few seconds, and then suddenly let go in one instant, releasing and relaxing all the muscles of the shoulders, jaw, belly, arms, and hands. Your body will take a beautifully deep breath and you will easily be able to feel the subtle pleasure and delight of relaxation course though your body in waves. In the same way, you can consciously (not mechanically) contract and relax the pelvic floor to increase your inner awareness and enhance the vitality of the area. If you wish you can contract on an in-breath to the count of four or five, and then relax on the out-breath to the same number of counts.

Returning to your body requires that you invert your attention on yourself. If you continue to scan your body throughout the day, making it a daily practice to do everything with as much physical awareness and relaxation as you can manage, you will become immersed in your body and develop a natural sensual grace and slowness.

Remember to honor yourself first; your inner connection to your own body is more significant than any connection to your partner's body. It may sound confusing to hear that you and your body are the priority, and not your partner, but this rerouting of attention will help both of you to be alive to yourselves right from the outset. Focusing too much on the other person would be like leaving home, abandoning your own fire tending, and instead going to ignite somebody else's fire to warm that person's house.

When you honor yourself first, you stoke your own fire. You don't depend on someone else to do it for you, and neither does your partner. The two individual fires join, they augment and enhance each other, and fueled by awareness, flames rise in splendid unison.

When our attention is split, partly on the other and partly on ourselves, we disempower ourselves by reducing our sexual potential. The simple act of attending to two or more stimuli at once can dramatically decrease the sexual metabolism. In sex there is a need to focus on yourself first and foremost to boost the fire of your own sexual metabolism.

Exercise: Going In and Down to Find Home in the Body
Identifying an Inner Center of Deep Relaxation

You can do this exercise right now, wherever and however you are sitting in this moment. Or experiment with it later when you are lying or standing. It's a simple way to connect to the inner dimensions of the body.

1. Close your eyes gently.
2. Scan your body and relax your shoulders, jaw, belly, or any place where you feel some tension or holding (see suggestions at the end of chapter 2). Take two or three easy, full breaths through the diaphragm and into your belly.
3. Then, with your eyes closed, begin to imagine that your eyes are looking backward into your body. Keep looking backward and use that inner vision to help you draw your attention into the body and then downward, so that you can sense yourself more from the inside.
4. Start to look around for a place inside the body that feels like home to you. A place that connects you to your body, the inner realms of ease, a place you can settle in to, one that makes you feel rested, as if you are arriving at home in yourself.

    Home can be anywhere below the head—spine, buttocks, belly, genitals, heart, breasts, low back, feet, or anywhere that feels good and right to you. Home can also be the entire body.
5. From home, wherever it happpens to be, however big or small, you can begin to spread your attention and link home to other parts that feel good, as if embracing other pleasant cellular sensations. Or you can expand symmetrically outward from the spine as the midline of the body.

An inner home acts as a resting place, a connection point, working like an anchor that roots the awareness within the body.

Exercise: Practicing Soft Vision with Your Partner

⊙ Using the Eyes as a Window into Your Being

The practice of being receptive with a tree or some aspect of nature, described earlier in this chapter, can be extended to a very nice practice with your partner.

1. Close your eyes and connect internally, as described in the previous exercise.

2. When you feel rooted within your body, you can begin to open your eyes fraction by fraction (without losing contact with your inner body—if you do lose this connection, please close your eyes again until you inwardly reconnect, then again slowly open).
3. When your eyes are fully open, gently meet your partner's eyes. Allow your partner into you through the eyes. Let your eyes be easy, soft, receptive, and inviting. It's okay to blink, this is not a staring exercise.
4. Gaze receptively at one eye at a time because trying to engage both of your partner's eyes simultaneously has a mesmerizing, unfocused effect. Perhaps you will notice it is easier to connect with your partner's left eye than the right. Or vice versa. Whichever eye feels comfortable for you, stay with it. Shift to the other eye at any time. If you have a vision deficiency, make any adjustments in distance that you need.
5. Take a deep breath into your belly and allow your eyes to receive what is there in front of them, rather than looking outward in an objective or judgmental fashion.
6. Take several deep breaths into your belly. Scan your body for random areas of tension, and relax them. Relax the belly and soften the muscles surrounding the genitals.
7. Enjoy another breath. Be present in your body, simple and easy.
8. Remain in receptive eye sharing mode for as long as it feels comfortable, and close the eyes whenever it feels necessary, either to reestablish an inner connection or as opportunity to sense yourself more deeply on the inside. Keep coming back to open eyes and being available to yourself on the inside as you receive your partner's soft gaze into you. Avoid keeping the eyes closed for extended periods.
9. When it feels appropriate or when there is a spontaneous drawing together of your bodies, move into a sustained embrace in which you can close your eyes; stay present and attentive to inner details as you relax your body and melt with your partner.

4
THE SEXUAL POWER OF QUALITY

Quality is born when we tune into the sexual intelligence lying within our human bodies. Quality is born when we are aware and relaxed enough to experience the inherent vitality of the sexual organs. Quality is born when we slow down enough to allow the bodies to connect in their own way and at their own pace.

GENITAL INTELLIGENCE

While it may sound a bit strange, the genitals do have an innate wisdom. They know what to do, how to do it, and when to do it, but only when we create the appropriate atmosphere, surrender, and allow them to function on their own terms. When there is an intentional withdrawal from building to a climax, we offer our sexual organs the opportunity and space to communicate in their own language. The genitals have their own way of communing, of sharing and exchanging energy, and it's nothing short of a miracle. The intelligence built into the genitals can best be described as "biomagnetic" or "electromagnetic."

Man and woman are extremely similar on many levels, yet vastly different on others. We experience this divergence in various ways, but how deep does the difference between us really lie? Beyond our differences in gender, physical appearance, and associated reproductive functions, what is the crucial distinction between man and woman?

On a profound energy level, the basic difference between us is one of polarity. A difference in polarity implies a difference in potential, and this polarity, embedded as an inherent capacity, is lodged as a powerful cellular intelligence in the genital tissues. There exists a polarity difference between the penis and the vagina that gives rise to a spontaneous flow of life force, vitality, energy, chi, prana—call it what you will.

MALE DYNAMIC FORCE, FEMALE RECEPTIVE FORCE

In essence, the male force is a dynamic force (but not a doing force), and the female force is receptive (also not a doing force). So in this sense both man and woman need to refrain from too much doing or activity in sex so that they can open to and access their essence. When we relax back into ourselves and become more aware, we come to exist as opposite forces in relation to each other. One organically gives, flows, or channels, as the other receives, takes in, or absorbs.

These equal forces are fundamentally opposite forces. (See chapter 5 for elaboration on this theme.) One is not less and one is not more; they are in perfect balance and harmony. Too easily we think of receptive as passive, floppy, and lifeless, or dynamic as action and accomplishment, but dynamic and receptive are equally powerful. These qualities are states and not something that can be achieved, except by falling back into your body and being to touch your natural essence.

Male and Female Forces Are Complementary

These two forces are equal yet opposite, and that implies that they are deeply complementary. Without one, the other does not exist. The male force is one half, the female force is the other half. Dynamic can only be dynamic, start to become a stream, or flow, when the container is inwardly prepared to receive such emanations. Receptivity is a powerful state of vitality and presence in which true passion is a surrendering to the genius of nature's ways. Without the quality of receptivity there is little chance for man to respond in true male dynamic fashion. In this way man is relatively dependent on the female environment that surrounds his penis, the quality of relaxation, awareness, and receptivity in the vaginal tissues. Similarly, when a man is present and aware in his penis, woman is more easily able to relax into herself, and in so doing, increase the capacity to receive the dynamic force.

"Positive" dynamic and "negative" receptive complement each other, and when joined together, the two forces become one unit, whole and complete. The complementary quality of the male and female poles is understood to be the source of our strong intuitive attraction to the opposite gender. And why sexual union appeals to us, calls us, and draws us.

Everything in existence that is not complete seeks completion. And in sex we find completion between ourselves through joining with the equal and opposite force, merging and melting into one integrated whole. The dynamic and receptive forces of the genitals are elements that cannot be seen, even under a microscope, but can be plainly observed in action.

EMBRACING POLARITY HERALDS A CHANGE IN DIMENSION

When you relax into the polarity level of the inner reality there is a shift to an altered state, to a new dimension where you perceive expansion, space, light, love, beauty, eternity. For such a spontaneous effect to take place, you (as individuals) have to position yourselves both physically and mentally.

I recently gained a fascinating insight into the word *dimension*. I was talking to a friend, sharing my personal observation that when I make very simple physical shifts of body position and adjust my alignment, a space opens up and presence and awareness is amplified. He surprised me by saying that he had fully investigated the ancient Greek, or Hellenic, language derivation of the word *dimension*. *Dimension* is rooted in the Hellenic ΔΙΑΣΤΑΣΙΣ, or *thiastasis*. There are two parts. First, ΔΙΑ (*thia*) which means "through" or "to divide." Second, ΣΤΑΣΙΣ (*stasis*), which comes from the verb ΙΣΤΑΜΑΙ (*istame*), which literally means "to place the body in a posture of stillness." At the same time, *thiastasis* means "the size of something when it is still." And the related *ekstasis* means "what comes out of the body's stillness." Embedded in the language lies the intelligence that position, stillness, and dimension are inseparable. A shift of position is required on two levels—mind and body. If we start with the mind, the body usually follows suit. There needs to be an intention to create a situation in which the complementary qualities of male and female come into play as dynamic and receptive forces, wherein man gives and woman receives. The basic direction of the flow is from man into woman, but the container needs to be in a state of poised receptivity to draw the flow of the dynamic force into itself.

The dynamic and receptive functions of the genitals are very clearly attested to by their physical shapes. Nature is very precise, not at all haphazard. The exterior male genitalia is designed to enter the interior female genitalia, and by virtue of being in the appropriate or "right" position in relation to her, has the capacity to channel vitality into her when she is in a correspondingly appropriate position to receive.

LUBRICATION OF THE GENITALS

To facilitate a slow journey into the vagina, it's recommended to begin with lubrication every time you get together. Apply lubricant generously around the entrance and lips of the vagina, as well as over the entire length and head of the penis. Unscented pure oil is recommended. A pure thin vegetable oil, such as almond oil, works well because a little goes a long way. The sensual slipperiness of oil allows for a silky smooth slow entry that can last several minutes as the vaginal canal is gradually probed open. If more oil is needed it can be added at any time. Sesame oil is used in ayurvedic preparations for the genitals. Olive oil can also be used but is a thicker type of oil, better for emergencies rather than for regular use. Oils that are commercially available will usually have natural fragrances added, however a pure unscented oil is advised. Almond oil is usually available over the counter in drugstores. Commercial synthetic lubricant preparations are not made of natural ingredients and can have side effects, such as clogging the deeper part of the vagina and affecting menstrual flow. Important to remember is that oil should *not* be used in conjunction with condoms; instead use a water-based pharmaceutical gel.

SLOW CONSCIOUS ENTRY

The initial approach and very first entry into woman's body is of great significance in keeping excitement to a low level. How a woman is entered sets the atmosphere or tone and will have a tremendous impact on whatever follows. This applies equally when a woman is having sex for the first time and every time thereafter. When man has an erection (see later section for when he does not), the actual entry and subsequent penetration should be done with extreme awareness, and therefore extreme slowness, extending into the vaginal canal millimeter by millimeter, and the slower the better. He should stop any time he feels resistance in the vaginal tissue, which needs time to warm up to receive and absorb the penis.

There are a variety of positions from which to begin. Figure 4.1 (on page 38) shows the most basic and obvious possibility for the very first slow penetration. A thick flat pillow can be placed under the buttocks of the woman in order to raise the level of the pelvis and bring the vagina closer to the penis. The raised pelvic position will also change the angle of the vagina slightly, which enhances and deepens the connection between the penis and the vagina.

Eye contact is easily managed here and will have a strong impact on the experience of gradual penetration. Lovers can allow their eyes

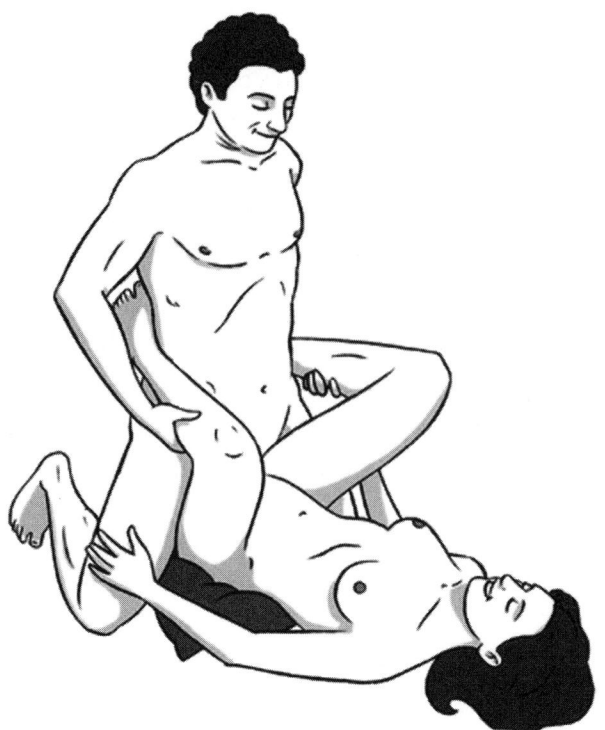

Fig. 4.1. Middle position, man kneeling
(with pillow to raise woman's pelvis)

to meet in a soft, inviting way as described in the exercise at the end of chapter 3. Eye contact can be held for the duration, although partners may close their eyes any time they wish to feel more attuned to the interior of their own bodies. One partner can have eyes open, the other closed—choose whatever brings more awareness into the situation. Do note that with closed eyes it is possible to drift away a little, and become slightly absent. It's also easier to get lost in sexual fantasy when your eyes are closed.

After a time, when the man has entered the woman fully, he can at any time change position, as illustrated in figures 4.2 and 4.3. In slow and gradual steps the man can eventually come to rest gently lying on top of his woman. In this position eye contact is often possible, other times not. It really depends on how you lie and the relative position of the two pairs of eyes.

The Sexual Power of Quality 39

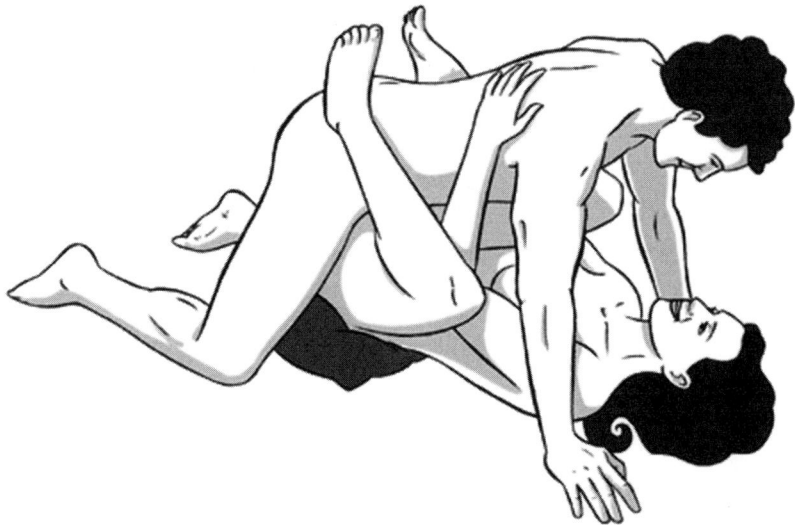

Fig. 4.2. Middle position, man on hands and knees
(with pillow to raise woman's pelvis)

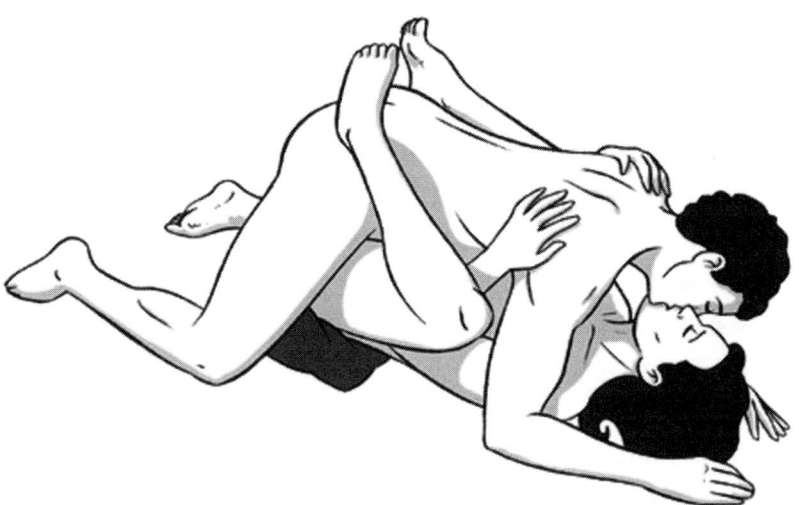

Fig. 4.3. Middle position, man lying forward, half kneeling
(with pillow to raise woman's pelvis)

Figure 4.4 shows another position option for extended slow penetration, in which both man and woman are lying on their sides. The man is actually lying between the woman's legs. In this position it is easy to make a slow, conscious journey and at the same time hold eye contact.

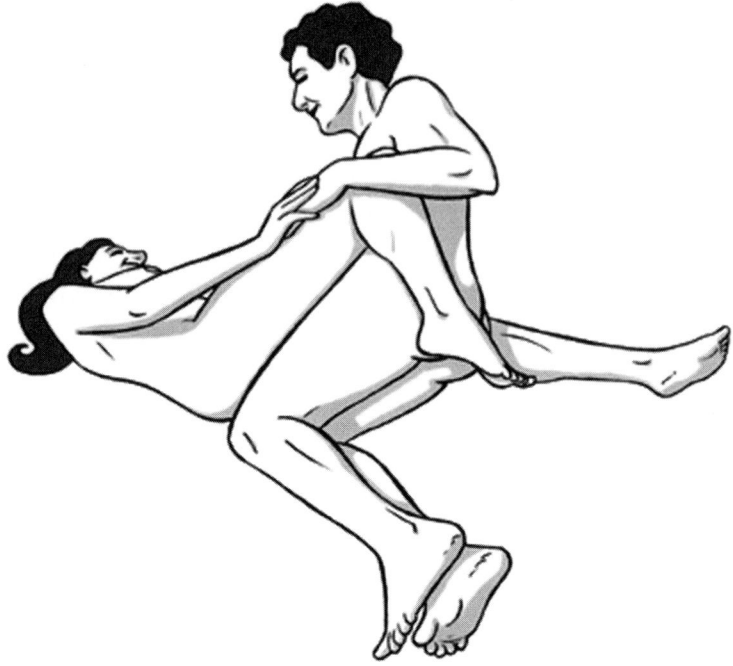

Fig. 4.4. Couple rolled to one side

Pain or Burning Sensations

It may be that the woman experiences some pain, even at the very entrance or perhaps just an inch inside the vagina. If a woman experiences any slight (or severe) sensation of burning or stinging in the tissues of the vagina as the man travels slowly inside her, she should communicate what is happening and ask him to stop in that uncomfortable place for several seconds. It is strongly advised that when he stops, the man also then pulls back a fraction so that the burning sensation or tension is reduced. This fraction of space allows tensions to move. In any case, stay with the penis head wherever pain presents itself.

Many men report that when they are slow and sensitive they can feel exactly what is happening within the vagina. The head of the penis is able to sense when and where the vaginal tissues are tight, hard, soft, receptive, defensive, relaxing, or melting. (This aspect will be addressed in depth in chapter 8.) It may take some time until the vaginal tissues relax sufficiently to allow the man to continue the entry. The time it takes is the time is takes. There is no hurry and no place for speed when it comes to entering a woman's body.

The woman can support herself by breathing deeply into her belly, taking her awareness and inner attention deep into the vaginal tissues as she relaxes and widens the canal. As she does so, the vagina becomes more receptive and welcoming, and man will immediately perceive this internal invitation, a giving way or yielding in the tissues. Buried feelings can also come to the surface for release and expression, which is a significant aspect of healing that we will address later.

STILLNESS AS AN ASPECT OF SLOWNESS

Slowness includes stillness. Slowness can transform into stillness and nonmovement at any point in which discomfort is experienced, when the "end" of the canal is reached, or when the man has arrived as far as he can go. There should be no pushing into or pressure on the cervix, which is the very sensitive entrance to the womb. Pressure can be very painful for a woman, so man must take care to pull back a fraction of an inch until pain is not experienced so that woman is able to relax and be open and receptive to the penis.

Moments or minutes of stillness can be extended to hours, if that is what both people wish. Space allows for the interplay of dynamic and receptive forces, and time allows them to respond to each other more fully. Sustain and stay with the stillness of the penetration before resuming movement. Man can hold (or intentionally direct) his awareness into the root or base of the penis and also into the head, which is like a highly sensitive and powerful magnet (see chapter 8 on healing).

To support his dynamic qualities man can imagine light energy, or gold, or love emanating from the root of his penis. While you are paused, consciously take a breath into the belly. Then scan the body by relaxing the shoulders, jaw, belly, genitals, and so on. Scan the body from head to toe and release tensions, because these cause a contraction in your energy field. Conscious relaxation of any body part will usually trigger a delicious deep breath as a wave of fine cellular sensation courses through your body in celebration. Enjoy and value being in the sexual experience without having the feeling that you have to do something. Enjoy simply being. All that is needed in the sense of doing or effort is to inwardly direct the attention to the body, and particularly into the genital tissues. Direct your awareness not only to the external surface and head of the penis but also into the very cells that comprise the tissues and muscles of the penis. For woman, move your attention from the clitoris into the tissues and muscles of the vaginal canal.

Pause for a little bit to enjoy the "now" before moving on, and then, when you sense it's the right or fitting moment, continue onward or move very slowly in the opposite direction. Halt every so often and feel into the experience; feel what you feel. Give the genitals space to become alive to themselves and alive to each other through your inner attention. Remember again the maxim, "Where attention goes, energy flows." The genitals are now "in a position" that makes inner sense to them, and the experience of new dimensions can become a reality.

Slow movements can be repeated over and over again, although you will discover that each move feels unique. What you feel and how you feel changes on each and every occasion. The bottom line is that we are wanting to establish a "correspondence" of genitals, and we put them in a position to behave according to the inherent polarities of receptive and dynamic. In normal sex the correspondence of these opposite forces is usually not happening. When we use the genitals in a mechanical, rubbing, friction-type way it certainly causes quite a stir, but at the same time it blocks access to the subtle inner potential. Through fast movement the genitals get overheated and overcharged, finally finishing up in orgasm. Being slow and still, however, allows a gently flowing cool stream of vitality to arise between them.

It is empowering to experience these subtle yet vital forces in the body, because individuals begin to feel more secure and authentic. Man feels and looks more man-like, more masculine; while woman feels and looks more womanly, more feminine. Both look younger, radiant, and relaxed. Having such experiences makes a qualitative difference to our lives with the feeling that we are stepping into a new relationship altogether.

ROTATING POSITIONS AROUND THE GENITAL CONNECTION

From time to time you will need or wish to move your bodies around to find new positions, and again relax into them. A part of the body, say the legs or back, will get uncomfortable after a bit, and when this happens, it's an appropriate time to move on. A change of position can be done at any time, after five, fifteen, or fifty minutes, whatever is required. It will bring fresh energy into the situation; you will experience yourself as more alive, alert, and sensitive. One of you will communicate your wish to move, and then you can move in unison according to the rotating style illustrated in figures 4.5 and 4.6 on pages 44–47.

Physical discomfort can be a major distraction. Instead of tuning in to the pleasure of sensitivity, your awareness is dominated by pain or discomfort. Or sometimes you may feel sleepy, a bit uninvolved, or a bit absent. A shift in position is a good remedy in these kinds of situations.

Whenever you move together the penis stays in the vagina, and you both move around with this connection as the focal point. You do not disconnect. If the penis happens to slip out, simply slip it in again. The intention behind rotating positions is to maximize the correspondence of the penis and the vagina, to keep them connected while changing position, and to bring more variety and quality into the exchange.

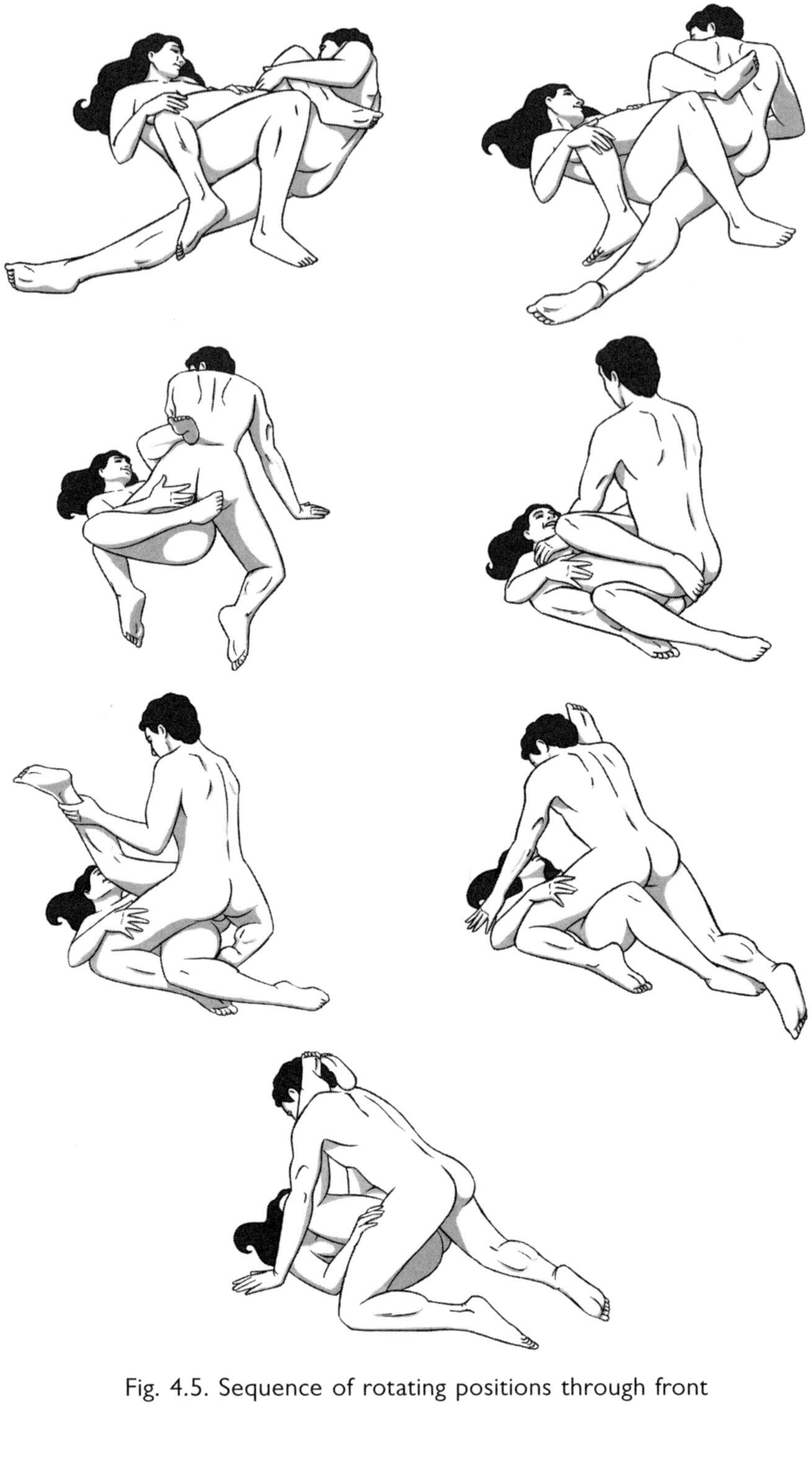

Fig. 4.5. Sequence of rotating positions through front

The Sexual Power of Quality

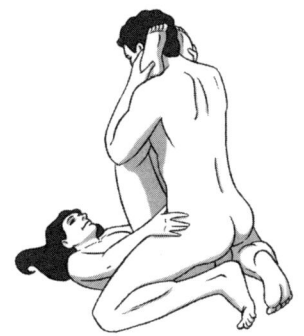
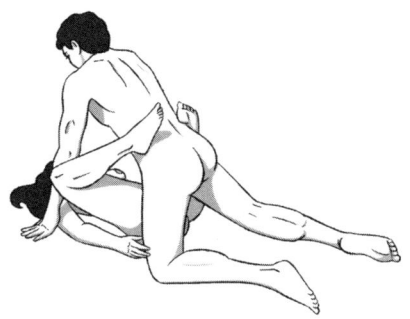
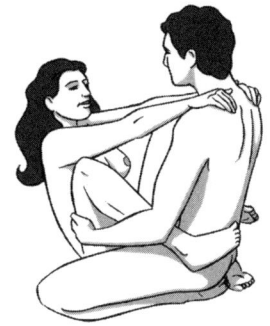
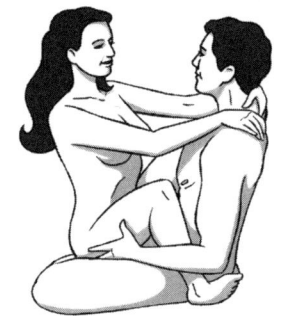
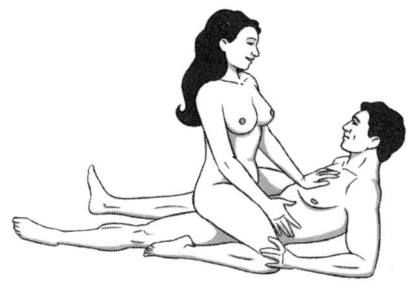
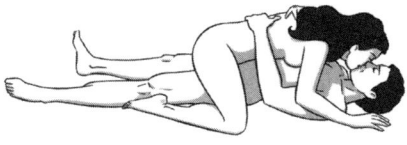

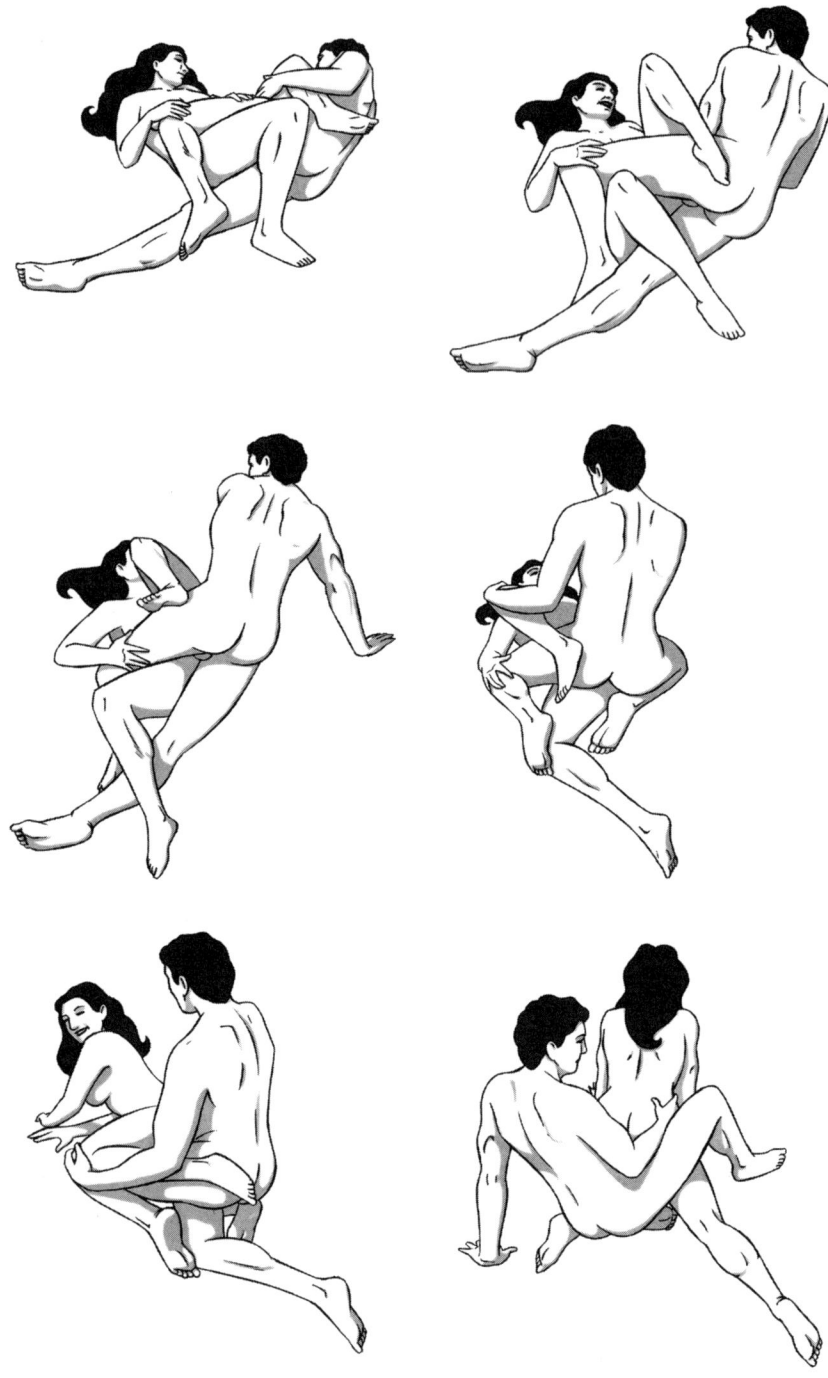

Fig. 4.6. Sequence of rotating positions through rear

The Sexual Power of Quality

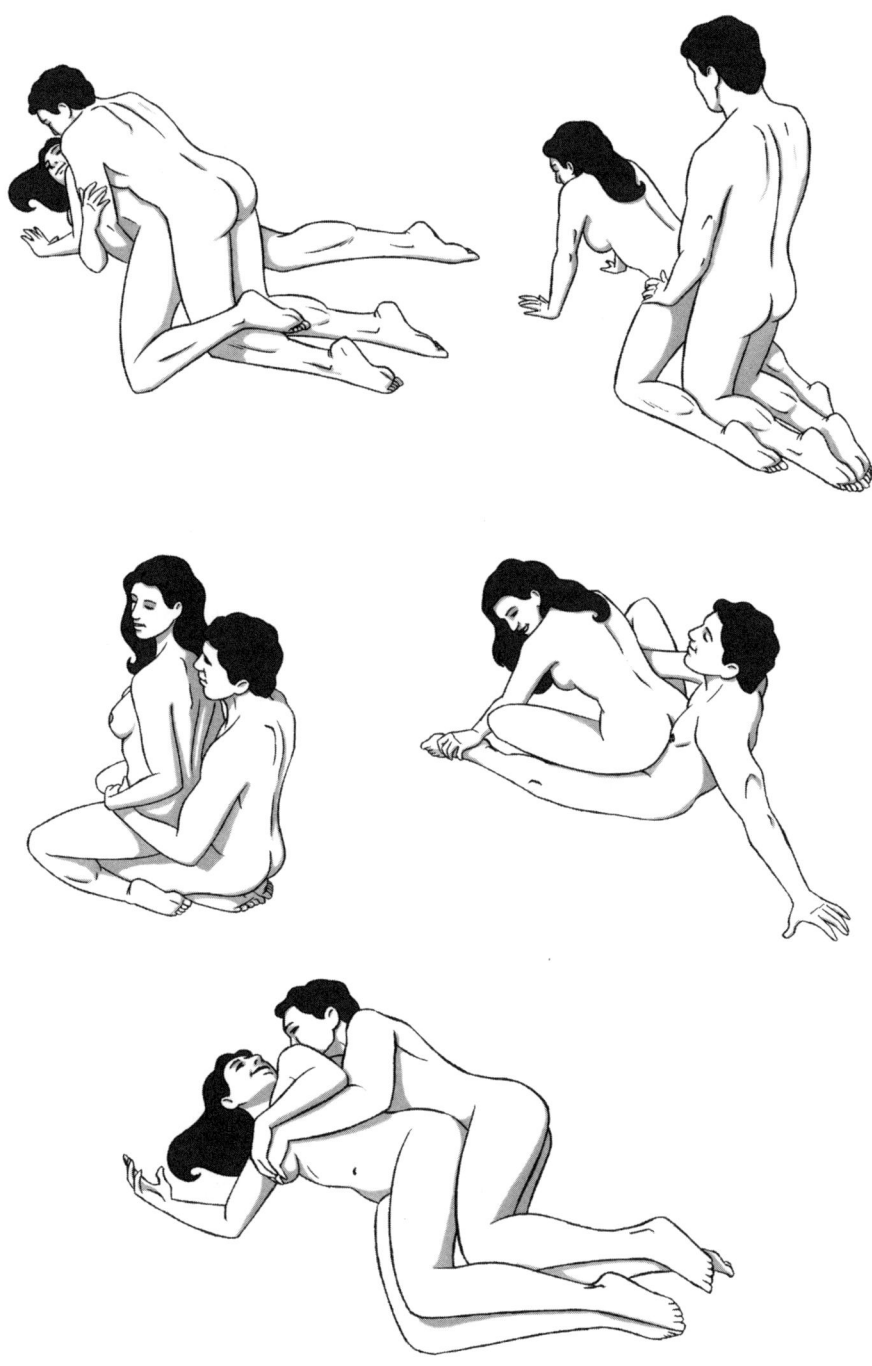

SOFT PENETRATION, ENTRY WITHOUT ERECTION

At times, especially when there is an intention to keep the temperature cooler through reducing excitement, it is not unusual to have no erection. In the usual approach, having sex is not an option without an erection—when erection fails, sex fails. However, in slow sex union is always an option because putting the penis in while soft and relaxed has great value, is easy to do, and comes highly recommended. A soft start to sex can become a regular thing, and you may find yourself choosing it as the optimal way to proceed with slow sex. A slow soft approach takes the pressure out of the situation because you can unite at any time you choose. Union is not dependent on stimulation, excitement, or erection.

Figure 4.7 illustrates the easiest position for penetration when there is no erection. Man lies on his side while woman lies on her back, and their legs intertwine in scissors-like fashion. It is recommended that this position be explored from both sides, with man lying first on one side of his body and then on the other. One side is likely to feel more familiar, cozy, and comfortable for you. The other side may feel more challenging in the sense that more is demanded of you in terms of awareness.

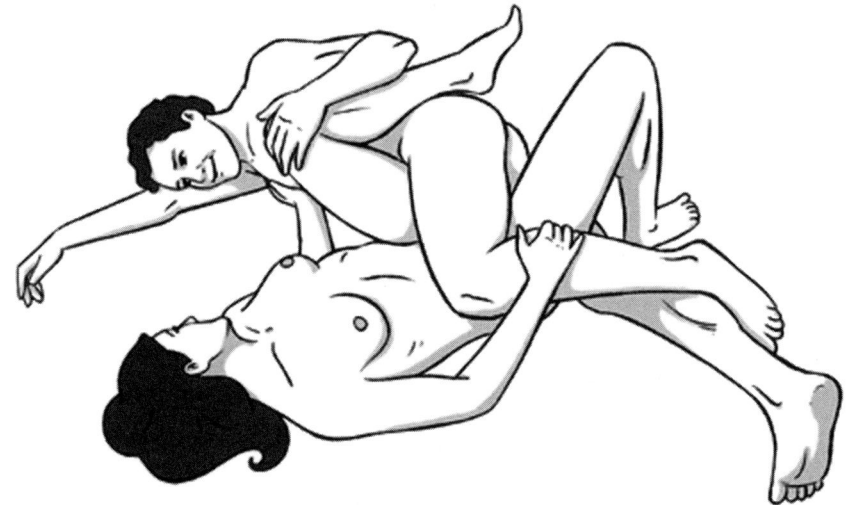

Fig. 4.7. Scissors position for soft penetration

This side-scissors position is only a suggestion for an easy starting point. The position per se is of no great significance, except that it is a very relaxing position in that both are lying down and no one is on top. It's a curious thing that the person taking the position on top generally feels compelled to do something in order to justify being in that upper position. This is man's basic sexual reality because he is more frequently on top, the missionary position being very popular. But if a woman is sitting on top of a man, she will notice a similar performance pressure, an escalated need to do something. When lying on their backs or sides, both women and men do not feel such a clear, strong drive to "do." In the scissors position man is, in fact, lying on his side, which is similar to the sleeping position, and can easily remind him of sleep. When the side position is mantained for quite a while it's not unusual for a man to drop off to sleep on occasion. Women on the other hand, who are lying directly on the back, will find it less easy to fall asleep in this scissors position. A short sleep can be regenerating, so this is not a matter for concern. If the sleeping becomes a habit, though, it's good to do some exercise before getting into bed, and to change position more often.

The side position is one from which many other positions can gradually be reached, through delicately rotating around the genital connection as illustrated earlier in figures 4.5 and 4.6. Yes, it's usually possible with a soft relaxed penis, and remember, should the penis slip out it is easy to slip it in again and continue. Other suitable positions for managing soft penetration are those suggested earlier in figure 4.3, where man kneels in the middle, and figure 4.4, where the couple is rolled over to one side (see pages 39 and 40).

Woman Inserts Man's Penis in Scissors Position

Before you move into position, it is recommended that you gently lubricate your own genitals, as described earlier in this chapter, or lovingly lubricate each other's. Do whatever feels right in the moment. As soon as you are oiled up, move into the side position as shown above and bring your pelvises close together, with the vagina opposite the penis. From here the woman can proceed by taking the penis in her two hands and gently rolling back the foreskin or any tissues around the head of the penis, pulling down toward the root of the penis. The idea of this is to expose the head's magnetic surface as much as possible in order to bring increased awareness to the radiant, dynamic qualities inherent in the penis.

Then, as shown in figure 4.8 below, woman (who should have short, rounded fingernails so that she does not scratch the vagina or penis) makes a two-pronged fork with the first two fingers of both hands. Place one finger fork (try the left hand) firmly at the base of the penis and hold the fingers there to stabilize the penis. Place the forked fingers of the other hand (the right) directly on either side and behind the rim encircling the head of the penis. Squeeze the fingers together so that you have a gentle, yet firm grip on the penis. And then pull the penis toward your vagina. When the head arrives at the entrance of the vagina you can push it a little way into the vagina. Pull the fingers back a little, then take another gentle grip on the penis, and walk or feed the penis even farther into the vagina. And then repeat the walking or feeding movement until you have pushed the whole length of the penis into you. Naturally, to do the insertion in one smooth, seamless move will take practice, so at first you may manage to get only the head, or a couple of inches, inside you. This is an

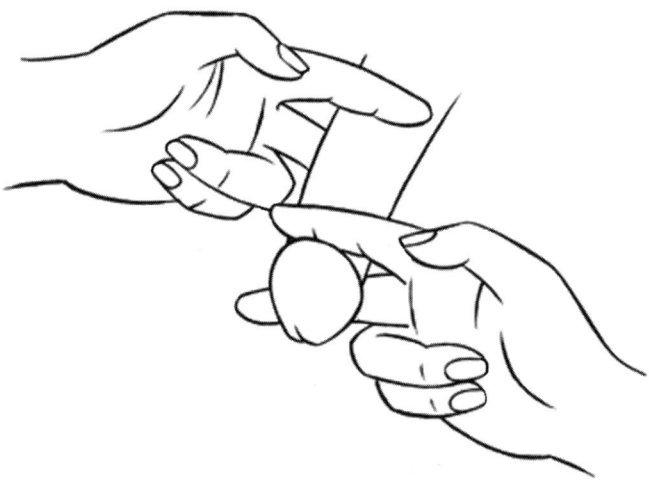

Fig. 4.8. Woman's finger position holding penis for soft insertion

excellent start and in time, when you get the knack of putting a relaxed penis into your vagina, doing so becomes second nature.

It is important to note that woman must keep her vagina relaxed and wide as she inserts the penis. Often her head is raised to look between the legs at what her hands are doing, but this move of the head tightens the abdominal muscles and the vagina. Once the fingers are in position, then woman should lie back and relax before she begins to insert the penis. When the insertion is complete and genitals are connected, wrap your legs around each other and bring your pelvises firmly together.

Bringing the bodies together in this limited-excitement way opens up all kinds of other possibilities during the sexual exchange. Just leave it up to the genitals, supported by your consciousness, and they will know how to communicate in a way that may even surprise you. It is important not to expect anything like what you have known before, and to share in words what you are feeling within. For instance, when a man hears from his partner that she can feel energy radiating from his soft relaxed penis, that is a great relief to him. Discovering that the penis has certain qualities, even if he himself cannot feel them, is very reassuring and relaxing. And instead of worrying about erection and performance, he can relax the anus and buttocks and fall back into his body and pelvis to become aware of himself from the inside out.

SPONTANEOUS ERECTION

The possibility of spontaneous erection through magnetic intelligence is built in to the genitals. The opposite forces have an effect on each other, and the penis has the capacity to wind up inside the vagina in a snakelike coiling, probing way, without any stimulation or excitement. A spontaneous erection is a by-product of the magnetic attraction and requires no effort—it happens. You can't *expect* a spontaneous erection, because it's spontaneous. It transpires when there is a constellation of invisible factors, such as when a man and woman are innocently in their bodies and merged with the inner cellular experience. Spontaneous erection is more likely when love is in the air, or where there is an element of polarization in the field, such as when man anchors his awareness in the root of the penis, the perineum, and woman connects internally with her vagina, widening and receiving.

Man will easily be able to feel the difference between spontaneous erection and intentional erection. One will feel inwardly potent and does not need movement or stimulation to maintain, while the other will feel more hollow and disconnected from the inside and is easily lost.

QUALITY IS BASED ON SLOWNESS ARISING FROM CONSCIOUSNESS

In exploring the vagina, you can again and again ask yourself a relative question: How slow is slow? It can become like a Zen koan. The answer depends on how conscious and aware you are willing to be in each and every moment. More awareness will bring more slowness. Perhaps you will be slow as a snail with one penetration taking several divine minutes, as in millimeter . . . pause . . . breath, millimeter . . . pause . . . breath. Slowness can also slow all the way down to the stillness of nonmovement, nondoing. This is not a state of deadness, but an immersion within the cellular aliveness and vitality of the body, feeling and being utterly present to what is.

When sex is cultivated with respect, love, awareness, sensitivity, and slowness, the reward is elevated, beautiful experiences of ecstatic pleasure that bring joy, love, and an increased sense of well-being.

Exercise: Become Sensitive to the Quality of Your Inner Landscape

Resting in Consciousness

Set aside twenty minutes for yourself and take a conscious rest. It's as simple as this: Lie down on your back, close your eyes, invert your attention, and reside within your body.

1. First, place a rolled blanket or pillow directly behind the crease of your knees, so that the legs are slightly bent and the feet/toes turned slightly inward. This support creates a softening at the knees that helps the connection to the lower body and is a great aid to deepening relaxation.
2. Then lie back and get your head, neck, and spine into one precise line. Tuck your chin slightly toward your chest so that the back of your neck lengthens. This physical alignment is crucial, because aligning yourself in this way increases the capacity to be present.
3. Lie with your hands open, palms facing up, arms lying close to your body.
4. Close your eyes, inhale a deep breath into the belly, scan and release any tense parts of your body, and then simply be present and aware in your body. You can also use the home in your body as an anchor, as was outlined in an exercise at the end of chapter 3.

Just be in your body for twenty minutes or so. It may happen that at a certain moment you sort of slip into yourself, then beyond yourself, and become taken in by your inner world into a space of timelessness. Resting in a conscious way is refreshing and rejuvenating, and turning inward gets easier with practice. This can also be used as a form of foreplay and attuning to yourself before coming together with your partner.

Dynamic/Receptive Pole Variation

The preceding exercise can be slightly varied by moving the hands and placing them over the groin area, palms down on either side of the pubic bone. Then follow the steps for the aligned body position as outlined above, resting at home in your body, alive to the vitality in your cells.

After a while, man can focus his attention internally to the perineum, a knot of muscle at the root of the penis. Imagine a thread of light or warmth connecting this area to the inner home. And in the same way, woman can draw her attention into the vaginal canal, soften and widen the muscles, and rest easily with the awareness within.

5
THE SEXUAL POWER OF RHYTHM

Rhythm is an integral part of the universe, nature, and human beings. There is rhythm in the seasons and as a pulse, in the ebb and flow of life. The very same pulse beats within each of our hearts, no matter how different our individual realities may be. We are similarly subjected to the rising and setting of the sun, and the waxing and waning of the moon. In the absence of rhythm there will be an absence of life. There are many rhythms in the human body, in addition to our basic heartbeat. Each of the visceral organs, such as small and large intestine, liver, gallbladder, stomach, and so on, has its own individual and precise rhythm and repeating pattern of movement. There are even rhythms in the brain and spinal cord, as well as three subtle levels of respiration in the body.

Perhaps the rhythm most overlooked—and therefore most neglected, even in our twenty-first century—is a rhythm truly basic to human sexual expression, the different rhythms of man and woman. In sex it is generally assumed that we have the same rhythms, that our bodies get turned on in the same way and at the same time. But this is not true. On occasion, most of us have experienced meetings or phases of being totally in tune, but as a general rule, we are different.

MAN AND WOMAN HAVE DIFFERENT RHYTHMS

Men's and women's bodies open up, or warm up, at varying speeds. Man is fast and woman is slow as a direct result of the bodies being equal and opposite forces. The discrepancy is not psychological, despite the myth that men enjoy and want sex more than woman do.

Nature designed man and woman as complementary forces of dynamic and receptive. Dynamic is "positive" and ever ready, as most men will agree, but this is not necessarily true for women. The reason for the slowness or lack of immediate readiness on the part of woman is that the quality of receptivity is an "absorbing" force, one that can also be described as passive or "negative" polarity. A receptive force will come alive when time and space is granted for the sexual temperature to rise and equal that of man. This is a basic requirement for the full sexual metabolism to be mobilized into existence. Only then does woman become alive as a force, equal, and truly in her feminine power.

In the early stages of a relationship there is more likelihood that woman will be present with a full "yes" at the same time as her man. Everything is fresh and new, so she is naturally propelled into the moment-by-moment experience—the mysterious present. Another basic reason for this increased rapport, or woman's yes to sex, is that she is in love and her heart is alive, vibrant, and open. The heart/breast area plays a significant role in woman's general readiness for sex, as will soon be discussed.

WOMAN'S LOSS OF INTEREST IN SEX

As the initial weeks and months of wonderful sexual spontaneity in a relationship span into years, and the situation settles into a routine, it is extremely common for women to feel an increasing reluctance to get involved in sex. And as already mentioned, the avoidance of sex by a woman is usually not something coming from her mind, in the sense that resistance is something she chooses for herself, but a very physical response in which the body just closes down and loses interest. The female body begins an involuntary and gradual withdrawal from sex because the essential quality of receptivity is not honored and given space in which to thrive. The fundamental qualities of man and woman, and the opposite qualities they bring to the sexual exchange, are totally ignored in fast sex, and the reality is that as life gets busier and the novelty wears off, sex tends to get faster and be over more quickly. As a result, in the course of time a woman will find herself hardening, losing her femininity, and becoming slightly male as a by-product and kind of defense.

I know for a fact (through the personal histories of so many couples that I meet while teaching) that the majority of men would like to have sex more often than their partners would. Yet woman is unavailable to man on the "instant" basis that he has been conditioned to expect. Instant sex is the reason for the existence of the oldest profession in the world—prostitution—because it represents to man the possibility for instant sex. Sex on demand, no fuss, no foreplay. I also know for a fact that when women have slow sex, when everything is taken with ease and leisure, then women want more sex. The solution is so simple. Some of us will remember the well-known words of an old song—that a woman likes a man with a slow hand—it is true.

So the whole issue of woman's apparent lack of availability is due to a lack of understanding of rhythm and how male and female bodies open in different ways in sex. A woman is definitely capable of a superficial opening without being fully involved and alive to the experience, without participating as a fully energized and willing body. For a woman sex can, and usually far too often does, take place inside her body when she is not really involved, except as the location. For countless centuries women have yielded to the pressure of sex, gone unwillingly into sex, without particpating and sharing equally in the act. Sex starts and finishes with such speed that for a woman's female body, there is not enough time to awaken and connect with her inner receptive qualities. Embracing the female force of receptivity is fundamental to elevating the sexual exchange.

THE OPPOSITE POLE IS CARRIED WITHIN EACH INDIVIDUAL

The secret to awakening or equalizing the sexual energy of woman, and thereby her interest in and wish for sex, does not lie in the clitoris or vagina. The route to woman's sexual source and innate vitality is via her breasts, which, on an energetic level, are very connected to the heart.

Earlier, in chapter 4, man's penis is explained as a positive, flowing, streaming force, while woman's vagina is seen as the complementary negative, receptive, absorbent force. Over and above the specific polarity we carry in our genitals, there is an even higher level to the intelligence of our human bodies—within each individual lies the equal and opposite pole. This means that in the male body there exists a female pole that is receptive, and in the female body there exists a male pole that is dynamic. Man is part woman and woman is part man, an inner design that has been proven by chromosome studies within the past hundred years. Our bodies must have always carried this astounding higher intelligence and vibration embedded in the cells of our sexual organs. Even though humanity has been following other patterns in sexual expression since the dawn of time, the creative potential of sex and its numerous benefits continue to remain alive within us as a source of vitality, inspiration, and spiritual elevation.

The body can be visualized as carrying an inner magnet with north and south poles. Or plus and minus poles, positive and negative poles, yang and yin poles . . . name them as we wish. In man the dynamic pole is the penis and his equal and opposite negative, receptive pole is the heart and chest area. In woman, as equal and opposite force to man, the receptive pole is the vagina and her dynamic pole lies in the breasts (including nipples).

Energy Is Raised from a Positive Pole

The problem with the common approach of going directly to a woman's genital area in foreplay and sex is that the vagina is a receptive pole, a passive organ, and energy cannot be raised from a negative pole; energy can only be raised from a positive pole. So for woman this means the breasts are the true source of her sexual awakening, while the clitoris and vagina are secondary. When attention (by woman herself, and also by man) is given to the breasts there will usually be (after some time) a kind of answering or response in the vagina, which is experienced as vibration or vitality, an inner awakening, together with an increasing wish to receive the penis. Awakening the positive pole in woman gives birth to the quality of receptivity in the vagina. So any inner connection a woman has to her breasts has a remarkable influence on erection, especially spontaneous erection, as described in the previous chapter.

The Role of the Clitoris Is Not Central

In my understanding and experience there is a better sequencing of events, and that is to leave the clitoris in the background until well into the lovemaking, if indeed you want to give the clitoris any direct attention at all. Again, there are no rules, but some women feel more relaxed and serene when there is no direct contact or stimulation of the clitoris; finding it preferable when pressure happens more indirectly, for example, through the position. Many women have highly satisfying sex lives without any clitoral engagement or climax-type orgasms at all. Some women find a quick peak orgasm will act as a link to the inner regions of the vagina, increasing their sensitivity. Others will feel a loss of interest. Each woman must explore the impact the clitoris has on her ultimate sensitivity and presence, and what is true for her.

The clitoris is not central to woman's higher sexual experiences. Stimulating touch of the clitoris causes sexual excitement and makes a woman full of desire. This has the effect of tightening the vagina as it gets tense with expectation. Most men have had the experience at times of entering a woman and the vagina feels hungry, demanding, or greedy, and it's an instant turn-off. The needy quality in the vagina can sometimes cause a loss of erection in man, or an immediate ejaculation. The tension of excitement and stimulation disturbs the receptive environment and throws the two equal and opposite forces out of balance.

Some men correctly observe that in their experience some women do, in fact, like, or even demand, to have hard and fast sex. Yes, this is true, some women have adopted and display man's basic attitude, but this reflects our sexual misunderstanding. Women are usually not familiar with the inner workings of their own bodies and their essential quality of receptivity. Many women have intuitions about how their bodies function, but these signals are usually discarded and the normal style of sex chosen through fear of not being loved, fear of losing a man, fear of not being sexually satisfied, or fear of being different from other women. These fears cause a lack of trust in the body, because we do not know ourselves very well. Recently I was with a group of sixty women where I asked the direct question: "Who has recognized that you have become sort of male in the way you have sex?" Every single woman in the room raised her hand. I also asked: "Who would wish for more time before being entered by man?" Again all hands were raised. The other pertinent question I asked was: "Who has observed that clitoral stimulation affects the quality of receptivity in the vagina and the impact of the penetration?" And again all the women raised their hands. The fact is, we all know the same things about our individual bodies, and yet as a group, as womankind, we continue to move forward under a collective hypnosis, repeatedly going against the truth of our bodies.

Women have yet to discover their receptive essence and the sense of arriving home to themselves that comes through honoring the body's wisdom. I have witnessed some women in my couple's groups begin in great resistance to a less active, less clitoral approach, and usually their softer, more feminine side will feel very remote because of the conditioned identification with the harder, more male side. Our personality is formed around the sexual image that we carry. The ego is, therefore, bound to fight for its rights initially, but once the experimentation gets under way, the transformation of a resistant woman is remarkably fast. Within two or three days of first having slow sex, the hardened facade begins a meltdown, the features soften and sweetly glow, and eyes shine with the light of love. And only because the vital, slow sexual rhythm and response of the female body has been acknowledged and honored. Women are, by birth and by nature, sexually slower than men and there is nothing to be done about it. It leaves us with no real choice other than to accept, respect, honor, and be grateful for the intelligence of our complementary inner designs and rhythms.

ALLOWING TIME

Respecting bodily rhythms requires granting time. Slowness in sex means allocating real time—several hours instead of just a handful of minutes. Make a date to have slow sex, and plan on at least three hours. Don't try to squeeze sex into a busy schedule, but make getting together a high priority of the day or the week.

The three-hour time proposal does not mean you have to be sexually engaged the entire time, although you may sometimes find yourselves doing so. Pauses and breaks will occur naturally. The extended time frame creates a valley of relaxation, giving birth to a slower rhythm, one where you have time to arrive in your bodies and gently flow with the experience. Start from zero and slowly warm up, instead of going from zero to a hundred in just a few minutes. With plenty of time allotted, the exchange can flow organically, with no pressure, no goals, no onward plan. There will be moments in which natural pauses occur—for adjusting position, pillows, or bedding, having a glass of water, using the bathroom, or whatever. You can stop any time for a shower or a cup of tea. And then come back to bed, connect, and give it another whirl.

Extending the Experience

Honoring sexual rhythm also implies taking it easy in the sense of extending each element of the actual sexual experience. Take the awareness and attention to the subtlest level you can manage. Any enhanced inner perception will make you more sensuous and sensitive, as if sipping and savoring each second with delight. When you enter the very moment, time and ego disappear. If you are alive to yourself at the outset and not lukewarm or detached, you get totally caught up in another dimension, fueled by an inner power. Bodies are capable of quite extraordinary and unimaginable energy events when tuned in to and trusted to flow at their own pace and in their own rhythm.

REGULARITY AND FREQUENCY

Rhythm also relates to how frequently you make love. More often is better than less often, especially when talking about quality, life-enhancing sex. Regular is better than irregular. Like many things, the more you practice with regularity and frequency, the better you get, and the more you want to practice. The more you experience the beauty of slow sex, the more you will want to partake. When good intentions and honorable wishes lose priority, complacency and laziness can quietly slide into the equation. Then, all too easily, you are out of practice, out of rhythm with yourself and your partner. In some ways the body is like a musical instrument, and if you've ever slacked off on practicing an instrument for six months or so, you know that getting back on track looks arduous and daunting; postponement and delay become the easier option. The impetus for adventure and the desire to explore the unknown are lost, as is the opportunity to be transformed in the process.

RHYTHM AS BREATH

Breath is vital to the metabolic power of sex, as it literally breathes vitality into the moment. In one sense we have no control over our breath—our bodies automatically breathe themselves. However, breath is a rhythm that we can easily influence to great advantage.

When attention is given to the breath—the very act of breathing—you are held in the present with enhanced alertness, which will further deepen and slow the rhythm of the breath. There are several ways in which the breath can be playfully explored to varying effects. You will, however, need to stay alert to the trap of the mind, which can get distracted, caught up with what's going on and with getting it right, thereby causing a certain degree of absence.

Simultaneous Breathing

In simultaneous breathing, you both breathe in at the same time and out at the same time. The breaths are deep and slow into the belly, in the direction of the genitals (use visualization if you do not feel any sensation of breath actually arriving in your genitals), and you stay as much as possible in breath synchronicity with each other. It's best to allow the breaths to be of a similar duration. You can even extend the duration for four or five counts, for instance; not aloud, of course (except at the outset, perhaps, just to mutually set the pace). If you slip out of rhythm, which can easily happen, relax for a few breaths and then slowly begin to pick up the rhythm of your partner again. Be light and easy and avoid making the breath into something stressful.

Alternating Breathing

In this type of breathing, one person breathes in as the other breathes out. Alternating breathing gets you very involved in the body and in what is happening, as it is happening. Alternating breathing can also be connected with so-called circular breathing, which uses visualization to awaken and support the electromagnetic circular flow of energy between the bodies, as in the exercise below.

Exercise: Rhythmic Circular Breathing with Visualization

◯ Circular Breathing with a Partner

In this exercise you can use visualization to accompany the breath. The excercise can be done with or without music.

1. Start with yourself, open eyes or closed eyes, and take the attention in and down, anchoring your awareness in the body.

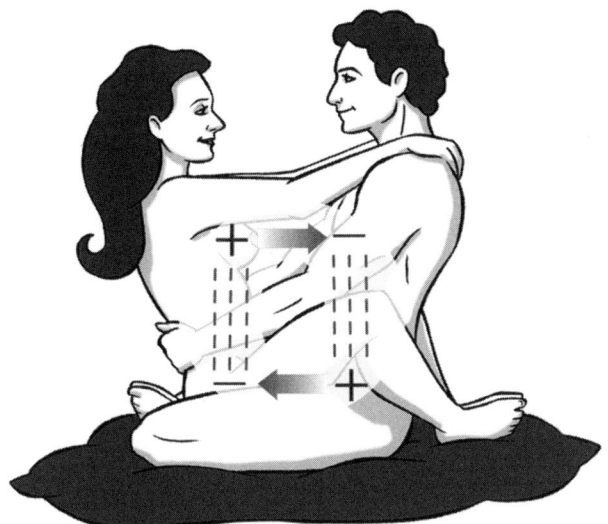

Fig. 5.1. Opposing female and male polarities
with inner magnets in alignment for circular energy flow
(in yab yum position)

2. Then bring awareness to the positive poles, man downward to the perineum (at the root of the penis) and woman upward to her breasts and especially into the nipples.
3. When you feel ready and in tune with yourself move into the yab yum position (making all suitable adjustments for comfort) and then bring your chests together (eye contact optional), and also line the nipples up so that they correspond with and directly touch each other. This can be done (and the effect felt) with or without clothing.
4. Once you are in a comfortable position, woman should imagine that light and breath is entering through her vagina on the in-breath, and flowing out of her breasts and nipples on the out-breath. She radiates light and life force into her man's chest.
5. Man can likewise imagine that he is receiving a vital force from woman on his in-breath, and in turn breathing consciously out of his perineum and penis as he radiates light, gold, and love into woman's vagina. Continue this alternate breathing and visualization for as long as you wish.

↻ Individual Variation of Circular Breathing

By using the flame of a candle, the breathing exercise described above can also be done alone by an individual.

1. Breathe the light from the flame in through the receptive pole (the vagina for woman, the chest for man).
2. On the out-breath, return the light to the flame through the dynamic pole (the breasts for woman, the penis for man).

You can keep a circle of light flowing between you and the flame for several minutes, synchronizing the direction of your breath with the visualization of a flow or perhaps you even feel the inner cellular sensation of flowing or streaming expansion.

6
THE SEXUAL POWER OF PLEASURE

Opening to more pleasure can spark metabolism and return the body to its natural state of balance. . . . What I would like to suggest to you is that health, and by extension any action that promotes health, is inherently a deeply pleasurable experience.
MARC DAVID (*THE SLOW DOWN DIET*, PAGE 110)

SENSITIVITY, THE SOURCE OF PLEASURE

Sex can be deeply pleasurable and can also benefit the health of body, mind, and soul in many miraculous ways. Pleasure in sex is generated through giving highest priority to the rhythms of nature that are reflected in our bodies, and giving value to, and enjoying, the innate sensitivity that arises as a result. Sensitivity is born through awareness, relaxation, and quality. Sensitivity and sensuality allow an intense aliveness as a by-product of honoring the differing rhythms of man and woman. More sensitivity creates more pleasure. With a connection to, and awareness of, our mighty senses we find ourselves in the optimum position to experience profound dimensions of pleasure. The pure pleasure of sex is a human birthright and one of the joys of living in a physical body.

Sensitivity indicates an awareness of, and inner connection to, the cellular aliveness inherent in the body. Sensitive does not mean ouch! this hurts or that hurts. Yes, this type of reaction is a reflection of a type of sensitivity, or in some cases a hypersensitivity, which is more related to memories in the body as a residual emotional tension or defense. However, the sensitivity required to experience pleasure at its deepest level requires an internal connection to the flesh—an awareness of the inner cosmos and all the magical sensations that can be experienced there. The key to activating the metabolic power of pleasure is to trust your body and your ability to experience pleasure.

SLOWNESS ENHANCES SENSITIVITY

The undeniable reality is that as soon as you slow down you become more sensitive. One of the remarkable things noticed by the men in our retreats is that after three or four afternoons of slow sex practice, their penises very quickly get more sensitive and perceptive. They can feel into the tissues much more deeply when their movements are slow and conscious; the penis has a much finer type of magnetic sensitivity, perception, and intelligence—different from the intense sensations experienced through stimulation. I am so often awed by the body and how quickly it responds when awareness and intelligence are brought into the sex act. Through awareness and its by-product of slowness, the tissues heal and become resensitized in a very short space of time, in both men and women. When asked, most women will admit that their vaginas are more sensitive and receptive after just a few days of making love in a more relaxed (and not focused on orgasm) way. The body regenerates as soon as it is granted the space and the trust. Pleasure loves slowness. Pleasure loves sensuality.

THE SHIFT FROM SENSATION TO SENSITIVITY

To increase pleasure we need to increase sensitivity, slowness, and sensuality. We need to tune in to our many senses: breathing as a sense of smell, touch as a feeling sense, eyes as a receiving sense, and awareness as a witnessing sense. Sensation as we commonly understand it is not truly sensitivity. Sensation is often the response of an erogenous zone or sensitive area to some form of external stimulation, but this is not cellular sensitivity. To become more sensitive requires that we make a shift away from sensation, which is based on stimulation and excitement, involves the other (the stimulus), and includes the buildup of tension. Certainly sensitivity can also be sensational, but not in the usual sense. Sex today relies almost entirely on stimulation and sensation, which actually leads, in the long term, to less sensitivity.

It has been scientifically proven that long-term overexposure to sensation leads to an ultimate loss of sensitivity. At the end of a couples retreat several years ago, a scientist who had participated told me that the loss of sensitivity in the face of intensity of stimulation had been scientifically proven in the second half of the nineteenth century by German physiologist Ernst Weber and physicist and psychologist Gustav Fechmer. Their research, formulated as the Weber-Fechmer law, is the theory of the relationship between stimulus and experience. Their research showed that the change in intensity of a sensation varies in increments proportional to the relative change of the stimulus. Today this is known to be true for every sensory channel within its range of dynamics. A simple example would be to light a match in the darkness. In this instance the light is like an explosion, but if you do the same in bright sunlight, it is barely perceptible. More sensation correlates to less sensitivity, and less sensation correlates to more sensitivity. Instead of habitually seeking more and more sensation, you can begin working on your senses so that you become capable of feeling the subtle, yet vital life force moving through you.

Fast, hot sex desensitizes the body, and especially the penis and vagina, because it is mechanical and extroverted, dependent on sensation. The more sensation is increased, the more innate sensitivity is lost. This probably accounts for the widespread problem of impotence. Impotence represents a loss of sensitivity and awareness. A man through overstimulation slowly becomes dead to himself, and then to others, eventually unable to respond to the sensation of a strong stimulus.

Very often the fear of not feeling (in man or woman) can be the impetus for seeking sensation. At least you know for sure you can feel *something* in that particular situation. With relaxation everything is wide open, and the fear of not feeling or the fear of the unknown will keep many of us in sensation-seeking patterns. The important thing as you begin to explore is not to expect the same things as you have known up to now. You begin to experiment and gather your own body of experience. You need to become more sensitive, relaxed, and open, and thereby more capable of feeling into yourself. And you need to discover the value of the subtle. There is a shift from mind to body, from sexual desire where the focus is up and out on the periphery in extrovert style, toward the opposite—a full inversion, diving in and down into the body. Finding rest at home. The more aware, relaxed, and present you become (where true relaxation equals aliveness), the more sensitive you will become. Sensitivity creates presence, so they go hand in hand.

SLOW SEX IS COOL SEX

Slowness is always kind of cool, and yet not cold. There's a kind of distance, but not disconnection, when you are inwardly absorbed by more subtle happenings in your body, and not caught up in making sex hot and exciting. For sure, fast, hot sex can have the immediate appearance of satisfaction—and that's its curious appeal—but over time its stresses and goals can easily give you the sense of going around in circles. Eventually nothing exciting beckons on the horizon. Sexual boredom, or eventual lack of sex, is one of the main reasons why it becomes difficult for a couple to sustain a relationship over many years, and these days the frequent change and exchange of partners is considered the way to address such an unsatisfactory situation. Sexual frustration and sexual desire underlie the increasingly high demand for pornography, which is invariably focused on stimulation and sensation. When sex is equated with heat, excitement, and stimulation, it can make a man numb to himself, encapsulated by a world of sexual fantasy.

Believing that sex is based on the heat of excitement, we keep looking down the path of sensation when, in fact, we should turn in on ourselves and look at (and feel) the ecstatic sensitivity of our inner cellular vitality. But you need to cool down so that you can bring the focus back to yourself, where you are rooted in your body and your being, not focused on excietment, orgasm, or on your partner. The thing about coolness is that it is eternal, it does not burn out and come to an end the way jumping around in excitement eventually does. Being hot all the time will eventually become exhausting! A cool stance gives you some centering and repose, and at the same time will have you gently plugged into something much vaster than you. There are no rushes, rises, or falls.

Staying cool is easily done by holding your attention in your own body. Find an inner home to anchor your awareness and attention, as described earlier in the exercise at the end of chapter 3. From this sense of rooting yourself in your own body (you can also include the whole spine as your midline) comes an absorption in the enchantment of your inner cosmos. From here, from your very center, you can expand endlessly outward into the beyond.

INCREASING THE CAPACITY TO PERCEIVE THE SUBTLE

Sensitivity is pure pleasure and increasing our sensitivity makes us increasingly capable of feeling the subtle. Sensitivity requires that you give yourself the opportunity and space to perceive subtle sensations. And to identify them as a source of pleasure. You tune in to yourself on a much finer level and doing so makes the body more porous; the cells become more vibrant and fill with light. With accumulated tension over years, the body becomes tight, and eventually hardened, which makes it dense, less porous, less sensitive, and less receptive. Relaxation and the inner expansion that follows is basic to the quest for more sensitivity and pleasure. Relaxation implies turning inward and getting closer to yourself, first and foremost, on an inner level. And it is this closeness to yourself, your own inner friendliness and familiarity, that will bring you the experience of greater closeness and intimacy with another person. The other doesn't change; *you* change. And because you transform your own approach, your partner usually follows suit and responds with sensitivity and presence.

It's an incredible and mysterious alchemy. The pleasure and delight of nature's genital intelligence and sensitivity is something that will usually grow with time and exposure, meaning that you actually make love and open up to experience deep fulfilling pleasure. Not a pleasure that leaves you wanting it again and again, but a pleasure that nourishes, fulfills, and uplifts you. When you are turned on by sex, when you experience sex in full-bodied pleasure, there is an impact on the entire sexual metabolism. A fast sexual style and fast lifestyle close a doorway of perception that decreases your pleasure threshold. There is a fascinating mind-body-spirit connection linking sexual metabolism, pleasure, and beauty. Opening to the finer pleasures of sex presents a thrilling arena that invites love and transformation.

7

THE SEXUAL POWER OF THOUGHT

Many years ago I heard it said that a man thinks about sex every two to three minutes, and a woman, every five to six minutes. Whatever the real statistics are, there is no doubt that sexual thoughts tend to dominate our minds. Even when we don't generate the thoughts ourselves, sex-related thoughts are continually provoked through advertising, media, films, pornography, jokes, and fashion. It is safe to say that the majority of us think about sex more than we actually have it.

The sexual domain is powerfully influenced by pleasant, painful, fantasizing, guilty, lustful, desirous, angry, disrespectful, disappointing, frustrating, or insecure thoughts. For many, the associations with sex are neither positive nor pleasant, and sex tends to be blanketed by a mantle of disappointment and discontent. In some individuals, searching for satisfaction can reach the level of an obsession or addiction in an attempt to fulfill seemingly endless and unfulfillable urges.

People think about sex more often than they engage in it because humans are not really having enough sex of the fulfilling and sustainable variety. As a result, our sexual energy is repressed and becomes diverted, sometimes in unhealthy, unloving ways.

THOUGHT AS DISTRACTION

The problem with our thoughts is that they are an aspect of the mind, separate and distinct from the body, where sex physically takes place. However, thoughts can have a strong impact on the body and alter the ensuing experience. Thought basically disconnects us from the inner subtle experiences of the body. I noticed how easily I slipped into irrelevant thoughts right from my first sexual experiences. I remember being shocked to notice myself having arbitrary thoughts during sex, thoughts that were not necessarily sex related. Any old thing would pop up and disturb my involvement in the present. In my innocent virginal imagination, sex should have been an all-consuming, overwhelming event that would somehow take control of me and obliterate my thoughts. But instead, when I found myself "still thinking," I remember being quietly devastated.

The propensity of the mind to drift off into thought and away from the body is something I have continued to observe, both in daily life and during my exploration of sex. It's like a lateral shift. The mind slides in sideways, distracts, and effectively darkens the inner light and subtle sensations present in the body. However, the instant the shift to mind is detected or observed (using the awareness), the reverse shift can be managed very easily. The inner connection to the body can be reestablished and the inner sensations resumed. It is not as if the inner sensitivity actually goes away in those moments of thinking. The inner cosmos continues to spiral and swirl in spite of us, but the finer level of subtlety and sensitivity moves out of the awareness and becomes swamped by thoughts.

THOUGHT AS SEXUAL CONDITIONING

Unsatisfactory sexual experiences and unhappy associations with sex are not due to sex per se. Definitely not. Sex in and of itself is God-given and divine, and we will explore the sexual power of the sacred in chapter 8.

The negative associations of sex are more a result of the way in which sex is used by the human race. It's focused on the spilling of semen and continuation of the blood line, and this has many consequences, some visible, others less visible. The stresses of survival and the ensuing speed with which we live our lives disconnect us from the cellular vitality of the body. As humans we generally turn sex into something profane by not being able to manage our magnificent sexual force with wisdom and insight.

The subject of sex is seldom directly addressed. Regularly I ask the participants in my groups, "Who received a sex education?" Only on occasion will one or two, out of a total of fifty people, raise their hands. And when I then ask, "And was it helpful?" the raised hands are slowly lowered. Not always, but usually. At school we are taught biology and the basics, the sexual organs and process of reproduction, but nothing is said about how to actually engage oneself, express oneself, and share of oneself during the sexual act. The sex education we receive is accidental.

In truth, anatomical and biological reproductive information about sex is of no real support to us, and at the same time, sex is a vital force that nobody can really avoid. Instead, we are directly influenced and affected by the powerful sexual vibrations in the atmosphere. We hear things, we see things, we feel things, we imagine things, and so become unconsciously conditioned by these mighty, yet invisible forces. The style of sex that we know is an acquired condition, and it is not necessarily how we are born to be in sex.

This unconscious conditioning has altered our minds and our psyches, and penetrated the very cells of our bodies. The orgasm urge holds us firmly in its grip, almost as if we are under a certain spell, which is why it is virtually impossible to conceive of another style of sex. Especially as we get a bit older and more settled in our sexual ways. My observation so far has been that the young couples (ages eighteen to thirty) who come to our seminars are noticeably more open to exploring and finding new ways than couples in their forties, fifties, and sixties, who are more identified with their sexual personalities.

When we are young we are more innocent, and our bodies and

psyches are more pure. We are not encumbered by a sexual history that has accumulated over years. Younger people need only a small shift; it feels natural and easy for them to be aware and relaxed, whereas for someone older, incorporating these aspects into sex can feel like an imposition on their expression.

This situation is a by-product of our sexual conditioning and a lack of insightful sex education. We are not to blame for the limitations imposed on our sexual expression, and at the same time it is good to realize that the situation is a direct result of blindness to our true sexual design. It is as if we have been looking through glasses that restrict our vision, so we cannot see the wider or higher purpose of sex. And perhaps our sexual approach is understandable, because until a certain point in time, humans were compelled to reproduce and master their environment to ensure their survival. Their whole orientation has been to focus their attention outside of themselves. There has been neither opportunity nor encouragement to explore the inner workings of human sexuality. And most of those who have turned away from the material outer world to the inner world have been religious groups promoting withdrawal from the body and denial/repression of the relentless urges of the flesh. Sexual energy cannot be tamed or contained, so it has been forced underground to become something secretive, impure, and guilt ridden.

When sex became a sin it was swept under the rug and reappeared again as secretive short-lived sex and thoughts circling around in our heads. The thoughts persist because of the relative lack of sex. When you don't have satisfying sex you fantasize or dream about it, you pervert it, or you masturbate. When we have eaten a fully satisfying meal we stop thinking about food. When we are hungry we look at the object of our desire in a very different way from when we are satiated.

THOUGHT AS DESIRE FOR ORGASM

Orgasm as the goal of sex is a reflection of our sexual conditioning. Some men and women who have explored sex in depth have shared their observation that the thought of orgasm is needed before there is the desire for orgasm. In other words, the goal is basically a mindset, and the body can be talked into it. I have observed this as well. Thought precedes compulsion, desire, and orgasm, and the exciting-climax fixation is, in fact, part of our inherited conditioning in sex and becomes a great disturbance in true human sexual expression.

THOUGHT AS SEXUAL FANTASY

For many people sexual fantasy goes hand in hand with sex. Fantasy can fuel sex. It turns you on, sets you on fire, and keeps you burning, especially when the actual reality fails to do so. It is considered totally acceptable to use sexual fantasy as a stimulant, and even encouraged as a way to find sexual satisfaction. Fantasy has become the trigger for the physical responses of the body, but fantasies are a projected world and not happening for real, so therefore have absolutely nothing to do with the inner reality of the human body. In fact, fantasy makes us absent to the present. The function of pornography, which is a type of fantasy, is to stimulate the imagination and inflame the body. Regular use can cause a dependence on sexual stimulation and excitement, and slowly the body's true sensitivity will be lost and become unresponsive, going kind of numb through overuse and misuse. Impotence is a sign of the body losing its innate sensitivity to the pressure and tension of stimulating sex.

Eyes open or maintaining receptive eye contact is the best way to reduce sexual fantasy. Eyes open anchors you in the present, in your immediate situation, and helps you to avoid drifting off into a world of fantasy.

POSITIVE THOUGHT AS VISUALIZATION OR IMAGINATION

Thoughts directed in a positive way can anchor the mind in the actual bodily reality and counteract the "absence" of fantasy or distracting thoughts. Our minds have a tremendous influence over the body and its responses, often to our detriment, but fortunately also very much for our benefit. When there is a change in mind about sex, followed by a new kind of experience, there will be a corresponding change in the nature and content of the thoughts one has in relation to sex.

The power of thought in the form of visualization or imagination (as opposed to fantasy) can be used with intention to connect with the inner realms of the body. This is a world apart from sexual fantasy and stimulation. Visualization or the imagination can help to cultivate "right thoughts" in relation to the body, so that its inner wisdom can be awakened and expressed. You imagine and support what is—something that *does* exist, and not something that does *not* exist, as is typical of fantasy. Imagination awakens energy or energy follows the imagination, and soon these extraordinarily delightful subtle inner sensations actually will begin to be felt.

A few examples of how visualization can be used: Visualize light vibrating in your cells, the color gold streaming and flowing through your body, or connecting your own positive and receptive poles. Or man can visualize energy, love, light, or gold flowing from his penis as a positive pole. And woman can imagine receiving these golden light emanations into her vagina. Woman can use her imagination in the same way and visualize love energy radiating from breasts and nipples, where her positive poles lie. Man can imagine the love and light being received into his heart and chest.

RIGHT THOUGHT AS INTENTION

Making a change to our sexual patterns usually does not happen accidentally; it requires intention and commitment. Any intention and commitment should not become a tension; it's more a matter of the willingness to pay attention. It's a relaxed orientation that includes intentionally using the awareness in order to make a shift from being mechanical and routine to being conscious and spontaneous—to going with the flow. The attention is being "inverted" and shifted back to the intelligence of the body. To help support any intention, a willing spirit, curiosity, and a sense of adventure are definite assets when stepping into the unknown.

Some kind of intention is needed because what we are attempting to do by breaking sexual patterns runs counter to centuries of collective beliefs and experience, so there is very little available in the way of external support. With the new understanding that the intelligence already lies within your body, that the secret lies inside you, there will be a slow evolution of experience that brings many benefits and blessings, and these will support a corresponding gradual shift away from fixed sexual habits.

POSITIVE THOUGHT AS REMEMBRANCE

The practice of remembrance requires awareness. Remember that first and foremost you are a body—and give it a loving thought. The body is so close it's easy to overlook its significance. It's the key, it's the bridge to the higher self. Instead the body is taken for granted and we search for a connection to the Divine outside of ourselves. Certainly the human is more than just a body, but that more follows later on as a by-product, or as a consequence of being rooted in the body, living in the awareness. At any moment during any day, fall back into your body with your awareness, scan your body, and release any tension or holding. Breathe deeply and slowly and just be suspended in the moment, as you hold the awareness within your body for several seconds. Remember, you are more than the mind; your basic truth is the body. The body is not there simply to escort and carry the mind around. The physical form is given to us to serve as a bridge to divine realms. Through intention and with awareness, humans naturally move on to higher spiritual dimensions.

The inner remembrance of any previous ecstatic experience (it is recorded as light in your cells) can be used as a very powerful means for continuing inner transformation and deepening sexual practice.

8
THE SEXUAL POWER OF THE SACRED

Sex has long been associated with the spiritual and the sacred, in the East as well as in the West, as mentioned in the introduction. Statues and paintings in thousands of ancient temples and places of worship reflect the spiritual orientation of earlier cultures. Sex in its sacred phase is transformed into a generative, creative spiritual force, which is a higher expression than its reproductive aspect. Sacred sex is focused on generating more vitality and life for oneself and maturing as an individual, rather than using sex to produce another life. Sex becomes sacred when you honor the intelligence of the body and create the situation and space for the Divine to enter. To receive the Divine you will need infinite nothingness inside you, because you are inviting the whole of existence into you.

ENGAGING THE METABOLIC POWER OF THE SACRED

Slow, sensual sex is a direct passage into the gentle and sacred arms of the Divine. The miracle is that each and every person who wishes to is able to gain access to the sacred. Sex is made sacred through intention and honoring the God-given wisdom of the body. We simply have to create the right environment and incorporate the universal metabolic enhancers, such as awareness, relaxation, rhythm, pleasure, and so on.

Marc David writes:

> Sacred metabolism is the chemistry ignited in the body when we are infused by the Divine. Because the Divine is the source of power behind all powers, the chemistry created when we experience the Divine supercedes all known laws of the body. Sacred chemistry is a meta-chemistry. Its effects can include or incorporate familiar psychophysiologic states, such as the relaxation response, brain-hemispheric synchronization, pleasure chemistry, immune-system mobilization, and others. (*The Slow Down Diet,* page 159)

ECSTASY IS BEYOND PLEASURE

Our innate bodily sensitivity opens the door to the Divine, easily, gently, and organically. We are designed by nature for a natural biological ecstasy, a dimension that can be described as being light-years beyond pleasure. Ecstasy is pure bliss, a sacred state of utter contentment, peace, and harmony in which the being merges with the whole of existence and falls into harmony with all that is.

The essential components of blissfulness or ecstasy are timelessness, egolessness, and naturalness. Ecstasy and bliss exist beyond the ego and the "I" that normally wants or needs something from sex. Without the "I" there is no need for orgasm and the body can drop back into the here and now. The energy is contained by remaining present to each moment. There is no moving forward, no pushing through to a climax and release in orgasm, so the vitality remains in the body.

Avoiding a climax applies equally to man and woman. However, with woman there is one difference. When a woman is able to have an orgasm easily and with no effort at all, while in a state of relaxation and being (and not doing), then orgasm is perfectly beautiful. But when a woman works with effort and intention to reach orgasm, first, she will be lacking in presence, absent through a focus on the goal. Second, she is likely to cause her man to ejaculate. And third, there will be a buildup and crescendo of physical tension, some of which is discharged in orgasm and some of which remains in the woman's energy system. These tensions can later give rise to a negative swing either on the physical level (such as vaginal irritations or menstrual pains) or an emotional level (feeling insecure, unloved, abandoned). Woman loses a geat deal of energy through the tension of much effort, just as man does. It is very interesting for a couple to begin to observe themselves hours and days after having sex, to watch their mood swings in relation to their sexual choices. When the choice is habitually excitement and orgasm, often there will be a certain level of tension between the two of you, perhaps evidenced by many emotional ups and downs that get in the way of the love you feel for each other.

When the vitality is not discharged and is allowed to gather at the base, the life force will (in time) start to rise upward. And of its own accord. This rising is not something that one can "do," as such. Actually the only thing you can really do in the situation is to stop doing the habitual orgasm thing. The situation has to be created, then the rising of energy happens by itself, as a by-product. The inner vitality is first contained, then it turns inward, a channel opens gradually, and the life force is able to spiral, or stream, or flow upward through the core of the body. When energy is contained and rises in this way, the spiritual or sacred phase of human sexual energy is stimulated into life as a generative uplifting force that nourishes the entire metabolism with life-enhancing effects.

Slow Sex Becomes a Sacred, Spiritual Practice

As sensitivity increases during sex, the exchange will become increasingly the experience of being here and now. Through remaining present and taking the awareness inward, one naturally engages with spirit and the mysterious sacred forces that breathe life into us. As many people have commented after experiencing slow sex, it feels natural and right, like a coming home to yourself.

THE INNER ROD OF MAGNETISM IS THE SOURCE OF ECSTASY

Containing the sexual energy and creating the situation for its rising involves taking a step over and beyond our inherited patterns and habits. Really what we are wanting to achieve is a shift from orgasm as a hurried event of a few seconds to the ecstasy of a timeless orgasmic state wherein the body loses sense of its physical boundaries and exists as pure, vibrant, vital energy.

The simplest route to the sacred is to take the body into consideration and honor its inner polarity. The potential for the ecstatic or orgasmic state lies within each individual because of this inner polarity, the equal and opposite poles of male and female carried within each individual, as discussed in chapter 4. Between these two opposite poles there exists a difference in potential that gives rise to an electromagnetic streaming of inner vitality, aliveness, chi, prana, or life force. There is an invisible but palpable "inner rod of magnetism" that forms a channel or passage for the flow and expansion of the subtle, electromagnetic energies that are the source of each person's orgasmic and ecstatic states.

SENSITIVITY IS THE BRIDGE TO ECSTASY

Ecstasy is not excitement. Ecstasy lies way beyond the pleasures of exciting sensations. It could rather be described as a state of pure pleasure, pure delight, and pure bliss. Through being intensely conscious and rooted in the sensitivity of the physical body, you can dissolve into a state of ecstatic bodilessness. I have found that the words from a well-known song, "you gotta get in to get out," reflect the truth. You need to merge first and foremost with your own body in order to travel and expand beyond your physical boundaries. You are born with a built-in mechanism for a natural biological ecstasy and you need to know how to harness its sacred qualities in order to move beyond the ego, time, and the physical body—to exist as pure vibrant energy.

Ecstasy Is a By-product of Coolness

Ecstasy is a cool experience. It is a state of intense inner vitality, and at the same time it is a cool and serene state. Ecstasy is definitely not hot and not at all overwhelming. Heat can and will eventually lead to some kind of a discharge of energy, whereas in coolness there is automatic retention of energy. Coolness results in an implosion, not a heated explosion. Coolness is oriented around relaxation instead of building up tension. All the contributing movements and actions are more conscious and much slower, and at times there can be stillness, too.

To invite new dimensions requires a shift of position; when you change your position you change your experience. The position can be physical, mental, or both—the two are strongly intertwined. Our conditioning is such that the body follows the mind more easily than the mind follows the body. So it's easiest to start with the mind and change our basic ideas around sex, to change our orientation to one in which the body is honored. A good physical position will have awareness at its base; the most important thing is that you have the capacity to observe yourself as opposed to being identified with a certain pattern or position. To shift your point of view on sex you need to have the capacity to step into the sexual unknown, which means finding the courage to drop the ideas you have held on to in sex, to question the identification you have with a certain style of sex. Letting go, relaxing, being present to whatever is, will pave the way to sacred dimensions.

DEFEMINIZING EXTERNALIZATION OF THE GENITALS

Slow sacred sex is a spiritual experience because it's an inner experience. Any turn inward, away from the outer world, is a feminine movement.

Outward moving is male, inward moving is female. Our culture has conditioned us to be more outward and extroverted in so many ways, including sex, that both woman and man have lost access to their true receptive feminine qualities. This loss of the feminine is increasingly represented by what I see as an externalization of the genitals in epidemic proportions, one that is oriented on stimulation and sensation—the almost compulsory fashion of removing all the soft, silky, sensitive pubic hairs that form a glistening halo embracing the male and female genitals.

Pubic hairs are designed to protect sensitive tissues, and their complete absence represents a dramatic loss in sensitivity. Each single hair acts like a portal to the inner world of sensation because it is connected to sensory nerve pathways via its root. When hair is lightly played with or softly stroked, or even better, when the hairs are pulled gently one by one with the fingertips, there is a subtle, yet thrilling, internal sensory response. A very little can go quite a long way. Constant low-level friction with no hair to act as a buffer between the genitals may also literally desensitize (callous, if you will) external nerve endings.

This popular trend of hair removal is a very strange and distorted perception that reflects the prevailing sexual confusion. Hairlessness appears to be an attempt by adults to imitate sexual immaturity in order to send out sexual signals, which somehow depreciates adults and their behavior. A woman without her stabilizing, balancing, integrating triangle of Venus is not a mature woman. How can she be? Instead, the inviting, compelling, and appealing triangle that symbolizes the female in all her glory is trimmed into a minimal rectangle, standing almost military in beefeater style. Or often the triangle is erased completely to reveal a childlike provocative slit, with the sensitive, tender inner lips open and delicate tendrils exposed.

Exposing and externalizing the genitals through interference with pubic hair is a visible sign of a lack of self-knowledge and evidence of a sexuality that has not embraced the inner feminine. And this is equally true for both men and women. A penis that is not nestled in a glistening halo of frothy pubic hair looks unbalanced, exposed, and vulnerable. The general idea, of course, is to make the penis look larger and more impressive; however, these forms of externalization ultimately displace awareness away from the biomagnetic source of our sexual vitality.

The fashion of piercing different parts of the body, such as the testicles, penis, clitoris, navel, tongue, and nipples, also reveals an extroverted sexuality. It is another way of looking to the periphery for stimulation and sensation rather than toward the center of our innate sensitivity and the source of the feminine receptive aspect.

Wise people observe that the real reason why the world is filled with so much chaos and fear is that the primordial forces of male and female are drastically out of balance. The way to heal this radical imbalance and return to harmony is to honor and respect the powerful receptive female force for what it is, giving woman her place alongside man, and encouraging man to honor his own female side, which is inward, receptive, and embracing. Male and female cannot exist without each other—we are conceived together as one. However, the female aspect of humankind in almost all cultures in the world has suffered a loss (and abuse) of the feminine. The graceful, intuitive, loving, flowing, sweet compassionate qualities are ignored and become masked by distortions.

The imbalance between man and woman is very clearly seen in conventional sexuality, and a new understanding and vision of sex would initiate tremendous healing and balancing. I would even go so far as to say that any vision for a harmonizing shift between male and female forces would have to include at its very root a more enlightened form of human sexual contact, one that turns away from the periphery toward the center and tunes in to the design of the inner body.

THE SACRED BALANCES AND HEALS

One significant aspect of sacred sex is the profound healing that is possible for mind, body, and spirit in ways we can't even imagine.

Reciprocal Cycle of Purification

Accumulated tension, fear, memories, and wounds from our individual sexual history are stored in the cells and can be liberated and purified from the system during slow conscious sex. As the body becomes more flexible and porous, man gradually encompasses his more positive, dynamic essence of male, and woman encompasses her more receptive and absorbing essence of female. A reciprocal cycle of purification exists between penis and vagina as a result of the interaction of dynamic and receptive forces. This means that a conscious penis will purify the vagina, and in so doing, the penis itself slowly becomes purified—more flexible, sensitive, radiant, and beautiful.

The Head of the Penis Is a Powerful Catalyst

The head of the penis is very similar to a highly sensitive magnet and when present (supported by man's consciousness) in the vagina, it acts as a powerful catalyst. It has the innate power to displace old memories, feelings, or tensions that are obstructing full receptivity. Cleansing of the poles makes the vagina more relaxed, receptive, and able to perceive the subtle. Similar tensions will also be displaced from the penis, increasing its ability to be a sensitive snakelike channel for dynamic energy.

Purification through Deep Sustained Penetration

A woman is most receptive and feminine in the deepest regions of the vagina, especially around the cervix—the entrance to the uterus. I like to refer to this place as the "Garden of Love." When woman is touched here her heart is also touched and great love arises in her body.

Purification happens with or without an erection, so a soft penis definitely has potency, but if a man wishes to travel deeper into the vagina, into the Garden of Love, he needs to have a half erection to a full erection. This can be achieved by just a little movement and avoiding getting into excitement. There should be just enough arousal for a soft, supple erection. Or an erection may arise spontaneously within the vagina, as mentioned in chapter 4.

After lubricating the penis and the vaginal entrance, woman can hold her labia open as man places the head of his penis at the entrance, waits a few moments, and then enters her slowly, stopping after a half inch or so, waiting for a few breath cycles, continuing in a little more, waiting, breathing, with man continually being present in and to his penis. Continue penetration as deep as the penis is able to manage, or until the man feels some resistance against the head of the penis. Usually a man will be touching the entrance to the uterus (the cervix) or the walls and upper boundaries of the vagina. In this area, the Garden of Love, woman is most capable of experiencing divine ecstatic energies through contact (and thereby man too). Do not use hard pressure against the vaginal tissues; this is important—pressure can compress the tissues, causing them to become defensive and closed. Once the man feels he has reached his depth, he must pull back a fraction—a hairsbreadth—so as to take pressure off the vagina and create a more porous and airy contact between the magnetic penis head and cervix. This fraction of space will enable an exchange between the male and female poles, the dynamic and receptive forces.

If a woman feels pain *at any point* during the journey of the penis deeper into the vagina, she must communicate this fact immediately and ask her man to stop and to stay exactly on that place where pain is experienced. The contact needs to be porous, so man must always pull back. Pain is a doorway in the sense that pain often reflects old memories or tensions that are held in the tissues. Hold the penis in this area for several minutes and see what wants to happen—there may be throbbing, pulsating, or electrical feelings. If any sadness or other buried feelings rise to the surface, they should be given space and expression, and honored as part of the purification process. It is not necessary to understand the source of the feelings, why and when, just allow them to pass through you. Feelings that surface should really *not* be repressed and reswallowed. By allowing old and unexpressed feelings to flow out of you, if and when they arise, there is a profound cleansing and purification on a cellular level. Over a period of time a man should explore and visit all angles and corners of the vagina, which will gradually soften, heal, and become more receptive.

Man may also experience pain, in the testicles, groin, or penis. It is very healing for a man to allow tears of sadness, insecurity, and vulnerability or whatever comes up, and gradually his penis will grow to be more sensitive, perceptive, and supple.

Positions suitable for deep sustained penetration are shown in chapter 4 in relation to man making a slow, conscious initial penetration. (See figures 4.1 to 4.4 on pages 38–40.)

SACRED SLOW SEX SUSTAINS AND STABILIZES RELATIONSHIPS

When we relax away from doing and into our being, we get in contact with the source of love—our essence—lying within ourselves. An endless source of love resides within each person. We are born in love and love is alive as light and pleasurable sensations in each cell of the body. Anywhere you feel good in your body is a place where love lives inside you. Relaxation into the being implies an awareness of, and involvement in, the body, because the body is the bridge. Awareness easily opens the way to transformation, a sacred alchemy in that awareness itself creates love. Slow sex is, therefore, by its very nature (conscious and aware) very loving sex. The awareness brought into the sexual exchange can transform the commonly repetitive act into a sacred act of love. You begin to love and respect yourself more, and this radiates to include your partner (and others), embracing them with more love, respect, and acceptance.

In the many years that my partner and I have been teaching slow sex to couples, we have been astounded to see what a powerful healing and balancing force it is and how quickly it seems to work. Sometimes couples on the brink of divorce or separation come to our retreats as a last resort to see if we have anything to offer that will help them stay together. All that we have to offer is, in fact, awareness. And this awareness is based on a new understanding of the human sexual system and how male and female are designed to unite.

We also create space daily for individual couples to have sex in privacy (always), so that they can put theory into practice. We don't need to hear from the couples how they are responding to a slow style of sex (some couples wish to share, but not all) because we can see its regenerating effects within two or three days. It's as if a breeze of light and love enters the room. The eyes shine and the faces are relaxed and radiant. The couples feel connected, while at the same time there is a unity lying within each individual. There is a simple undemanding presence and intimacy as each person settles into his or her own body. Through this awareness, self-love increases and naturally overflows onto the other. We do know as a fact that many couples remain together after being with us for this week of exploration, because they write to us afterward to say how important and life changing this education has been. Naturally the success rate is not 100 percent, but high enough to be impressive, and therefore, worthy of note. Our approach is not foolproof; rather it depends on individual awareness, curiosity, and an interest in change. Slow sex can be talked about endlessly, but it has to be tried out—put into practice so that it becomes your own experience and you feel its benefits and healing effect directly and personally.

Over the years we have witnessed a steady trickle of people returning to our retreats with a new lover. Actions are said to speak louder than words, and the return of so many, particularly men, is their living endorsement of the immense value of changing the way one makes love. Once a man has been fortunate enough to have a taste of his male potency flowing into and through a woman and being received by her, he naturally hopes to create similar experiences for himself in the future.

Basically slow sex makes sense for any couple that wishes to stay together and continue to have sex in the years after the honeymoon high fades, especially as they begin to mature and age. Classically, sex is often the reason for a separation, whereas slow sex creates a bond and a union that is beyond the need for excitement and change. It's like a ripening process in which the flavors become more refined and dimensional. And even if you separate for any reason, the experience you have had together, the learning and reorientation you have made, will stay with you and give you a good foundation for the next time you enter a love affair.

INNER SEX AS THE MOST EVOLVED FORM OF SEX

The human body is designed so that each individual is fully able to have "inner sex" and circulate magnetic vitality. Inner sex is the highest and most evolved form of sexual expression, in that it returns to individual completion and fulfillment and is beyond, but not against, sexual union. Each of us has the capacity to circulate vitality or energy between the male and female poles in our own bodies *using the power of the awareness*. Inner sex is not self-touching or self-stimulation or masturbation. Conscious touch can certainly be used as a way to increase awareness in the positive, life-giving pole. In woman by cupping and holding the breasts, and in man, by laying the hands on the groin area or lovingly holding the penis and testicles while placing attention on the perineum. Attention on the positive pole will eventually and in time awaken the opposite pole and both will become vibrant with life. There will also be a streaming of vitality between them. And, in theory, when sensitive to ourselves, we all have the capacity to access the source of the orgasmic state lying within because we are all of similar electromagnetic design.

Many highly sensitive individuals have been blessed with the experience of the orgasmic blissful state in aloneness; for example, while out in nature or enraptured by music or dance. They are suddenly touched and graced by the Divine because of such an intense (but not tense) immersion in the body through the senses that they dissolve into the present moment. When at one with our senses there is an openness, an invitation and receptivity to the encompassing sacred forces of Divine creation.

When we have a regular long-term partner we have an opportunity to make love with another person frequently. This is the way we can help each other to access our inner orgasmic potential. We engage the inbuilt resources of the body (represented by dynamic/receptive forces) to assist ourselves in rising a few rungs on the inner ladder of growth. One thing to note is that one partner having an orgasmic experience does not guarantee that the other partner will move into the same ecstatic space or share the same experience. It may happen, but not necessarily.

Remember that the source of the orgasmic state lies within each individual and is not really dependent on another person. In a couple constellation one partner may, in fact, be more sensitive on a cellular level than the other partner, which can lead to a discrepancy of experience while having sex. For example, after some hours of making love, one partner may be entering an orgasmic state while the other is partially alseep or generally absent. The initial contact of the vagina and penis, and the ensuing inner electromagnetic circulation, initiates the process and acts as a trigger; however, the ultimate elevated experience will often be that of one person only.

Marc David writes that, "What we oftentimes label as anomalous or miraculous are simply latent biological traits activated once we are touched by the hand of the Divine" (*The Slow Down Diet,* page 160). He believes that we are at the frontier of what we know about the capabilities of the human form, and that what we know is but the tiniest fraction of what is possible. Is it possible that the fulfillment of your metabolic destiny is to be found inside you, intelligently seeded there and awaiting your discovery?

As I see it, the missing link for humans, the seed of intelligence and ultimate source of our health and well-being, lies in how we have sex, how we use our bodies and share ourselves sexually. The metabolic powers of the sacred become engaged during slow sex because there is an honoring of the eternal wisdom lodged in the body.

Marc David writes:

> . . . the sacred has its own terms that are available to all in this time and place, and whose terms are these: love, truth, courage, commitment, compassion, forgiveness, faith, and surrender. These

eight sacred metabolizers—and no doubt there are more—are sacred because such soul qualities bring us closer to the heart of the Divine, to the intelligence that created us. By embodying them we become more like the source from whence we came, more of who we are meant to be and who we know, somewhere inside, we want to be. And I'm suggesting that when activated in our system, the eight sacred metabolizers can produce profound healings and powers, metabolic breakthroughs, and rejuvenating effects on body and spirit. (*The Slow Down Diet,* page 161)

In slow sex, where relaxation, awareness, quality, rhythm, pleasure, and right thought is incorporated into our way of having sex, we begin to find ourselves naturally aligned with the eight sacred metabolic forces of love, truth, courage, commitment, compassion, forgiveness, faith, and surrender.

> *Love:* When we enter sex with awareness we touch the being as the source of love lying within. Love is the alchemical by-product of awareness, and ordinary mechanical or routine sex can be transformed into love through engaging awareness.
> *Truth:* When we enter sex it is our intention to live the truth of our bodies, honor and respect their intelligence, and create a situation in which we embody and appreciate our human sexual design.
> *Courage:* When we enter sex a certain courage is needed to be curious enough about ourselves and be willing to not know. We need courage to challenge and be creative with our habits and patterns in order to live according to a higher sexual vision.
> *Commitment:* To make a shift in consciousness, as is required in slow sex, requires commitment to the now. Commitment is part of personal and spiritual transformation. It is not an obligation, but more a sense of seeking to find out who we really are, and to make time and space for the sexual exchange as often as possible.
> *Compassion:* With a new approach we are able to enter sex with compassion and understanding for our bodies and for each other.

We have compassion for the crucial complementary differences between male and female systems.

Forgiveness: To enter into sex requires that sometimes we have to forgive ourselves and/or others. This will usually entail releasing, through forgiveness, certain events or acts from the past.

Faith: It takes faith to leap into the unknown and trust that such elevated experiences are available to a human being.

Surrender: To approach sex in a spiritual and sacred way requires that we surrender ourselves to the intelligence of nature by relaxing into our bodies and giving way to forces greater than ourselves.

Exercise: Using Prayer to Invite the Divine

Blessing Your Union

One beautiful way to begin lovemaking is with a blessing or prayer, silent, spoken, or shared.

1. Kneel or sit opposite each other and bring your hands together in prayer position in front of your chest and heart. Begin by closing your eyes, taking a breath, and relaxing into yourself.
2. When you feel ready you can open your eyes and hold a soft eye connection with your partner for a while.
3. Speak your prayer (or say it silently), and then lean forward with lowered heads and bow to each other, letting your foreheads rest together.

When you bless and pray you invite the Divine to participate in your love creation. You attract unforeseen supportive forces into the electromagnetic field around and beyond you.

Exercise: Using Ritual to Invoke the Sacred

Create an Atmosphere of Love

Ritual is a powerful way of creating an atmosphere for the sacred. Following certain steps or protocol helps you to crystallize your intention and focus your awareness with the senses tuned in to the present moment. There are many ways that a ritual can be performed and many different elements that can be included. The ritual space (the bedroom, for instance) needs to be prepared and beautified so as to invite the spirits. Spirits love beauty so if you don't know many details about creating ritual, then let pure beauty be your guide. Flowers, low lights, candles, beautiful embroidered cloths, crystals, treasured or sacred objects, fragrance, and music can all be incorporated into the ritual arrangement. Having your heart in the right place is what counts most.

Focus Your Sacred Intention with an Altar

An altar can be created as a focus for your intention to invite the sacred, perhaps on a small round table or in an alcove. You might like some of the following suggestions for how to arrange your altar, or perhaps you already have some ideas of your own.

- Place crystals as the centerpiece of the altar to represent and channel a certain quality, such as love or compassion, into the atmosphere.
- Arrange three crystals at the center to honor, give gratitude to, and ask for blessings from Mother Earth (the feminine), Father Sky (the masculine), and the Great Spirit that breathes life into this union.
- Flowers or a candle can also be placed in the center of the altar.
- Set any other precious, meaningful, or high-frequency objects around the central piece in a way that is energetically or visually meaningful to you.
- Photographs and pictures can also be used to invite particular energies into your sacred space.
- A glass of fresh drinking water is nice for the spirits, too.

Use Ritual to Come into Your Body in the Present Moment

A ritual will usually begin with (or along the way include) some kind of prayers or blessings, as mentioned in the previous section. You may wish to work out a specific sequence of words accompanied by certain movements that you engage in as a way of beginning every time you make love. Ritualized steps function to bring us step-by-step into the body and into the present. A part of a ritual (or the whole ritual) can also take the form of a meditation, dance, or breathing exercise. There are a variety of ways that can assist us in bringing the body, the awareness, and the senses into focus and alignment.

Select something you enjoy that is meaningful to you. Even something simple like bowing down to each other and then lying down separately and relaxing into your bodies, resting in the awareness for ten to twenty minutes, is a good preparation (as described at the end of chapter 4).

Move Consciously into Physical Contact

Then stand and move very slowly and deliberately toward each other, maintaining eye contact. From here you can slowly come into an embrace, kiss if you wish, then lie down together. You can also take some time to communicate to each other what you feel in your body and your heart.

Sharing your internal now experience (like a brief weather report) will help to amplify the inner experience. The acknowledgment or the recognition of what is—what exists in the present—is rewarded by the sensations expanding delightfully through the body. Speaking aloud about inner sensations also lets each one know what the other is feeling, so no guesswork is needed. This is very relaxing and supportive. Any kind of preparation that gets you more involved and engaged with the body and its sensitivity will be a tremendous support for experiencing sex in its elevated form.

9

THE SEXUAL POWER OF THE STORY

Each individual, regardless of who we are or where we were born, has two basic stories with sex, simply by virtue of having arrived in human bodily form. There is the personal story and the human story. The personal sex story very often contains many stories, and some of them may be not so pleasing or worthy of remembering. This is not because of sex itself, but because the how of sex is based on an absence of true bodily respect, understanding, appreciation, and insight.

THE HUMAN STORY IS A SEX STORY

On the human level, the story is that sex is the most basic expression of our bodies. It is determined by our DNA and the biological programming that is set for continuation of the species, as is true for all living species on Earth. At its most superficial level, life is focused on procreation and nourishment.

From day one we live in a human body and are all similar, not at all individual. The bodies and psychologies do get influenced in many ways by different experiences and exposures, but in our essence we are all one and the same. This similarity means we have to embrace the sexual story endowed by our Creator and lying inherent in the body.

The story of the body is our three-dimensional human story and the urgent need to follow our inner electromagnetic design, so that humans can experience an evolved style of sex. Slow sex, and that means sex that has awareness as its base, represents an evolutionary step for us. There is no need to elaborate on the sexual distress and malaise present in our culture. The evidence is all around us as we witness a massive escalation in abuse and pornography, plus a sharp rise in the rate of divorces and separations based primarily on some sexual reason: boredom (and finding someone new and exciting), lack of interest in sex (woman's body closes down when her body is entered too fast), lack of fulfillment (because energy is repeatedly discharged), and so on.

Each of us, whether we know it or not, like it or not, is in an intimate, lifelong relationship with sex. Sex is a relationship that really cannot be avoided because we are genetically programmed for it. Our bodies (with amazing speed) become sexually mature in order to reproduce the species. Fortunately, if we don't have sex we don't die, but all the same, most individuals will have an ongoing relationship with sex in some form or another, whether they want it so or not. Sexual energy can be diverted and the force of it repressed, but there are significant negative consequences to repressing nature. We cannot really choose whether or not we are sexual beings, but we are definitely in a position to choose when and how we act on it.

THE PERSONAL SEX STORY

The human story all too quickly becomes a personal story, especially with the prevailing lack of insight and information about sex. Millions of people suffer as a result of negative sexual experiences. Countless lives are traumatized as a direct result of an absence of respect for innocent human beings that leads to sexual abuse and the overstepping of personal boundaries. Abuse takes place because a sexually repressed individual is controlled by sexually demanding urges (and fantasies), desires that harm others when acted upon.

Sex can be the source of tremendous personal pain, guilt, and confusion, as well as a source of attraction and great pleasure. It is indeed, then, a blessing from the Divine that slow, sensitive sex has powerful healing and balancing effects. Deep pain and confusion exists on the collective level, too, so culturally sex continues to be shrouded in a veil of darkness and secrecy that separates us from the deeper reality (and need) of the human body. We have almost no meaningful or creative insights into the true function of sex. Tremendously high levels of frustration, suffering, distress, anger, and even rage exist as a result of "unholy" sex, even if we do not necessarily recognize the connection between these emotional consequences and sex, or the lack of it.

As far as sex goes, humans are more or less on a starvation diet. Insufficient sex, as well as the briefness of most sexual interactions, leaves us undernourished on profound metabolic levels. Our quality of life is dramatically affected and reduced to the minimum. When the sexual energy is flowing (within oneself or between two people), then creativity flourishes and love ignites and spreads. Sex "rightly" used is known to boost the immune system, stimulate creativity and intelligence, and increase happiness throughout adult life. In the current state of affairs, sex comes to a standstill and many people abandon sex when they get older.

Many people take sex to extremes of sensation and stimulation (and insensitivity to themselves) while endlessly seeking "satisfaction." Pornography and visual stimulation is at an all-time high. Exploitation of children is tragically acute and on the increase. For many, masturbation, fantasy, and virtual sex are becoming more of a reality than real-time sex. Many men need pharmaceuticals, such as Viagra, to give them potency because they have lost innate sensitivity. Most men cannot control their ejaculation and many women struggle to have a climax.

SLOW SEX, A STEP IN HUMAN EVOLUTION

As humans we are caught, without intention but by an unconscious conditioning, in the reproductive, biological, and extroverted phase of sex—brief and hot. Is this truly all that it is meant to be for us? What is our actual potential and our deeper story with sex? Slow sex enables us to step into the generative, creative, uplifting aspect of sex in which the feminine and inner workings of the body are honored and embraced. It becomes essential to our health, well-being, and sustainability at the deepest level of reality.

Couples who have done our "Making Love" retreat often return two, three, and even more times to repeat the week-long experience so as to deepen their inner exploration. The human sexual story is an unfolding; it's not something that can be fully grasped all in one shot. You have to live sex and transform its expression step by step. What usually happens is that people will begin to change and transform themselves, through the very practice itself. The whole process of transforming the sexual energy into a spiritual sacred expression is the process of becoming a witness and observer of your experience. As you go along you will begin to understand more, see more, have insights and revelations, and one by one the pieces of the jigsaw will fall into place and you'll find yourself standing in a totally different world. All the same elements will be there, but the constellation will have changed dramatically. There will have been a revolution in the way you see your personal sexual story, realizing it has become a human story that brings you back home to yourself, and returns you to your electromagnetic place in the universe.

10
YOUR PERSONAL SLOW SEX PRACTICE

Slow sex is a journey in which today counts, and each and every day counts. It's a slow journey that can extend over many years and into old age. Or so it is happening for me, and I can definitely say that I did not plan for it to be this way. Very slowly, one thing has led to another through curiosity and practice.

Practice brings about change and transformation much more effectively than just thinking about doing something.

Below, slow sex is defined as an actual practice. I have synthesized information from the previous chapters (and cross-referenced it) to explain how to get started in your own personal practice. You can change the guidelines at any time. Feel free to trust your intuition and improvise!

The vital thing is to take it slow, without having great expectations or waiting for a grand display of inner fireworks. Expectations stand in our way of perceiving what actually is; they make us consider what is *not* happening, rather than what *is* happening. Changes are likely to be subtle and gradual, but not necessarily. Great changes can also accompany one single vital insight gained while practicing slow sex. In general, it is a bit like going back to the beginning, being prepared to be an infant again, feeling wobbly and finding a way to walk on two legs, not knowing what's coming next.

The Benefits of a Slow Sex Practice

There are many positive outcomes to the practice of slow sex.

- First and foremost, you become more loving as a human being. Within you lies a deep sense of contentment, of having arrived home, and of self-love. Through the inner connection to yourself the intimacy with the other is deepened.
- There is more harmony and understanding within the relationship, less fighting and controversy between egos, and therefore, fewer emotional ups and downs that disturb love.
- Life seems lighter and much brighter. The sense of well-being deepens. Joy and enjoyment accompany each day.
- Embracing sex in a conscious, slow way is truly transforming and gives rise to deep insights, inspiration, and creativity. When sexual (life) energy is in nature's flow, living gets easier, the outlook is optimistic and positive.
- Reducing the pressure and tension in sex (especially the habit of forcing the body to a climax) boosts the immune system and enhances general health, an effect that becomes more apparent over time.
- The love and awareness generated between two people overflows onto their children and their life as a family unit. The rapport improves and children become more easygoing and self-contained. This relaxation happens because they can sense immediately (and they definitely can, from their earliest moments on Earth) the reassuring fragrance of love in the air.
- Essentially, when a couple decides to be more conscious and

> slow in sex they are doing peace work at home, and what they create radiates outward into the world, not only to the immediate family, but also to all those with whom they associate. A couple has the innate power to become tremendous generators of spiritual and positive loving energy in their community.

WHAT KIND OF PRACTICE IS SLOW SEX?

Slow sex can best be described and approached as a loving spiritual practice in which awareness rests in the body and the genitals. We gradually discover how to be present in sex, rather than actively doing sex.

> **When we have sex with sensitivity and slowness, sex transforms itself into a spiritual practice that creates love and deepens the experience of the present moment.**

Any spiritual practice needs to be given time and space in order to feel the benefits. At the same time, even after the first few times you try a more conscious sexual approach, you are quite likely to feel some fulfilling "results," and often in unexpected ways. You may suddenly notice you feel more connected to your partner, more in love (with your partner and yourself), or you feel uplifted and joyful, open, relaxed, and more alive to your senses.

In slow sex practice the attention is rooted in the body generally, and especially in the genital connection—the penis and vagina. Slow sex makes it possible for them to develop their very own language, to exchange energy according to their intrinsic dynamic and receptive qualities. It's a practice that takes time to get the hang of and master, as with any other spiritual practice, or most practices in general. Just as when mastering a musical instrument or a sport, practice and repetition in slow sex lay the foundation for more sustaining and fulfilling experiences.

In certain practices there may be ideals or goals of perfection to be reached, but in slow sex, there are no goals. We immerse ourselves in our bodies and become involved with the unfolding present moment. We see what our bodies want to do, and we watch how they respond intuitively with their own sensual language. We do not interfere and come between the bodies with our minds and preconceived ideas.

At the end of the day, it is ultimately the capacity to turn *inward* that plants in us the roots of our blissful experiences. Bliss and ecstasy do not arrive on demand, but will arise when we give up all mental goals or expectations and relax into a profound acceptance of the body and its inner polarity design. Using the body as a stepping-stone, we can experience the timelessness of the present moment, in which all boundaries evaporate and everything rests in pure peace and harmony.

A Shift in Consciousness, Not a Special Technique

Slow sex is definitely not some kind of special technique, as in a-b-c leads to x-y-z. It is not something that you *do,* but rather something that you become. You enter yourself so as to meet your own body from the inside. Slowing down in sex is based on a shift in consciousness, where the emphasis is on *how* you do something, not *what* you do.

> **To become slow in sex requires a mental reorientation, a new way of looking at it.**

You'll first want to understand the why and the value of trying something new in order to drop or transform the ideas and expectations commonly associated with sex.

Even with good intentions and a fresh orientation, the very first few times you meet you may feel at a bit of a loss as to how to begin. Perhaps you'll even feel a bit confused. This is what happened to me at the outset. I also realized how strange it was that I felt very comfortable with sex when I had a specific and known routine, but as soon as any unknown element entered the picture, I got shaky and unsure of myself. I didn't know who I was, really. When I was relatively unconscious I felt secure, but upon being asked to be a bit more conscious, I felt insecure and thrown into doubt. In reality, feeling confused or insecure is a very natural human response to many situations, so there is absolutely nothing wrong or unusual with any initial hesitation, shyness, or awkwardness.

As much as we live in a society in which sex is very evident in advertising, media, and the like, when it comes down to the reality of this very moment and divesting ourselves of our protection (clothing, the masks of the personality), there can be challenges. You may also feel shy or exposed. But these are not such big hurdles that you need to hold yourself back or prevent yourself from being interested in exploring your higher potential. Confusion and lack of confidence make one feel more vulnerable, open, and present, so any feelings of awkwardness also have positive value. And when feelings are admitted and communicated to the other person in simple words, such as "I feel lost as though I don't know anything anymore," as if giving an inner weather report, then you will immediately feel more relaxed, at ease, and lighthearted. You are being more honest, more authentic, more human. You begin to trust yourself. You will find some more specific suggestions on how to begin later in this chapter.

Slow Sex Is Most Suitable for Long-term Committed Relationships

Our Creator designed human beings for slow sex, so in this sense slow sex is suitable and appropriate for one and all. Simple evolution is available to anyone willing to explore taking sex to another level through being slow. Any person who takes it slow is likely to feel the heightened love and sensitivity that being conscious brings into the exchange, and usually the partner will have a similar experience.

In general, slow sex is most sustainable for heterosexual couples in long-term committed relationships. They have a stable partner with whom to practice over an extended period of time, which is, of course, a great advantage. An opportunity not to take for granted.

> **Many couples eventually are forced to give up having sex for a number of reasons—the most frequent being women's loss of interest or physical discomfort, or male impotence—so slow sex offers a wonderful opportunity to reawaken their sexual life and begin again within a "polarity" framework, a new understanding of the why and how of sex.**

For those couples who are having sex anyway, being conscious and slowing down in sex usually opens the way to a colorful mosaic of experience and expanded love and well-being. A partner is clearly required for the slow sex practice, and at the same time, much can be done as an individual to increase your own awareness and inner sensitivity. As mentioned earlier, inner sex—in which electromagnetic energy streams between the positive and negative poles within your own body—is the most evolved form of sex. Inner sex is valuable whether you are single or in a relationship. At the end of the day you are still a single, in the sense that you are left with yourself and your body. The more interest you invest in exploring your personal inner world, the easier it will be to tune in to the sensitivity called for in slow sex. Many of the exercises in this book are suitable for the individual and can be used as a foundation to grow in awareness and awaken to the cellular light essence of the body.

If you are single and meet someone with whom you wish to be intimate, be alert in your body and senses right from the very first sitting beside each other, bathing in each other's presence, the initial reaching touch, and any ensuing embrace or kiss. This alertness also applies if you are already in a couple and wish to start anew. Begin with being more conscious of what you are doing and how you are doing it. Incorporate awareness into your approach and physical engagement in general, and on each occasion, not just now and then. Small shifts in behavior, such as attempting to pay attention to your own body (and inner body) rather than focusing on your partner's outer body, will usually have a profound impact on the situation. A quality of silence and stillness enters the atmosphere, the senses are alive, and each moment is a jewel to be treasured and valued. Using the awareness in this way (for instance, scanning the body and relaxing tensions, being aware of the breath, relaxing into being rather than doing), you will experience for yourself the positive, transforming, uplifting vibrational influences of the universal metabolic enhancers.

Commitment to the Present Moment

Above all, the personal slow sex journey begins with you and your personal commitment to slow sex. This will be based on your desire, inclination, and willingness to explore new terrain by investigating sexual ways. Transforming or changing old sexual patterns requires a full commitment, not to another person or a relationship, but to oneself. It's not a heavy, burdensome yoke to bear; it's simply the commitment to make a shift, to become aware of what you do and how you do it.

There is an understandable tendency to postpone the sexual investigation for *next* time because you will find (as you have probably already noticed) that as excitement begins to mount, so does the desire for orgasm. That desire and urgency can easily obliterate all alternative intentions, so to make any inroad into the situation you have to take advantage of each and every opportunity presented to you, and not postpone until next time. Deferments will tend to continue, as tomorrow gradually turns into years.

> **So when can you really start anything at all? Only *now*, and *this* is the moment to begin.**

Just a little turn is needed and right around the corner lies the Divine, offering us a new track or direction based on awareness and relaxation andf listening to the intelligence of the body.

Awareness and Vitality
Replace Excitement and Arousal

The great thing about slow sex is that it does not take much energy and you can enter into it even when you are not feeling fresh. It is more a question of whether or not you are able to hold an awareness of the present. Sex can take energy and be arousing at times but does not depend on high energy or getting excited at the outset. It's an engagement with awareness, as has been described in a variety of ways in the previous chapters. Naturally, there will be moments where things will get a bit hotter, but the basic level of arousal (eros) is monitored and intentionally kept cool. At other times, of course, it may be that we get caught up in the excitement and take ourselves to a climax, but with awareness so that these events form part of the experimentation.

> **The significant thing is to do whatever you do with awareness. Nothing is implicitly wrong in orgasm; it's just the habit of running toward it and the tension that is built up to achieve it that is being questioned.**

You attempt to relax into the orgasm. Avoid becoming too tense and focused on the destination, but instead find a way to arrive there at a more leisurely pace. Using the universal metabolic enhancers in this way will transform the situation into something fresh and innocent.

GETTING STARTED AT YOUR SLOW SEX PRACTICE

Here I offer some specific pointers that may be useful as you begin to transform your sexual practice into a spiritually uplifting exchange. Pointers include information on preparation and foreplay, how to make and keep a sustained connection, physical penetration with or without erection, and how to conclude a slow sex encounter and resume other activities.

Make a Date to Make Love

We make dates and appointments for countless things, why not for sex? Human beings don't have enough sustainable and fulfilling sex, so setting a fixed time makes absolute sense. In fact, the best way to establish slow sex as a sustainable practice is to set aside times specifically for that purpose. It's of great value to establish a regular place and time for slow sex. Plan it and incorporate it into your life just as you would a yoga practice or any exercise regimen. Choose a date, choose a time, choose a venue. Sit down together and decide, and then write SS down on your weekly calendar. And from then onward, on a week-by-week basis, intentionally create space and make dates for sex. Just as we prioritize certain other activities, we can bring slow sex into the foreground and give human union a higher value.

Dedicating time to sex usually means that you will have to make fewer appointments with friends and family. You will also need to make appropriate arrangements if you have children at home, so that they will be looked after or kept otherwise engaged. Remember that love made between a couple radiates outward onto the children, so children should never be used as an excuse not to make time for slow sex. Be certain to switch off all phones and cellular devices so you can enjoy tranquility and peace without any interruptions or disturbances.

Creating a protected or sacred space leads to a deeper level of relaxation, awareness, and sensitivity. By making a date for sex you make yourselves available to each other; sex is not happening by accident, habit, or routine, or not at all! Instead the meeting and joining is a conscious choice by two consenting and willing people wishing to commune sexually with each other on a spiritual level. The intention behind the sexual meeting will automatically elevate the ensuing experience. You know what you are doing and why you are doing it.

Starting out with a fixed appointment might initially feel a bit unromantic or clinical, but once you get accustomed to it, these conscious meetings feel ordinary and completely natural.

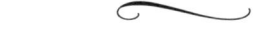

Plan a Time Frame That Is Realistic and Sustainable

There are no rules about how much time to devote to sex. What you can manage is what you can manage, and at the same time a certain level of commitment is required. Anywhere upward of forty-five minutes is advisable. When at all possible, try to give yourselves a basic minimum of three hours, because it does require time to warm up and enter fully into the situation. This is not necessarily true for men, but is certainly true for women, because female sexual energy takes longer to awaken. This difference in sexual temperatures and readiness is the vital difference between men and women, as explained in detail in chapter 5. When the underlying polarity difference is acknowledged and embraced, sexual communion is easily elevated; there is a shift that leads to a finer tuning. And when man understands that the more open woman is, the higher he himself will be able to fly, he is more than willing to grant woman what she needs.

At the start of our retreats we tell couples that they will be given a three-hour window for slow sex each and every day. Most of them look quite aghast and shy; disbelieving laughter usually ripples around the room. Within a handful of days, however, many are happily and confidently announcing that three hours are simply not enough. These don't have to be three hours of solid lovemaking, although this may certainly happen on occasion. At any time during slow sex you can simply stop (by mutual decision, or sharing your needs) to drink a cup of tea, take a shower, go to the toilet, change the music, adjust your positions, or whatever. And then afterward, you return to bed and begin again.

Each time will have its own flavor and fragrance. That's the beauty of slow sex—you never know how it's going to be. There's no set routine; it's always an unfolding according to the constellation of the moment and the presence and awareness of the parties involved.

Two hours, one hour, or half an hour will be fine if that is all you can accommodate. Periodically it is really worthwhile to give yourselves a whole day in bed, eating and showering and refreshing yourselves as needed, but continually going back to bed, lying around, cuddling and snuggling. The more you make yourselves available for experience, the more surprising, spontaneous, graceful, and flowing the bodies become—joining in relaxation and ease.

The slow sex approach includes a version of the famous conventional sexual quickie, too. Does this surprise you? Remember that slow sex is all about *how* you do something more than *what* you do. So the slow sex quickie is a conscious, harmonizing get-together or gentle congress for some minutes, anywhere from ten or fifteen to forty-five, depending on your time frame. The quickie is a gentle fusion of the genitals as described in chapter 4, in the section on soft entry without the need for erection and excitement. If there is arousal and erection, you penetrate extremely slowly, then just flow with or be with what is present.

A quickie suits occasions when there is not as much time as you'd like, but ten or fifteen minutes is feasible. Quickies can be enjoyed any time of the day—morning, afternoon, evening, or all of the above. Mornings are a perfect time to come home to yourself and anchor yourself in your inner reality before you engage with the outer world; this simple type of energy exchange has a subtle yet profound impact on the quality of your day. You will feel more positive, more alert, more alive, more happy. Quickies are also perfect for afternoon siesta hours, and a quickie at night can help send you off to a more peaceful sleep.

Frequency of Slow Sex Appointments

Slow sex needs to take place on a relatively regular basis if there is a wish to develop more sensitivity and experience its beneficial rewards. Two or three or four times a week is good, and every day is, of course, the optimum.

> **The more loving sex we have, the more we wish for it. The more we practice, the more insights we receive, the more we learn and understand.**

If we don't make love often enough it is easy for complacency and laziness to overshadow our good intentions, as we forget the positive effects of slow sex and how inwardly uplifted, more connected to our partner, and appreciative of life it makes us feel.

As far as regularity goes, maintaining the same time of day every day (or on designated days) will make it easier to sustain a slow sex practice. And any time of the day or night is suitable—dawn, morning, afternoon, sunset, and moonlit midnight are all perfect times. Each part of the day brings its own quality, and experimenting with time of the day or night will introduce more variety and spontaneity into the exchange. It may be easier to be fully present at certain times of the day or night, so decide on a time that works well for both of you. Personally, I have always favored mornings and fortunately my flexible schedule allows for this. It's a juicy and inspiring way to start the day! I find my mind more empty (less cluttered by daily thoughts), my body more fresh and open, and it's easier to fall into the innocence of being. Some men may prefer mornings as well, because at that time of day testosterone levels are said to be higher, which is something to consider if there is difficulty getting an erection. However, the option of entry without erection makes union possible at any time.

Impotence Poses No Barrier to Slow Sex

Many aspects of impotence have their basis in man's mind. Often man equates or identifies his ability to achieve an erection with basic manhood, so when erection is lost he feels so insecure and unworthy that his whole identity can crumble. Without a hard penis, who am I?

When the causes of impotence are understood (as an excess of stimulation leading to loss of sensitivity and numbing of tissues and nerve responses), then a doorway is opened for great healing, penis rebalancing, and a slow style of sexual interchange that is based on sensitivity and not sensation. Impotence is not a dead-end road, as most people imagine or experience. I heard on television the other day that an estimated twenty million men today are regularly taking Viagra! This is a sad situation. It's sad that so many men have erection disturbances (and certainly there are more who are not taking Viagra), but also, Viagra serves only to satisfy man's mind (not the body, the body is simply used). Viagra fulfills the man's psychological need to experience himself as virile and hard, even if it's chemically orchestrated. The body is simply used as a vehicle to satisfy one of the deepest insecurities in a man—the fear of losing erection and not feeling like a real man.

From the slow sex perspective, true male authority arises through man's capacity to be present to himself and his penis, and present to woman when he is inside her, and has nothing to do with erection per se.

In these circumstances erection or half erection may spontaneously arise (even when man is reportedly impotent) because the interplay of dynamic and receptive forces creates the erection. Not stimulation. A magnetism arises within and between the bodies. Certainly men who have shared about their Viagra experiences with me are aware that its main value is psychological—they say having a hard-on gives self-confidence, a sense of self. At the same time, I have also been told that when using Viagra the sensitivity of the penis is not particularly enhanced, that there is not that much genuine feeling. I also understand that sometimes the erection continues after sex is over—it just won't go down and can sometimes become painful or disturbing for the man.

Preparing the Sacred Space

As a venue for slow sex your own bedroom is perfect. If you have an extra room in your house, you may want to turn it into a love temple—specifically reserved.

- You'll need a big comfortable bed and privacy. Sometimes couples will move their bedroom furniture around and clear away clutter so as to create more space and a fresh awareness of their surroundings.
- Many couples buy a new mattress. The comfort of the bed is vital if you are to spend many hours in it beyond your usual sleeping hours. A large bed with a relatively firm and supportive mattress is best. Mattresses that are too soft cause the bodies to roll toward the middle (which means the mattress gives no support), and the changing of positions and so on becomes more awkward and cumbersome.
- Do not restrict yourselves to beds, either. Sofas, tables, and the floor also offer suitable places for bodies in semi- and fully horizontal positions.
- Make your room beautiful by adding flowers, lighting candles, and spraying fragrance.
- Lighting can play a significant part in creating atmosphere. Use well-placed lamps in corners of the room, for example. Some level of lighting is necessary in the sense that you want to be able to see your partner's eyes and face. Sex in the dark can also be magical sometimes, but you'll mostly want to maintain contact with your partner's eyes. Soft, receptive eyes are also a significant tool for remaining in the present.
- Music is enjoyed and valued by lovers because of its powerfully enveloping qualities that help us to relax into our bodies, enter the present, and go with the flow. At the same time, and depending on the piece of music selected, it is pos-

sible for a person to get carried away with the intensity of the music, slip out of awareness, and get caught up in making something happen. As the music gets more dramatic you may also get more dramatic. Experiment with music and no music, and observe its impact on you. Choose music that does not carry you away, but helps you to be present. Don't use music as a habit or crutch; from time to time allow yourselves to be surrounded by sounds of silence or nature, or whatever other sounds are present in the environment.

Preparation and Foreplay

When you look at your calendar on the agreed-upon day and see the 8 p.m. to 11 p.m. date scheduled, you are likely to inwardly notice a smile and feel the thrill of joy and anticipation. The "knowing" can act as a kind of a subtle foreplay that inwardly prepares you for the meeting. Throughout the day you can begin to tune in to your body, especially for man in the perineum, and for woman in the breasts and nipples. These are the poles that raise male and female sexual energy, so it builds energy and vitality if you maintain an awareness in these places. Again and again, go to these places and infuse them with your breath and your awareness, as if touching and massaging yourself on the inside.

Connecting to your body and feeling alive and well in your own physical being will enhance the experience.

> **Sex takes place between two bodies, so begin by entering your own body with awareness and connecting with your inner aliveness.**

Your increased inner vitality will have a big impact on your sensitivity and capacity to be present. You may want to take a luxurious warm bath followed by a cold shower, do some kind of exercise that you enjoy, dance a wild dance, massage yourself or exchange massage, sing a few songs, shake for fifteen minutes, maintain conscious breathing, or lie down and tune in to yourself. Anything will do, really. The idea is to channel your awareness into your body and there are a variety of ways to do so. Ritual and prayer can also be used as powerful forms of preparation to harmonize the energy and enter the present. It is not absolutely essential to prepare every time, but good to realize that preparation makes it much easier to tune in and come alive to the vibrant inner realms of the body.

Tools, Not Rules

There are definitely no rules about how to practice; just follow your feelings or intuition in each situation. Be guided by your body and listen to its gentle whispers. If you feel a spontaneous urge or pull arising from your body, follow it, flow with it. Don't hold yourself back with the thought that this is not how it is meant to be. If you hold back for even a couple of seconds the moment will be lost, the wave you might have ridden has passed through you and is now beyond reach. Any time I ever repressed myself in that way I was always the loser. Learn to trust the body and surrender to its language and undulating expression.

All the suggestions throughout this book are designed to help you keep your attention anchored in the present, to stay aware of what is taking place in each and every moment. The most significant aspect is that whatever you choose to do, you do with awareness; that is all. The guidelines offered are merely tools that can help you root yourself in your body, which is a prerequisite for experiencing slowness in sex.

HOW TO PROCEED—GETTING YOUR FIRST SLOW SEX DATE OFF THE GROUND

Here you are on your very first slow sex date and it is finally time to put theory into practice. For some of you, slow sex comes easily, almost as if it's your second nature. It is! You find it simple to enter into a shared awareness and fall into a sensuous, non-goal-oriented exploration in which you relate to each other's bodies in a relaxed, easy way. If this is the case for you and your partner, just keep trusting your bodies doing whatever they're doing, always being mindful to keep a clear, cool, and conscious connection alive between you.

For others, and perhaps for most, the first slow sex encounter is going to be a bit awkward. You may even feel embarrassed or shy, at a loss for what's supposed to happen next. This is to be expected. How can one know a language fluently without going through a period of practice, which includes much trial and error? It's important to give yourselves a big time frame, not to try slowness just once or twice. If it's difficult for any reason, people will tend to revert to their more familiar, tried-and-true sexual behaviors. The known becomes very attractive because it's a sexual "comfort zone" and it's not so comfortable to feel uncomfortable—at any time really, but particularly in sex where the ego is very identified with a certain sexual style.

At the end of some preceding chapters there are specific exercises designed to support you, as individuals and as a couple. Some are exercises to practice alone (although you can do them in the company of your partner, both perhaps doing the same thing simultaneously), while other exercises are shared experiences. Practicing any of these will direct you to the delights of your inner world and help you be more present in your body and present in the situation. That basic shift back to yourself is all you need to begin your slow sex practice. For convenience, the exercises are also described below (in somewhat less detail), which means that some repetition of suggestions is unavoidable.

Making the Inner Connection

The very first step is to make contact with yourself, within your own body. Sex happens between two bodies, so this initial step is more significant than having immediate contact with your partner. To get closer to another person you must first get closer to yourself—and literally closer to your very own body. Enter into the world of your inner body where the source of cellular sensitivity and aliveness lies. The awareness rises in your body before you begin thinking about, or turning toward, your partner. What follows with your partner flows and evolves from your initial inner connection. In fact, your inner rootedness makes it very simple to establish contact with the other person. You feel more confident and you trust yourself. The essential inner connection can be made by practicing the following exercise.

⏺ Exercise: Finding Home in Your Body

You can either practice this exercise alone before you meet with your partner or you and your partner can do the exercise together as a way to begin your slow sex date.

1. If you and your partner are doing the exercise together, sit, stand, or lie opposite each other and a little apart, without physical contact.
2. Close your eyes gently and take two or three easy, full breaths through the diaphragm and into your belly. Scan your body and relax any part that's holding tension.
3. Then each of you should take your attention inward and downward into your own body and look for a place that feels like a "home" in the body. It might be the heart, solar plexus, low back, belly, feet, genitals, or wherever—anywhere below the head—that will internally connect you to the realms of your flesh, blood, and bones.

An inner home acts as a resting place, a connection point, working like an anchor that holds your attention within the body. When you have made this inner connection you'll be more ready to open your eyes and meet the eyes of your partner.

Making Eye Contact with Your Partner

In slow sex, learning to keep soft, receptive eye contact with your partner becomes an important tool for deepening your connection to each other, while at the same time staying centered in your own body. The following exercise will give you some pointers on how to develop this skill.

⊙ Exercise: Practicing Soft Vision with Your Partner

1. When you feel rooted within your body, you can begin to open your eyes fraction by fraction (without losing contact with your inner body—if you do lose this connection, please close your eyes again until you inwardly reconnect).
2. When your eyes are fully open, gently meet your partner's eyes. Allow your partner into you through the eyes. Let your eyes be gentle, soft, receptive, and inviting. It will be easier to gaze receptively at just one of your partner's eyes at a time.
3. Take a deep breath into your belly and let your eyes receive what is there in front of them, rather than looking outward in an objective or judgmental fashion.
4. Continue to breathe deeply, relaxing the belly, and softening the muscles surrounding the genitals. Be present in your body, simple and innocent.
5. Remain in receptive eye sharing mode for as long as it feels comfortable, and close the eyes whenever it feels necessary, either to reconnect inwardly or to sense yourself even more deeply on the inside. Keep coming back to open eyes and being available to yourself on the inside as you receive your partner's soft gaze into you. Avoid keeping the eyes closed for extended periods.

This special soft and receptive way of using the eyes has the advantage of enabling you to connect with your partner and, at the same time, keep your attention on the inside of yourself. Your attention within your own body can be seen as your priority. You embrace, kiss, and make love with the body, so there has to be some sort of process to enter into it. If and when the inner connection is lost (which can easily happen at first), simply close your eyes again and relax back into your body, retreating into the suggested "home." Open your eyes again when you feel more rooted in yourself.

The First Physical Contact with Your Partner
When you get the feeling of being able to stay with yourself on the inside, and at the same time be open to your partner on the outside (and this may require practice), then you can move consciously across the space separating you and generously extend your arms or your hand or your lips, moving into whatever contact feels right in the moment—an embrace, touching and caressing with sensitive hands, or a kiss that is sustained by keeping the lips soft, relaxed, and sealed together.

Avoid choosing a position that is your habitual cuddle position, because it's already so familiar to you both that it won't be easy for you to feel any difference or make any difference. For instance, a woman should keep her head straight when embracing a man, instead of turning it to the side and resting it cosily on his shoulder or chest. When the head, neck, and spine are in one line, it's easier to turn the awareness inward. Physically you are further away from your partner, but you will feel yourself more present and more connected energetically. Likewise, a man should not collapse forward over his woman during an embrace, but keep an alignment through head, neck, and spine. If a man is much taller than his woman, he can stand with his legs wide astride so as to lower his height, rather than bend forward over the woman. Or the woman can stand on a stable cushion, or on a step to increase her height. Standing on tiptoes can work, but it is not easy to sustain for longer periods.

Another Way to Begin:
Establish Polarity within Yourself
All human beings have an internal magnet within, with a positive pole at one end and a negative pole at the other. Woman's positive pole is her breasts. Man's positive pole is his penis. When each partner brings their own positive pole to life before the individual bodies move together, the meeting will be filled with a special circular energy.

Exercise: Establishing Personal Polarity before First Contact

1. Stand or lie down without physical contact, three or four feet apart.
2. Close your eyes and take up an inner connection with yourself. Take the time to drop within and establish yourself in your inner body.
3. Then, after some minutes, man places his attention on the perineum (the area at the root of the penis in front of the anus) and woman places her attention on her nipples. The idea is not to concentrate or focus on these parts, but to melt into them and bring them to life. Visualize the tissues filling with love, light, and vitality.
4. Take some time, and when you have the feeling of being connected with yourself, alive to yourself, turn gradually toward each other and, inch by conscious inch, close the space separating you, bringing the bodies into their first contact.
5. Don't push your bodies into each other in a hard physical way; let there be some inches of space between you so that contact is porous and fluffy and ensures that the energy bodies remain vibrant and expanded.
6. In your own time move ever so slowly into an embrace or kiss (or whatever) with eyes closed or open, whatever feels right.

Some Alternative Approaches

Another approach is to lie (or stand) with your bodies several feet apart, and before you physically connect, allow your eyes to meet for several minutes in a receptive vision connection, as described earlier. Or man can gently lay his hands on woman's breasts while she gently lays her cupped hand over his pubic mound and penis. Or the testicles can be gently lifted from beneath and held warmly and lovingly in the hand.

> **The orientation is toward aliveness and awareness rather than stimulation and excitement. You are looking for what helps to open and expand your partner's energy field, rather than what turns them (or you) on and causes the energy field to contract.**

This is a basic guideline for any type of foreplay, that it should lead toward sensitivity and *expansion* of energy rather than excitement and *contraction* of energy, which can easily give rise to restlessness and the desire to go after orgasm.

THE FIRST SLOW SEX PENETRATION

It is possible that your very first date or dates will not progress as far as actual sex, so it is important to keep pace with what unfolds and feels comfortable for you both, rather than feel compelled to get somewhere specific. A childlike, innocent approach is a great support. If and when you feel ready to get your bodies together, then you can do so in ways described below, or follow your intuition.

There are two basic scenarios that you are likely to be presented with: when man has an erection and when he does not. So man should not be overly concerned about his erection. If it's there, you enter woman in one way; if it's not there, you enter in another way.

At this stage or at any earlier point, you can both oil or lubricate your own genitals, or each other's, bearing in mind the touch must not be a very stimulating one. Lubrication is covered in more detail in chapter 4; it is really helpful if you use lubrication every time you make love.

With Erection:
Make the Initial Penetration Exceptionally Slow

The value of an exceptionally slow entry into woman's body is described earlier in chapter 4, and is particularly significant for women if they are virgins, and also later in menopausal years. When man enters woman slowly (and with lubrication), she usually will not feel pain because man is being conscious and honoring her receptive feminine environment. The missionary position is perhaps the most suitable for slow penetration, but it can also be done in the side-scissors position and a number of other positions. In missionary position, woman can place a thick flat pillow under her buttocks to raise her pelvis and bring the vagina closer to the penis (see fig. 10.1).

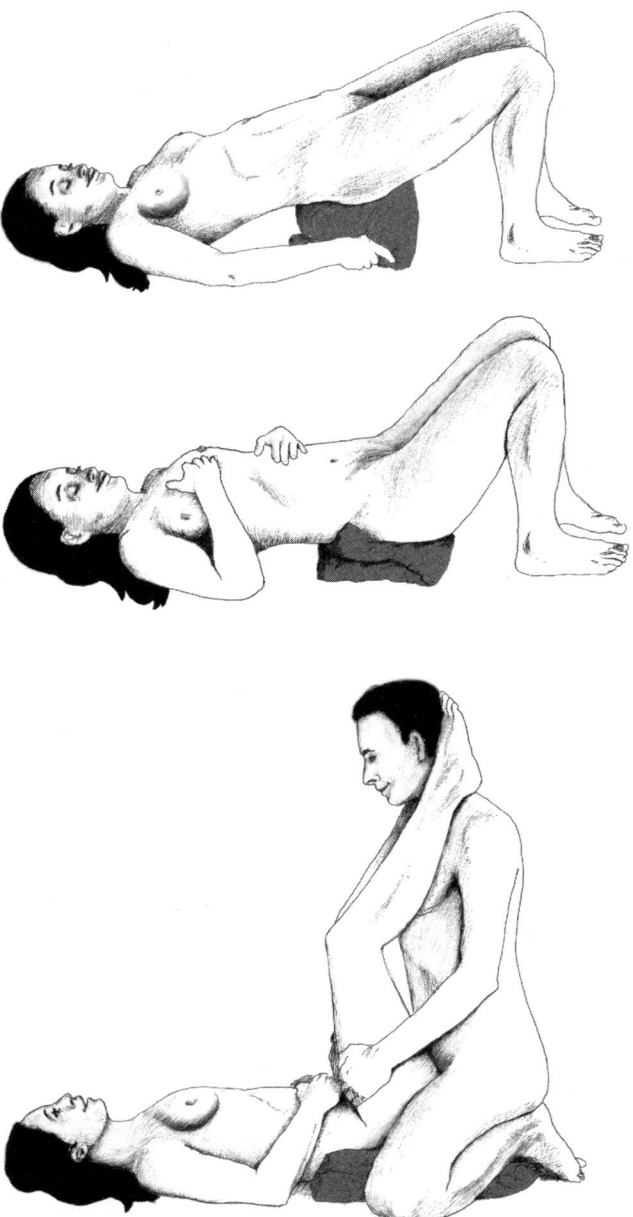

Fig. 10.1. When lying on her back, woman can use a pillow support under the buttocks to raise the level of her pelvis. In the first image woman uses her legs to raise her pelvis and place the pillow in position. Its final position is shown in the second image. The third image shows a nice variation of the missionary position with woman's feet resting on man's shoulders.

◉ Slow Penetration Step by Step

Step one: Woman must spread her lips and can keep her hands there for some time while holding the lips apart. This clearing of the pathway allows for unimpeded penetration, graceful and highly pleasurable, especially when lubrication is used. Opening the lips will bring crystal clarity into the contact and heighten the correspondence between the dynamic pole (penis) and the receptive pole (vagina). At a certain point woman may have to move her hands away because they no longer fit between the pelvises, however I strongly recommend that woman repeat this spreading action of the lips frequently during the union, and not be shy about doing so. Man will need to pull back a few inches to allow space for woman's hands, but the slight interruption has great rewards in terms of thrilling magnetic contact.

Step two: The next step is for man to place the head of the penis at the entrance of the vagina and wait for a few moments. Then you can make eye contact in a gentle way and, should you wish to, you can maintain eye contact for the duration.

Step three: And then man can, literally millimeter by millimeter, begin to glide in with utter consciousness, the focus of his awareness in the perineum as well as the head of the penis. Be aware that if woman feels the penis is entering her too fast or without a loving awareness, she will unconsciously (or consciously) tighten the vagina to prohibit deeper entry.

Stop along the way and feel the moment, as if you are pausing on a riverside walk and appreciating the waterfalls, the damp air, the silver bubbles, the silently streaming undercurrent. Slow sex enjoys and values the immediate present, what is happening for real, and not what the mind thinks should happen. The journey has a variety of moments along the way, and there is no real final destination in mind. The first (or any) penetration can last several minutes (or hours), and the penis can remain in the glory of the depths of the vagina (provided this is comfortable for woman; if not, please see chapter 8 on pain and the healing or purification of the genitals). There is no need to regularly move in and out of the vagina. When the moment feels right, all moves within the vagina should be done with consciousness and slowness. In general, rapid, friction-oriented movements are avoided, as these cause woman to shrink on a subtle level, lose her receptivity, and lead in exciting directions instead.

Through using the awareness the immediate instant is highlighted and you will find yourselves slipping into another realm, one in which you are invisibly yet powerfully connected to some higher force. You become totally engaged in, and utterly enthralled by, each and every moment. Seconds effortlessly roll into hours of flowing beauty and grace.

There should be no attempt to keep the erection going; if it fades away, then relax down into the side-scissors position (see fig. 10.2) and remain in genital union.

Without Erection: Connect Using Soft Entry

Soft penetration is suitable if there is no erection, and has been described in detail in chapter 4. Soft penetration is a perfectly valid way to begin. In fact, for many couples starting out soft becomes their standard way. From there many things can happen, including erection, but erection per se loses its significance. In fact, my lover and I had the curious experience over many years that he would usually go in soft to start and come out hard when we had finished. Everything turns on its head when the approach to sex is simplified. Obsessions and insecurities about the need for erection gradually fade, for both man and woman, and are replaced by the simplicity and innate sensitivity of the genital connection.

⊙ Soft Penetration Step by Step

Woman can help a man to enter her, and some positions are particularly suited for soft penetration, such as the so-called side-scissors position, shown on page 124. This is a position in which both partners can be physically comfortable for an extended period and it lends itself to relaxed nondoing because neither partner is on top.

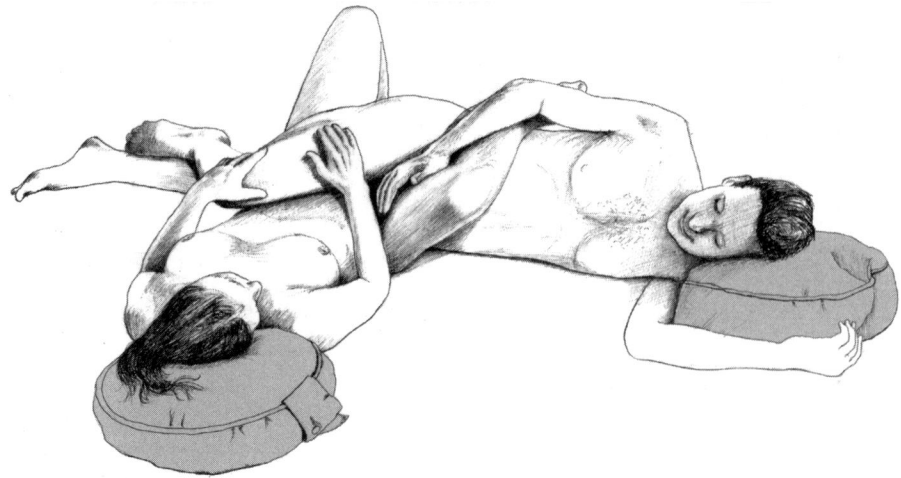

Fig. 10.2. In side-scissors position woman lies on her back and man lies on his side, their legs intertwined in a scissors-like fashion. Head support for both partners, as shown here, is helpful for sustained relaxation.

Step one: When you are both in position the very first thing a woman should do is open the vaginal lips by moving them aside to expose the vaginal entrance.

Step two: Then woman can reach behind the head of the penis, taking it between the index and third finger with a gentle yet firm squeeze.

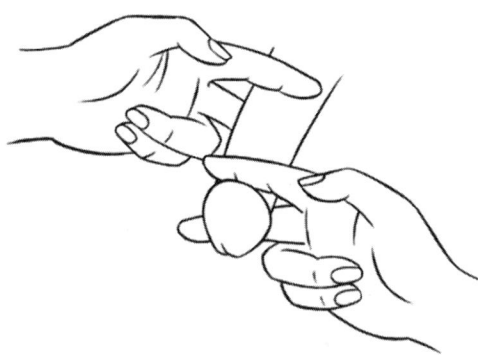

Fig. 10.3. Woman's finger position for soft penetration

Step three: Then she lies down on her back (to keep belly relaxed and vagina open) and guides the head toward the vaginal entrance pushing the first inch or so into the vagina; even just the head is enough to start. With a little dexterity, practice, and moving the fingers back a few centimeters, step-by-step the rest of the penis can be fed into the vagina.

Step four: Then relax back into yourselves, keeping awareness on the genital connection, breathing slowly and deeply and maintaining eye contact—not as a rule, but as a tool. You may want to close them now and then, perhaps to sink more fully into yourself.

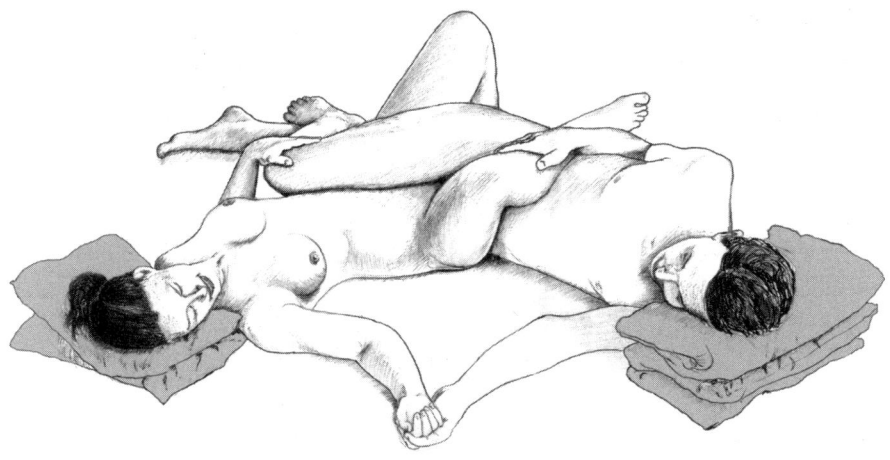

Fig. 10.4. In a nice variation on side-scissors position man and woman can hold hands and gaze softly into each other's eyes.

The side-scissors position is just a start and has value because both partners can relax simultaneously. However, you can alter your position at any time, according to what is needed. For example, if erection arises spontaneously, you may wish to adjust position to be more present and involved. Or you may feel movement will disturb what is taking place.

FINISH SLOW SEX BY RETURNING TO YOURSELF

Couples often tell us that once they get the knack of slow sex they sometimes find it surprisingly difficult to stop. And they ask us, "How do you, in fact, stop?" Indeed, in the beginning it can feel a bit strange to complete sex without having a climax to mark the end. An orgasm functions like a full stop at the end of a flowing sentence. However, once you become more accustomed to it, not "finishing" feels normal and not unusual in any way at all. We usually reply to such questions by explaining that you have to be practical. If you need to go somewhere or do something, then you must; just be sure to separate as you have been together—with awareness. So you simply disconnect the genitals and bodies gently and gracefully, bowing to each other, or find a way that completes the union for you.

Then take a few minutes to lie on your back and dive into your own body again, bringing all the wonder back home to yourself as an individual. I was interested to hear from a participant recently about the magnetic fields that surround a person because he had the capacity to measure such energies using a pendulum. He measured his own and his girlfriend's individual magnetic radiance prior to making love. And then he measured them while joined in sex and established that the magnetic field was greatly increased—and much larger than the sum total of their two individual fields. Then afterward, when they were physically separated, he discovered that each individual had retained the larger magnetic field. In union they become one large field, and in separation two identical twin energy fields remained. Fascinating!

I have always found it very important to finish a slow sex encounter by coming back to myself before leaping out of bed and getting involved in the next steps required of me. If I leave the sacred space of awareness too quickly, later I find I sometimes feel a bit wobbly, fragile, or oversensitive (slightly emotional—see later in the section on issues that may arise). If there is no real or urgent need to stop having sex, then don't! Why on Earth stop having sex? The bodies will naturally come to an easy completion in due course. When the bodies become fully engaged and get on a roll of their own, spectacular moments unfold between you, and before you know it you have been plugged in for hours on end.

How you finish is as important as how you start. Separate consciously, disconnect slowly, and come back to yourself and into your own space for several minutes.

Usually it is quite nice to have a period without physical contact so that you can reconnect with yourself as an individual. Lie down or sit and be with yourself, attention in the body and being present to the delicate sensations now streaming within you. Take fifteen or twenty minutes. If you disconnect too quickly and run off to do some urgent task, then you may later start to swing the other way. After an experience of expansion in consciousness it is good and appropriate to ground the experience in your own body, so that the opposite swing is not encouraged. When you take time for yourself and remain present in the awareness, there is a natural balancing force to any swings, and you are less likely to feel disoriented or vulnerable.

SUSTAINING YOUR SLOW SEX PRACTICE

Like any practice, slow sex needs to be sustained for a good period of time in order to reap its benefits and transformative powers. This means that to keep your slow sex commitment alive, you'll want to make dates to meet as often as possible. Below are some guidelines to keep you on track, comfortable, and curious in your exploration. Sometimes people say that the journey looks long and arduous, and wonder how long it will take to get there. The truth is that you never get anywhere! You only get more and more here. And this cannot be a goal because your body is *already* here. It's more a matter of appreciating your here-ness, getting your mind to pay attention to your body in the present moment, feeling rather than thinking, and generally shifting your perception from the outer to the inner.

For me personally, there has never been any resistance, conflict, or difficulty, and perhaps that is so because I have had absolutely no goal or objective all along. I have not tried to get anywhere or achieve anything. My intention at the outset and in my early thirties was to change the way I made love. As simple as that. No big theories. And not because I was dissatisfied or bored, not in the slightest. Just inquisitive. Actually at that time, in the situation in which I was living, there was an abundance of possible sex partners and many flavors to enjoy. I began out of sheer curiosity to know more about my body. I connected with one man in particular and we started from zero, from where we were, and that is pretty much the same place for each one of us—conditioned to have fast sex with orgasm as a focus.

My exploration brought me many understandings and insights. It's not that I knew all I know and understand today at the outset. Not at all. I was totally innocent in that sense. Clarity arises, insights descend, sensitivity increases, heart expands, body balances—all as by-products of practice, not as prerequisites to it. That is why I insist that slow sex is not a technique, it is not something you do and follow like a recipe, instead it evolves steadily.

> **Slow sex is something you enter and become, an ambience that you create through your bodily relaxation, awareness, and presence, and you change as a result. Profound personal transformation is possible simply by changing the way you have sex, shifting from being unconscious to conscious.**

Sex lies at the foundation of our system, the lowest major energy center. Any shifts and changes in the base will definitely ripple throughout and have an impact on the higher energy centers that lie above.

To encourage couples I sometimes tell them the truth about myself, that I am basically a very lazy person. And the only, and I mean only, reason that I am in a position to sit in front of them and share my experience with them is because everything happened lying down. I was comfortably horizontal in bed, so for me it was pure heaven. If it had been necessary to do the whole exploration in a standing posture, then I can say with certainty that I would not be in a position to say anything about sex today.

Remaining Present in the Sexual Encounter

To be in the present means to include any aspect of the metabolic enhancers as outlined in the previous chapters, such as awareness, rhythm, and relaxation—there are many subtle ways for you to remain present. For example, using awareness you can travel internally to different parts of the body—man might want to travel to his positive pole in the perineum, woman to her nipples. You can also experiment with relaxing other parts of the body—man, the anus and buttocks; woman, the vagina, and anywhere else too. Stay here and now with the unfolding moment, alert in your senses, aware in your body, playful and curious.

- Relax your body consciously again and again, scanning from head to toe, looking for tense places, relaxing and letting go. Release the unconscious holding in the shoulders, the jaw, the solar plexus, the belly, and the muscles around the genitals. Each time you intentionally relax your body you may notice that a spontaneous deep breath follows, along with a wave of subtle sensation moving through your cells.
- Engage each other's eyes as much as possible, with inviting vision, so most of your awareness remains rooted within your own body. Close your eyes when you feel the need to sink deeper into yourself. Speak about your wishes to your partner. This avoids giving them the impression that you are escaping the situation or somehow abandoning them. Sharing helps you to avoid possible misunderstandings.

- Keep your attention on your breathing. Breathe deeply and slowly. Breathe into the diaphragm and belly, imagine your breath touching the genitals. Breathing is a simple bridge that can lead you from thinking to a greater immersion in the body. Breathe in and out together, or one person breathes in as the other breathes out. These breathing patterns will often establish themselves on their own, but it's good to explore the effects of doing them deliberately.
- Kissing, caressing, and touching all keep us present in our bodies and senses. Touch consciously and without any demand, just a loving, generous touch.
- Smile a little, keep your lip corners up, and observe what doing that does to your facial feeling and present moment.

Notice how these small offerings, as acts of awareness, can weave together to become a significant contribution to the intricate tapestry.

Share the Experience of Your Now

The present moment can be greatly magnified by sharing what you are experiencing within yourself, how you feel on a heart level, and any subtle sensations and sensitivities you might be experiencing on a body level. Letting your partner know what you are feeling and where you are feeling it opens a window into your inner realms. Sharing literally brings you into a shared world, which is very helpful at the outset as you establish an unfamiliar style of sex. It's good to know what's going on inside each other. Otherwise you are both left guessing, which may give rise to doubts and tension, and these would not help or support your exploration.

On the other hand, just a few words reporting what you feel can be tremendously relaxing for you and your partner. Share small observations in a few words: "I feel a tingling" (or warmth, light, or whatever it is you happen to feel). Inner sensations are continually changing, shifting, moving, flowing, streaming, so there is usually something small to observe and share. No big discussion and your partner does not need to respond in any way, other than to also say what he or she is feeling at the time.

Extraordinarily, when inner cellular sensations are acknowledged, they amplify. Just by bringing attention to good feelings or good places in the body they will immediately respond by expanding.

When you tell someone about your inner experience, you are simultaneously communicating this to your body, your higher self, and especially to your brain, and this is very powerful. Speaking out reeducates you making you more conscious, more here, and more alert.

Give Space to Feelings that Arise

There is much pain and sadness associated with sex, either from personal experiences in the past or from collective pain due to the misunderstanding, abuse, and repression that has happened through conventional sex. Every individual has felt the impact of these pressures and tensions to a greater or lesser degree, whether we know it or not. It's in the atmosphere, and from our very earliest months of life we are affected by what we feel, sense, see, hear, touch, and imagine. We are shaped by invisible forces; there is no choice, it's a conditioning that grows in us unconsciously. It's a twist on the sexual picture that causes us to lose touch with our sexual innocence, our conscious nature, our restful beings, our loving hearts. Therefore, when consciousness enters the sexual frame, it is a deeply healing force that will begin to move unhappiness out of the system, so it is quite usual for tears to flow. It's a really positive response and highly beneficial to let tears move through you and out of you. In this sense, be open to yourself and yield to your tears, pain, or whatever comes up for you.

If you feel or sense nothing in particular in your genitals, and this is very common at the outset, say so. And also share how it feels not to feel. Admitting to this is taking a big step toward regaining your lost sensitivity. If suddenly tears begin to flow, let them flow; they will refresh your heart. Afterward, you will most probably observe an increase in sensitivity and an aliveness in your cells, especially in the penis or vagina.

When you observe the sensations of a rising feeling—and are able to catch it in the split second it arises—stay with the sensation and open a passage for it. Surrender to it and give way to the flow. Don't hold back or repress for an instant. When you stay faithful to a rising feeling you will often notice that it lasts only seven seconds or so. It passes through you like a wave, and afterward you feel more alive and open.

When buried things are on the move it's usually impossible to communicate to your partner what is happening without stopping the feelings or distancing you from them. At the same time, sometimes saying a word or two, admitting to yourself and thereby your partner, can initiate a healthy torrent of feelings, and it's cleansing to let whatever comes up emerge. Otherwise these feelings remain in the body and are stored as emotions, which generally numb and desensitize the system and also revisit us in destructive and habitual ways (see later section: "Separating Love from Emotion").

Giving free yet conscious rein to your withheld or repressed feelings is profoundly healing and refreshing, both physically and spiritually.

You may also experience unstoppable laughter from time to time, or uncontrollable shaking and shivering, or sadness and tears may reach deeper into heart-wrenching sobbing and wailing. You do not have to understand why you are weeping and wailing or whatever, just live it. Insights as to why may come, or they may not. But don't waste or miss healing opportunities by trying to analyze and figure out why this is happening to you. It is happening, so welcome it; don't try to control it through analysis.

Anger can also come up during sex, in both men and women.

Anger has certain golden rules attached to it and these rules *must be obeyed at all costs.*

Do not project your anger onto your partner. Immediately turn to the side and away from your partner before you let the wave of rage or frustration pass through, perhaps in one grand roar. Or leap out of bed and begin jumping up and down on flat feet, heels hitting the floor first. Keep the arms raised and shout out "Ho!" each time you land on your heels. Do this for several minutes until the wave of anger has passed. The source of all anger lies in accumulated sexual frustration, and most humans are frustrated sexually in the sense that we have not experienced ourselves as a unit of dynamic/receptive forces with an inherent circular movement between man and woman, fulfilling a divine cycle of giving and receiving. So it is very common to feel anger, even rage, arise during sex; take it as an encouraging sign that anger has risen as a way to purify the cells.

Changing and Holding Positions with Awareness

There are no special positions other than the ones that work for you and your partner. It is awareness that makes a position valid and valuable, and not the position per se. It's good to change positions. Once you have achieved genital union you can change position at any time to refresh yourself and become more alert to the situation. Positions and their significance were discussed in chapter 4, where figures 4.5 and 4.6 illustrate the two sequences of rotating positions that allow movement while the penis remains within the vagina (or if not, slip it back in). Or there are some positions that can be held for a longer time without much movement. The side-scissors position is particularly good for sustained penetration with or without erection. (See figs. 10.6 and 10.7 on pages 139 and 140, which illustrate some props that can make the position even more comfortable.)

Yab yum (fig. 10.5 on page 134) is a really wonderful position because

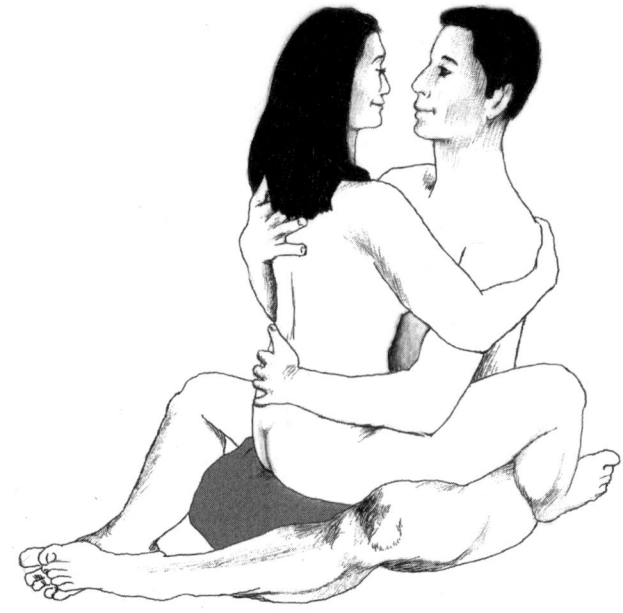

Fig. 10.5. In yab yum position a pillow under woman's buttocks helps to bring the bodies to a similar level so that they align at the genitals and hearts, which encourages circulation of energy.

there is a greater correspondence of the inner magnets within the bodies. The hearts meet through the chest and the breasts, and below there can be an almost magnetic lock of the organs, which then enables energy to ascend, circulate between the bodies, and expand beyond them. Yab yum can be sustained over a long period of time using different approaches to the breath, as suggested earlier. For instance, you can experiment with man breathing out of the penis and in through the heart, and woman breathing out through the breasts and in through the vagina.

Movement Is Part of Slow Sex

Movement is a blessing, movement is life. There is certainly no rule that says during slow sex there is no movement. It's more a question of how we move, as well as why. The basic inquiry is one of whether movement is mechanical or conscious, or if it is appropriate in any given moment, rather than the move being something habitual or deemed to be an essential ingredient of sex. In some moments stillness is appropriate, in others a slow movement is fitting, and in others a shift of position is required. What you do depends on the communication between the penis and vagina. Maybe an adjustment of the legs can deepen the penetration, or a small movement of the pelvis can open up a range of new inner sensations.

Movement is discussed in chapter 2, where it is mentioned, among other things, that an interesting aspect to explore is the basic motivation behind any movement. Why are we doing the movement? Is the movement for stimulating and building up excitement with orgasm in mind? Or do we move because we're wanting to increase awareness or physical comfort, or attempting to enhance pleasure through the correspondence of the penis and vagina?

Movements during slow sex occur in direct response to the present; they arise out of what is needed in the moment and are guided by the light of awareness.

Because they are not goal oriented (not moving toward climax in the future), slow sex movements are of quite a different quality than the movements in conventional sex; they are relaxed and leisurely, the moves evolve in a gradual, sensual, organic way. There is a sense of allowing it to happen, giving way and unfolding, rather than controlling the event according to our usual sexual routine or ideas.

Lust versus Passion

The difference between lust and passion is a matter of definition and requires some clarification. Many people think that in giving up orgasm they are giving up their passion, but this is not the case. Basically you are giving up lust. If you look closely at lust when you are caught up in it, it always has a direction. And this invites tension, expectation, and pressures that swamp the simple present moment. The movements will be building

> toward climax as the goal of the union. A fixation on the end point causes a lack of connection to the present, the orientation is in the future, sometimes subtle and sometimes not so subtle.

Slow sex is not lustful in the usual sense we understand (or experience) hot climactic sex. At the same time, slow sex can sometimes be full-on in a way that is utterly dynamic and involves big movements. But each movement comes from an inner place of stillness and is independent of the movement before it and of the movement after it. Each movement is complete in itself. The moves are not being stepped up to arrive at orgasm as final destination, but as a way of celebrating the present. This type of sexual experience is true passion—pure presence. Passion has no goal and leads nowhere.

You can be fully passionate and be totally unmoving. Or be utterly still and feel inwardly wild at the same time. Passion and authentic wildness are extremely conscious states that reflect tremendous inner vitality and sensitivity.

Sensational heat through the excitement of friction (repetitive in and out movements of the penis in the vagina) short-fuses the system because excitement so easily leads to orgasm. Friction for an extended time has to be used with caution in the sense that once we find ourselves on the roller coaster of excitement it's difficult (if not impossible) to find the awareness or wish to jump off the ride. That's why from the outset it's advisable to stay in the cooler zones of sexual connection where there is less excitement and stimulation, so you do not get hooked up with the need to climax. The coolness creates the sustainability. In addition, in the long term, mechanical friction between the genitals does, little by little, reduce their sensitivity. When sensitivity is lost, more sensation is required and then sensitivity suffers a further loss. To regain sensitivity also means to reside in the genitals in a cooler, calmer, more conscious way.

Instead of mechanical in-and-out movements there are an infinite number of subtle sideways or circular pelvic movements (especially of man) that will help the penis reach and probe into the deeper reaches of the vagina and touch all the surfaces, with very pleasurable effects. Woman can position her pelvis at interesting angles and then hold still so as to invite deeper exploration of the vaginal canal.

Recognizing the Urge for Orgasm

We all know intimately the urge for orgasm, but it is useful to be aware of it in the very moment the desire arises, when suddenly we become tense and switch into fast forward. It is not physically healthy to deliberately repress ejaculation or to repeatedly build tension up, then repress it again. So should ejaculation need to happen, let it be so. Basically orgasm is not wrong. What we are questioning is the conditioning that sex equals orgasm, and the habit of actively striving toward a climax. We are inadvertently creating tension and future goals when, in fact, we need to relax and be here to have elevated experiences.

There is an extremely creative option that you may want to try when faced with the desire for orgasm. When your desire arises, confront it with the totality of your awareness, the totality of your being. At the same time, relax the body utterly and completely. Breathe deeply into the belly and just be, alert in body and senses, present to the moment.

> **If you completely pull back from desire in the very instant it shows itself, a miraculous thing can happen. The energy that was moving outward is powerfully inverted and will implode within you, soon to rise up again through your core in a wave of vitality that becomes a tremendously empowering personal force.**

You ascend to a higher octave, a rarer vibration beyond thought, where the bodies become spontaneous flowing forms and configurations.

If there is a decision for orgasm, don't go into it mechanically and blindly, but consciously and slowly, relaxing tensions, breathing deeply, using your inner eye of awareness to remain present to the unfolding. That very awareness of following the process and relaxing into it, rather than getting tense about it, will fundamentally transform the conventional orgasm experience.

Physical Comfort
Helps Relaxation and Sensitivity

Sustaining your practice also means you need to be able to sustain lying down in bed for longer periods, so be sure to take care of your physical needs. If there is discomfort in the legs, knees, hips, or back, it is time to change position. Otherwise the discomfort becomes a distraction and prevents you from settling into your body and your inner sensations.

Have on hand a selection of pillows of different shapes, sizes, and densities, which can be used to aid and support the postures, as illustrated in figures 10.6 and 10.7. (Also see figures 10.1 and 10.5 on pages 121 and 134 respectively.)

SITUATIONS AND ISSUES
THAT MAY ARISE DURING PRACTICE

It's helpful to know of common hindrances and difficulties that a couple can run into when practicing slow sex. Maybe you got off to a good start and things were going well for a period of time, but then one of you is feeling less satisfied with the practice. Or you are having difficulty keeping a commitment to the practice, you're meeting less often and finding excuses to cancel. Sometimes unexpected emotions arise and get in the way or your expectations are a little bit high, which blocks your awareness of the present moment. Below are some situations that you may find yourselves in, with guidelines on how to deal with them.

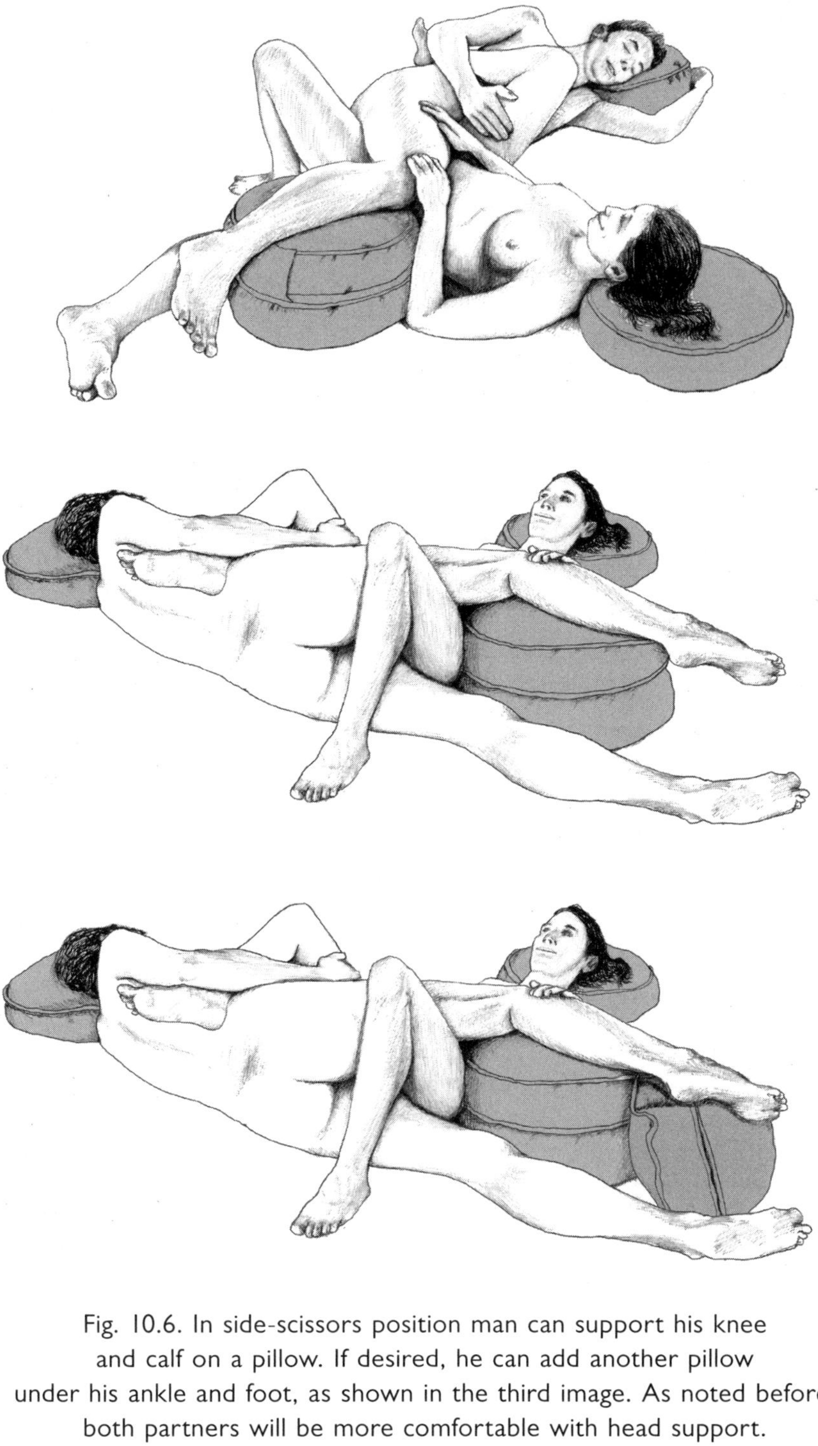

Fig. 10.6. In side-scissors position man can support his knee and calf on a pillow. If desired, he can add another pillow under his ankle and foot, as shown in the third image. As noted before, both partners will be more comfortable with head support.

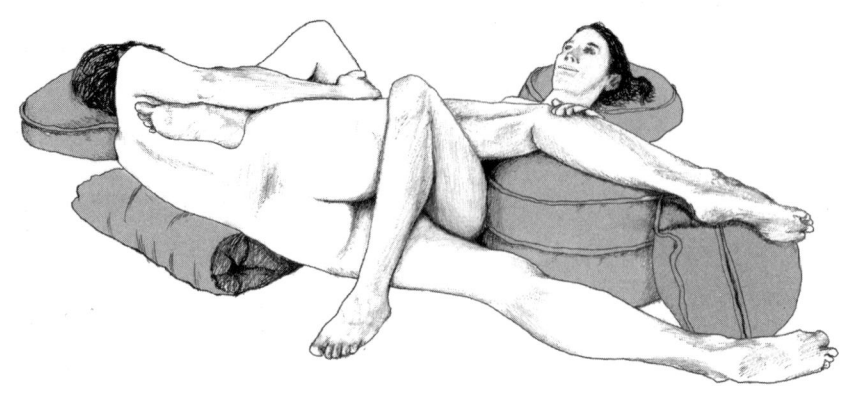

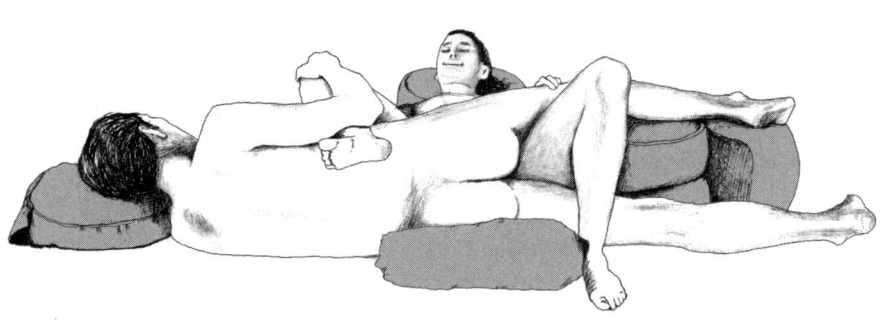

Fig. 10.7. To prevent himself from rolling backward in side-scissors position, man can wedge a pillow support under his back and pelvis. This is particularly helpful for sustained soft penetration. The upper image shows support under both back and hip; the lower image, hip support only.

No Sensitivity or Nothing Really Happens

Many people find that they don't have much sensitivity in the beginning, and the best approach is to accept the situation as it is. Look, it is going to feel different without the usual excitement or stimulation, so take that into account and don't expect to feel the same thing or even anything like it. Don't give in to frustration because you are not getting what you usually get. It's different, and that is all. It takes patience and curiosity to discover the delights of the subtle inner world. Accepting the reality that you don't feel very much will help you to relax, because all acceptance leads to inner relaxation. When we are fighting against something, resisting it, denying it, we create tension that stops us from feeling. If you allow tears of sadness to flow you will notice how your sensitivity improves.

> **Something always happens, even if it is nothing. Becoming aware of this nothingness is already something.**

Nothingness is not easy to accept because there is a deep fear of emptiness and not feeling anything. Fear is often the motivation for movement in sex, to build up feeling in the way of sensation. So when you go slow, and sometimes stop, it will be normal that you cannot easily feel into your genital tissues. In the past you have perhaps been more *around* your genitals, not really in them. In a way it can be difficult to believe that we are not fully sensitive in that part of the body, partly because we are pretty sensitive there for the purposes of conventional sex, and partly because it is difficult to believe that *you* might be insensitive.

In our retreats we always make a great effort to gently warn couples that they may not feel anything at first. We say so again and again during our talks so as not to create expectations and possible disappointment. Even so, after a few days individuals do come up to me looking really shaky and concerned, and share that they can't feel anything in their genitals. So even though we warn people, it is still difficult to accept (and take in) when lack of feeling happens to you.

Patience is needed. Not patience as a duty, tapping your fingers in the meantime, but patience as compassion, understanding, respect; honoring yourself, your body, your partner, your partner's body. With patience comes stillness and silence, relaxation into what is present in any given moment.

Confusion, Insecurity, Not Knowing

It's quite usual, as you start to change your style of sex, to feel that you don't know who you really are. You may feel confused and somewhat lost. When you are on a learning curve a bit of confusion helps, because it loosens up the ego, the personality structure, and you become more vulnerable. You can't expect to be fluent in something that has not been your experience, so a period of disorientation is a valid response to the situation. If you think back to when you first had sex, you probably felt insecure then as well. But now that terrain is traveled and you know your way around. Now you are learning a whole new way of having sex, and also having to unlearn many things you've learned accidentally, so it would almost be surprising if you didn't feel somewhat baffled.

Share your feelings of confusion and insecurity with your partner as soon as they come up. Don't postpone talking about them, otherwise you'll just feel more and more shaky. Once you express what you feel, having said it out loud will quickly make you feel more at ease and at home within yourself. With more slow sex practice and experience you will soon find yourself feeling more confident, clear, and secure.

One Person Feels Something and the Other Does Not

It easily happens that one partner can feel more than the other—usually the woman—and this is quite understandable. Woman as the receptive force, the environment that man moves into, is bound to feel what enters her environment. Conversely, man needs time and practice to orient himself in the new environment. Where woman feels something taking place within her body she can communicate that to man (or vice versa if the situation is reversed and man feels more than woman). She can briefly share what she feels with the presence of the penis inside her. Her feedback can be tremendously reassuring for a man—it tells him that at least his woman can feel him, a fact not to be underestimated.

One Partner Is Better at Communicating

It is often the case that one of the two finds it easier to share and express what is felt, where, and when. Their gift of sharing will support and encourage the other partner to express themselves in words. Do not make differences such as these into problems; rather see how you can help and support each other. The communication also acknowledges your inner body, so you are informing not only your partner, but more importantly, your higher self. Learning to talk about your inner sensitivity is an art that can be learned.

One tip is to start with what is. Often people are more focused on what they think should be, and begin to perceive a lack of something instead of directing the attention to what is present in the moment. Share about simple things you observe in the body. The feelings don't have to be momentous or extraordinary, just what is there. When you acknowledge what is present, you nurture roots of pleasure in the body, and your sensitivity will grow as these roots slowly spread through you.

You Don't Feel Like Having Sex

Bodies always love to make conscious love; the mind is less willing. Often, as in many other situations, there is a natural resistance to stepping out of the mind and into the here and now. It's the mind that will find all kinds of excuses. In this situation you need to acknowledge that you are in resistance, deliberately step over your mind, and connect with each other. Pretty soon you will find that your body is extremely happy to be in that situation. And if it really does not feel as if genital union is appropriate, then you can continue to enjoy an hour or two of intimacy—touching, breathing, receptive vision, being present to your body and each other.

It may appear on the surface that the resistance is a resistance to sex. But in reality the resistance is to being in the present.

I discovered this through the practice of massage, which has been a passion of mine for more than thirty years. In spite of how much I enjoyed it, shortly before an appointment I would often begin to hope that the telephone would ring and my client announce a sudden cancellation. Of course this did not usually happen, and soon enough there would be a knock at the door and I would simply have to accept the situation and proceed accordingly. As soon as the person was on the table and I started oiling their body, I would naturally bring myself into the present by connecting with the skin, flow of my hands, and movements of my body. Within five minutes I would be in heaven, slipping and sliding my way through ninety minutes with ease and timeless joy.

Some years later I was very surprised to notice the same type of resistance coming up with my sex appointments. And again the same realization—resistance to being present, not to sex. And again the same experience. If I accepted the situation and connected with my body in the present, everything flowed easily and the experience was a pleasure. So the guideline is to avoid listening to your mind, which is capable of a thousand and one excuses, and use your body as a bridge to the mystery of the present.

If you are genuinely ill it is wise to respect the state of your body and give it time to heal. If there is a fever or anything really debilitating, sex is probably not advisable. However, there may be some states in which you do feel weak and tired and yet capable of slow sex, especially as no great energy output is required. You will be surprised to discover that afterward you are likely to feel much better, with more energy and an increased sense of well-being.

It's a very good idea to keep your planned dates. It may be that your partner is really counting on that date, and if you make excuses or don't show up, the other person may be disappointed and feel let down. Causing this type of disturbance is really not worthwhile or supportive, as it can take time to get back into equilibrium.

You (or Your Partner) Are Falling Asleep

If you are in a relaxed position, such as the scissors position used for soft penetration, it's easy to feel sleepy or actually even fall asleep. This is especially true for man because lying on the side reminds him of sleep. Whereas woman lies on her back where it is less easy to sleep. It's fine to allow yourself the space to rest deeply for a short time; a short sleep can be regenerating. Some couples remain connected throughout the night, and this is also fine if you are able to sustain the position and sleep at the same time. It's something I have never managed.

In general, though, during sex it's time to be awake and not asleep. You have designated a place and a time and you have a commitment. If you arrive at your appointment exhausted from the other commitments of your day, tired and in need of some sleep, it is better to rest for twenty minutes or so before you begin. Your partner can rest with you. Set an alarm clock, bearing in mind that a twenty-minute nap is usually more refreshing than a two-hour sleep.

> **It's helpful to know that the urge to sleep can be due not only to tiredness, but also to avoidance.**

Overwhelming heaviness in the eyelids can sometimes be induced by reluctance to acknowledge deeper feelings that are coming to the surface, such as old unexpressed pain. The pull toward sleep is a defense mechanism to switch you off and keep you comfortable and undisturbed. When you notice something like this happening to you, the way through is to take a step deeper into yourself, delve into the buried feelings, and give way to them. Afterward you will feel much more present, alive, and loving. Prolific yawning is often another symptom of underlying feelings rising to the surface. The yawning reflex keeps feelings at bay.

One Wants to Move and the Other Doesn't

Sometimes during slow sex one person wants to be more still and the other wants a bit more action. It's generally more common that the woman is seeking stillness and the man wants movement, and this is probably because the female organ is a receptive organ and the male organ is a dynamic organ. However, the man has to discover how to be present and vital within the vagina as a dynamic, complementary force, rather than being dynamic in the way of literal activity, moving in and out. So there is a need for man to challenge himself a little in order to discover the true qualities of his penis. He also needs to develop compassion for woman and a greater understanding of her situation. Too often she has entered sex without her body being fully open, and she has pushed herself to please man to keep love in her life. Now finally, with a new understanding in hand, she is able to relax and receive—her true nature. Usually she will intuitively know this is the right way for her.

At the same time, and equally important, woman needs to understand that man is stepping down from a big performance program (as demanded by conventional sex), and have compassion for him. Also, he has been accustomed to a rubbing movement in order to feel his penis. Basically, when a movement is a conscious movement, it slows down and the whole quality changes including sensitivity. So you can agree on conscious movement, which is fair enough. After all, it's been the unconscious way that has usually made woman less available for sex in the past.

What a woman has to watch out for is her mind falling into resistance, repeating again and again to herself, "I don't like it." This attitude makes you internally tight and unreceptive, so for sure you will not like it! You have to dive into yourself and see what you can do to change the situation, rather than ask the other person to change, as in "Please slow down" or "Please stop." Too many instructions can make a person feel manipulated and controlled, which can lead to feeling wrong or unworthy.

> **I discovered that if I put all my awareness into relaxation, widening and receiving, especially in the vagina (instead of**

being caught up in the mind), the man would slow down enormously and even sometimes come to a wide-eyed standstill.

In this way woman does have a certain power as the receptive environment. A penis entering the space is immediately affected by the absorbent forces enveloping it, and it's better for her to direct her energies in this direction, see how she can directly transform the situation through awareness, rather than try to change her man.

You Feel Frustrated

Frustration can arise because things are different and you don't get what you are accustomed to getting from sex. Frustration can also happen because you expect too much or don't feel much. If so, definitely begin to do something with your own body every day, some kind of exercise that you enjoy. Become more alive to yourself. To increase sensitivity and awareness in your genitals you can also do a self-massage of your pelvic floor.

☉ Exercise: Pelvic Floor Self-Massage

1. Lying on your back, knees up, hands between your legs, make small circular movements with your fingertips circling deep above, on, and below the pubic bone, spreading sideways to the sitz bones. Then turn onto your side and reach behind to massage the coccyx area.
2. Then, lying on your back again, give a deep massage to the muscles around your genitals. Take about an hour to work on the area, and repeat the massage several times over the next few weeks.

A self-massage done with gentle, loving hands will help to release tension and increase circulation and sensitivity in the pelvic region.

It's important to find some kind of balance in the engagement between the two of you—you don't want to get so frustrated that you get turned off, so you need to keep it interesting. And at the same time, become aware of how strong the sexual conditioning is, how strong the urge to do something in sex is, and how difficult it is to just be floating in it. You need to be willing to challenge your patterns in order to access your higher sexual potential. It takes time and practice to learn the knack, so keep it interesting for yourselves and be patient, loving, generous, and supportive.

Loss of Erection

Loss of erection is natural when stimulation is reduced, so it is helpful to accept active and passive phases of the penis, and to accept soft entry as a viable alternative. Man carries a lot of insecurity and fear around the whole erection issue because it's fragile. Usually when a man begins to lose his erection he feels very awkward about it, even embarrassed, and the last thing he really wants is for his woman to realize it. So a man often tries to cover up a diminishing erection by exciting or stimulating himself or woman in some way. A relaxed penis is an equally valid instrument and it continues to have dynamic properties, however many men consider the erect version of the penis as being *the* penis. They believe a flaccid penis is of no real consequence, where soft sadly equals impotence.

> **Instead of feeling shame and fear around loss of erection (and trying to get it back), it is far better for a man to allow his penis to relax and stay within the vagina (or use soft entry), and at the same time connect with (be aware of and true to) his real feelings, which may be insecurity, weakness, or a feeling of helplessness.**

Feeling these feelings can be a kind of small death. There may be sadness and tears, or not knowing, accompanied by shaking and shivering. Expressing the deeper fears that underly loss of erection is a form of healing, cleansing, and empowerment that establishes a man more deeply in his authentic male authority.

Expecting Results

People often ask, "How long before we can expect ecstasy?" Such expectations show that you are standing in your own way. Ecstasy can never be a demand or an expectation; it's a blessing and a gift. You have to create the situation and be an invitation for bliss to descend upon you. It needs receptivity and preparation. There are some prerequisites to meeting the Divine—naturalness, egolessness, and timelessness. Ecstasy happens when immersed in the present, not absent through being expectant. And in any event, many thrilling moments of delight and pleasure are possible every time you get together.

People often think that ecstasy is something hot and overwhelming, but this is not really true. Ecstasy is, in fact, exceptionally cool and peaceful, and arises when there is a silent receptivity, porousness, and ease.

We cannot expect bliss from the first footstep we take on the journey. Many steps have to be taken, but these are not arduous; the way is one of fun, curiosity, and exploration. Become sensitive and attuned to yourself on the cellular level first. Put the foundations in place and build on that solid base.

Making Rules Out of Tools

A very common error is to turn tools into rules. When we get serious, tools become rules and exploration is no longer possible. Women, especially, tend to point their fingers—do this, don't do this. Loving, playful cooperation is absolutely essential, otherwise we don't get anywhere.

Trial and error is what you are after. Teach yourself, explore, and establish the truth of each tool instead of making it a rule. Finding the truth also means exploring tried and tested ways (as in conventional sex), so do not deny your past experience. Use the past as a bridge to the present. Return to known experiences in order to discover the truth, and don't rush to conclusions, as in, "It's like this because of that." Check it out again and again, and see if the same holds true over time. Only then is a truth truly your truth—when it has stood the test of time.

Lack of Time

The time factor is a common complaint from couples. Even with the best of intentions, between the joys and stresses of family life and work life there is rarely enough space for slow sex dates. In the end you simply have to carve time for yourselves as a couple and at least find time for the slow sex quickie now and then. Love has to be given some priority. Consciously creating love through slow sex will support you personally and as a couple, and put you in a better position to handle every other aspect of your life.

Arguing, Discussing, or Fighting

If you find yourself in some kind of argument, discussion, or blaming mode while supposedly having sex, then it's best to take some space apart from each other. Or it may be more subtle—you may notice some kind of negative or unloving charge (hidden or not) in your communication. If there's any kind of emotion in the air, then sex can easily move in the direction of excitement and discharge as a way of eliminating the emotional tension. Best is to tell your partner what's happening with you, using simple, first-person words such as, "I feel emotional," or "I feel disconnected from myself and you." Then separate physically (after agreeing that you will meet again later), find a place to be alone, and do something active with your body.

Do something physically strenuous, and with intention, to rid yourself of the accumulated tension. When you have come back to yourself and can feel your heart again, return to your partner. Usually there will be an immediate sense of connection, but if for any reason you continue to feel slightly separate, you may need to move a bit more. Whatever you choose to do, do it with intention and self-awareness, not in a halfhearted way.

The danger of staying in the same place, not separating, is that the talking and arguing will be prolonged, perhaps going around in circles for hours. The unhappiness and tension that has arisen (for whatever reason) has to be dealt with differently in order to protect and preserve your love. If you continue fighting, too easily things escalate and hurtful, revengeful things are said to each other, which is a much less effective way to rid the system of tension. So if you hear yourself using phrases like "you always" or "you never," this is a signal that you have moved from connection into disconnection. Or if you notice you can't look your partner in the eyes, this too is a sign that the connection is out of order. (For more on this subject see below, "Separating Love from Emotion," and the book *Tantric Love: Feeling versus Emotion— Golden Rules to Make Love Easy* by Diana and Michael Richardson.) Recognize what's happening, announce it, and separate briefly to get a handle on the situation without acting it out on your partner. And then afterward come back together again.

DEEPENING YOUR SLOW SEX PRACTICE

Your experience will deepen through regular and frequent practice, not just leaving it for now and then (although now and then is infinitely better than not at all). You may reach various plateaus, which is perfectly fine, and also rewarding and beneficial. Regular meetings give rise to a refining of the polarity within and between your bodies— male more male, female more female. You become more finely tuned as time passes.

> **Unlike conventional sex where the thrills tend to dry up over time, slow sex is sustainable over many, many years and encourages togetherness. Sex can be a cohesive force.**

This bonding element alone speaks loud and clear for the value of slow sex. I hear from so many couples after our retreats that the only reason they are still together is because they began practicing slow sex. Through the awareness required they came back into connection with themselves, and through that, with each other. The awareness made it possible and easy to be able to continue a loving relationship in happiness and harmony. When the level of awareness between any two people is raised, then love is the alchemical by-product.

PENETRATING INNOCENCE

Stay light, easy, and playful. These qualites of innocence will support you. A sense of humor is tantamount to a best friend when you explore sex. Very amusing situations can arise so the capacity to be light and see the funny side of things helps. A sense of humor gives you perspective on the situation; you are less identified with what is taking place. A sense of humor definitely means being able to laugh at yourself. When we are lacking in humor it may be because we are somehow trapped in the mind and identified with our sexual selves, our performance, or how the other person perceives us as a lover. Avoid taking yourself too seriously and don't get serious about what you are doing. Make it a play, a dance. Be easygoing with yourself and your partner. Life and love are an unfolding mystery and adventure, so it doesn't help to get too serious about them.

> **What is essential is sincerity of the heart, not seriousness of the mind. Sincerity keeps to the commitment, gives rise to curiosity and willingness, and knows the value of love.**

Entering the inner dimensions and realms of the body is basically a feminine search. The spiritual inquiry is a feminine one because it looks inward; both man and woman are engaging with the feminine. This is an essential balance to our very extroverted, masculine, outward-oriented society with its material, external values. As a general shift, humanity needs to turn back inward to access resources that lie within and have sustainable value beyond the material.

When the dynamic and receptive sexual forces resting deep within are allowed to express themselves in slow sex, tremendous healing and regeneration is possible, both individually and collectively. Engaging in slow sex enables your system to come into natural flow and balance. As you heal and harmonize yourselves you will generate a powerful positive energy that becomes a contribution to society at large.

Developing Presence

Our first effort must be to arrive in the present. The present moment is most easily found in your body. Through being aware in the body, the senses, the breath, and the inner world, you being to develop the quality of presence. This quality has the capacity to develop and grow to the extent that your presence begins to have an impact on others and alchemically draw them into the here and now.

> **Don't be concerned as to whether your partner is present or not; rather, look to see if *you* are present or not. And find ways to intensify your presence (using your awareness) so that it energetically draws and engages your partner.**

I found it a great help to always try to change myself first, before considering what I could ask my partner to change. It's not that you deny your needs or your truth, but first and foremost you turn back toward yourself and become curious as to what you can influence through your awareness and relaxation. For me, doing so has always had magical results.

A Shift from Doing to Being

The body is the bridge to the being, and when you relax into your being, you naturally connect with the source of love within yourself. The source of love is within you, not outside you. At times you may decide to drop verbal communication or close your eyes, because you have reached a stage where you can hold the awareness in the present and for a change wish to enjoy silence, closed eyes, and just being.

There are quite a few inner doings that can go on while you

are being in your body. You might want to experiment with some of the following:

- Bring your awareness to your perineum (man) or breasts (woman) and notice what takes place on a subtle energy level.
- Travel internally with your breath and assist it in reaching deep into the genital tissues.
- Breathe incredibly softly with your awareness at the nasal openings and see how you can enter into your breath.
- Curl the tip of your tongue upward until it touches the roof of your mouth, and feel what inner connection happens when you leave it there.
- Bring your awareness to the third eye (midline forehead, just above the eyebrows) and feel the inner expansion.
- Hold the awareness in the solar plexus and see how a certain spontaneity arises in your body, or in the connection between you and your partner.

Little tricks like these, connecting energy circuits or connecting to energy points (using the awareness), will often intensify inner sensations and sensitivities, and they are great to play around with and explore. At the same time, getting too involved with this inner point or that inner point can turn into a subtle form of doing and create a slight but significant level of absence. So this by-product has to be balanced by simply being present to what *is* in the body.

Spontaneous Erection and Orgasmic Experiences

Spontaneous erection, one where the penis spirals upward by itself inside the vagina, can happen at any time. This phenomenon is based on a magnetic type of interaction between the penis and vagina's dynamic and receptive forces, as we discussed in more detail in chapter 4. Avoid having expectations. It may happen, it may not happen. Maybe today, maybe tomorrow. But do not use spontaneous erection as any kind of measure of success. Do not expect anything to happen because expectations form subtle barriers that block your potential experience. Expectation involves thought and judgment and removes you from your inner connection to the body. Spontaneous erection will usually be a by-product of deep merging with body and senses; it can never be a goal because it is an outcome of a certain constellation of factors. You can only create the situation and settle ever more deeply into your body.

Orgasmic states can arise for both man and woman, but they cannot in any way be engineered or expected. In the orgasmic state you experience an expansion beyond the physical boundaries where you come to exist as pure boundless energy through a deep relaxation and inner merging.

SEPARATING LOVE FROM EMOTION

Love is not an emotion, it is a state of being. Love is tremendous insight, clarity, sensitivity, and awareness, and these intrinsic qualities grow when we relax back into the body to touch the source of love that resides in the being. Taking responsibility for negative emotions and emotionality is a big step in maturity that permits us to behave as adults and not five-year-olds. With taking responsibility comes a newfound freedom in which we are able to preserve love and leave behind unhelpful patterns. A slow sex practice will definitely bring more harmony and reduce the level of emotionality between partners.

Expressing Feelings and Sharing Your Needs

It becomes necessary to communicate your needs and not expect your partner to intuit them. Sometimes it is difficult to admit to our needs, let alone express them, but if you don't tell your partner what does or doesn't suit you, you risk feeling unhappy a bit later on—like a backlash. Not getting needs fulfilled is a big source of our unhappiness and emotions. By speaking up in sex it is possible to eliminate at least one source of ongoing unhappiness and discontent.

When feelings rise to the surface, give way to them, let them move through you. Or tell your partner what you are feeling, making sure to talk only about yourself and avoid any form of subtle blaming or making your partner responsible for what you feel. Releasing or sharing old unexpressed aspects of yourself is integrating and deeply healing. Through purifying the tensions of old feelings that are stored in your body, you transform like a caterpillar becoming a butterfly.

The Difference between Feelings and Emotions

If you don't express your feelings or share your needs it is highly likely that sooner or later you will get emotional. Feelings and emotions are not the same and knowing the difference is life changing.

> **A feeling arises for expression out of the present moment, but when it remains unexpressed, the energy can turn in to negative emotion.**

That means that feelings we do *not* express in the present get stored inside us, accumulate with time, and cause disturbances. You will know the moment you are emotional because there are certain distinct signs or symptoms that help you to recognize what is going on.

For the brief period of time when we are emotional, we are unconsciously caught up in the past, and not really anchored in the present and in reality. You begin to experience distance or a sense of separation from your partner (and also from yourself), whereas earlier you were feeling connected. When everything was rosy in the present there was the experience of connection—you were with the perfect person. Now, however, you may suddenly find yourself feeling far away and finding fault with your partner in some way, blaming them for this or that.

These swings in mood happen because from time to time our stored, unexpressed feelings get triggered, in and out of sex. And what leads us into trouble is that we have a *multitude* of unexpressed feelings, given that we live in a society where expressing genuine heartfelt feelings is not really okay. So most of us (and especially men) repress many of our feelings. As a result of centuries of repression, human beings have the tendency to be pretty emotional. All the unexpressed feelings remain in the system and go slightly sour, and when provoked in any way (even the slightest nudge can start a fist fight) they pop up and express themselves. The difficulty lies in the fact that the old unexpressed feelings have become toxins in the system, which explains why so often a person becomes so destructive or so vengeful when caught in the emotional state.

> **People sometimes do and say dreadful things to each other when they are experiencing a wave of emotion. And the toxic vengeful quality of emotion is the reason why whenever you recognize that you are emotional, you must literally tell your partner, "I am emotional." And then, to avoid further possibly hurtful words, leave the room.**

Instead of venting your emotion on your partner, do something physical to burn up the emotion that has become active in your system. This really simple solution may appear *too* simple, but it invariably works. Afterward, when you return to your partner, the wall that was separating you has probably come down. If not, that's your signal to go and do some more work on yourself. Taking responsibility in this way means that you save yourselves the pain of going through many emotional upheavals that are destructive to your love connection. After too many fights the repairs start to take more time and be more temporary. Love slowly begins to erode and slip out of our hands. The toxins produced by too many fights, or one fight too many, has been the cause of many a couple finally separating.

Love is precious and we have to protect it from the destructive effects of overwhelming and inconstant emotion. Knowing how to tell the difference between the two very different states of emotion and feeling can save your relationship.

Deepening Polarity and Healing of the Penis and Vagina

As a couple opens to slow sex, the genitals go through a purifying, refining, and balancing process. Pain in the male or female genitals is sometimes indicative of old tensions leaving the body, yet another expression of buried and unresolved feelings. Be aware that healing or detoxification happens at any time and in many forms. For instance, nausea or vomiting, loose stools, headaches or migraines, toothache, exhaustion, boils or pimples, irregular heartbeat, or feeling very weak.

It's common for some women to experience pain in the vagina during sex and, regrettably, they accept it as part of the package. Some women will even fake pleasure by making suitable sounds when in reality sex feels painful to them. As a woman gets older and enters menopause, she frequently will report pain upon penetration or dryness of the tissues, so much that she can no longer have sex. Slow sex, however, is possible and enjoyable.

Sometimes during sex a woman will become aware of hidden pains or numb places at the entrance, along the sides, or deep in the higher part of the vagina.

Pain and deadness usually represent old wounds or memories stored in the tissue. Pain is positive in the sense that it acts as a door to the past and the tension accumulated there.

The powerful and healing effects of conscious sustained penetration are described in detail in chapter 8.

Opening to and giving way to buried feelings can be an effective way to release physical pain in the body, especially pain in the genital region. If you have a pain that suddenly arises and persists, especially after sex, always look to see if there is an emotional component hiding behind it. Perhaps there is some sadness, anger, or anxiety that you are holding under the surface. Allowing old feelings heals, balances, and sensitizes.

Men can also experience uncomfortable pain when they start to have slow, conscious sex. Pain in the groin, testicles, or penis is usually an indication of previously held tension being released and purified from the system. (Please note that ejaculation control by repression is not recommended, as mentioned earlier. Repressing ejaculation will also lead to pain and tension, but this is due to congestion and not because of purification.)

Sustained penetration can become a style of sex, with or without erection. The opposite poles spend simple time together and gradually become more attuned and alive.

RAISING CONSCIOUSNESS

In many ways, mastering slow sex is really a matter of unlearning a certain behavior and learning another one. You are installing consciousness in a place where expression has been more automatic, mechanical, and unconscious. So transforming unconsciousness into consciousness is a great shift and gift for your life, a blessing intended for you by the Creator.

Afterward Is Your Teacher

Essentially you have to teach yourself the conscious way. Learning is not going to happen just by reading and thinking about it; rediscovery can only happen through practice—hands-on experience. What you learn from yourselves is revealed by how you feel after you have had sex. Afterward is your teacher and shows you the way.

Intentionally begin to observe yourself after you have finished making love. How do you feel? Pay attention to immediately after, a short time later, and even a couple of days later. The tendency is to evaluate the high point—the climax—but we do not really observe ourselves during the minutes and hours beyond the moment of orgasm. Watching yourself afterward helps you to put together a new picture of sex. If you notice after slow sex, even while you may have "missed" some aspects of the fast approach (such as orgasm), that you feel more at ease in yourself, more loving, more nourished, then this feedback is teaching you something about the nature of exchange. If you perhaps observe that you feel brittle, abandoned, or lonely, it's good to look back at that as well. What did you do and how did you do it? Do you notice a connection between what you do and how you feel afterward?

> **My partner and I tell people in our groups that "afterward" is their teacher, we are not. Both of us have certainly found that observation of the period of time after sex, even days later, has been the greatest teacher thus far.**

Teach yourself through asking, "How was it?" Teach yourself how as you go along, by trial and error. Starting happens by getting down to doing it, and in your own individual way. Approach it with a sense of adventure, interested in what lies on the horizon.

Becoming Messengers of Love

Slow sex is an inquiry; you begin to examine sex. Answers will come to you, like the slow dawning of the day; you don't have to know everything in advance. Wanting questions answered in full before being willing to step out is not realistic. You might hear something said, but to make it your own truth, the experience has to be lived, and the truth verified.

Sincerity and general sensitivity in the body, especially the genital union, can produce transforming higher states of consciousness.

> **Ecstasy is not, however, the new goal that replaces the old goal of orgasm. It cannot be seen in this way because ecstasy only shows itself when there is a dropping of goals, a diving into the present, and a dissolving into the infinite inner cosmos.**

Recall the three beautiful elements to the experience of blissfulness mentioned: egolessness, naturalness, and timelessness. Egolessness means there is no "I." Naturalness means you surrender to the intelligence of your body. Timelessness means you slip into the present, and therefore completely out of time. Bliss can also happen without a partner, such as when alone enraptured by nature, and many people have had such an experience. So we cannot do bliss, we can only humbly and reverently create the situation that allows bliss. Sex definitely offers the perfect situation for exploring these elements, and it is perhaps one of the easiest, because the central theme reduces itself down to how you do something, and not what you do. Attributes such as innocence, sincerity, compassion, and courage are the qualities to pursue in order to elevate consciousness.

You don't need advanced techniques. The ever-deepening experience of penetrating your inner world can accompany you for the rest of your life. It's an experience that evolves with time and practice. Sex gets more simple, sensitivity grows, and you transform as time goes on. Slow sex becomes a practice involving a finely tuned awareness with positive, uplifting, long-term benefits that generally increase the quality of love and of life. While slow sex encourages togetherness, it also encourages aloneness and independence. You begin to feel complete, whole, and integrated, happier in and with yourself.

As you grow together you also grow as individuals, and your male and female poles come into balance. And the curious thing about the inner balancing of masculine and feminine energies within yourself is that you don't need to do anything with the opposite pole. You need only live and explore your male qualities as man, or your female qualities as woman. Living these aspects will alchemically establish the equal and opposite pole within you. Man by being more male accesses his feminine qualities, while woman through being more female accesses her masculine qualities.

Your inner flow of magnetism comes to life in such a way that energy can stream within you as a form of inner sex. This means you can circulate energy within yourself and continue the inner process of transformation that you have started together. The capacity to circulate vitality within yourself is the most evolved form of sex given to human beings, so it is something that can be done alone or in each other's company. You may already feel some streaming within; if not, visualization works very well, as it helps to awaken the energy.

Through practicing slow sex you will come to see and understand that sex is not what it seems to be on the surface. Any inherited preconceptions and ideas of sex are mostly false, and these misunderstandings form a screen between you and the real power of sex.

Through sexual exploration you will discover that the true function of slow sex is to bring more love into being. In this way each and every person can be a messenger of love by creating love and offering it to the world. Likewise, a couple can become a positive force in the community as generators of love and light.

Man's deepest wish is to be loved by woman, just as woman's deepest wish is to be loved by man. When you discover the how of love, then love is easily sustained. Couples begin to value, support, and appreciate each other as equal yet fundamentally opposite and complementary forces.

If there is any hope for humanity, perhaps the only genuine hope is that man and woman find peace with each other. Practicing sex in a conscious, slow way builds bridges of communication that kindle the flame of peace, enabling them to live as a cohesive force enjoying physically and spiritually uplifting lives.

The end of the story is that there has to be a drastic turnaround in the way people use their sexual energy. A few innocent, simple sexual steps are all it takes to initiate a journey back home to oneself, in accord with nature and the cosmic plan. There has to be a ripening and maturing process, whereby sex incorporates the universal metabolic enhancers so that the higher dimensions can easily be accessed and revealed. Slow sex is simple, sustainable, and life affirming, and enables us to be radiant purveyors of light, love, and peace on Earth.

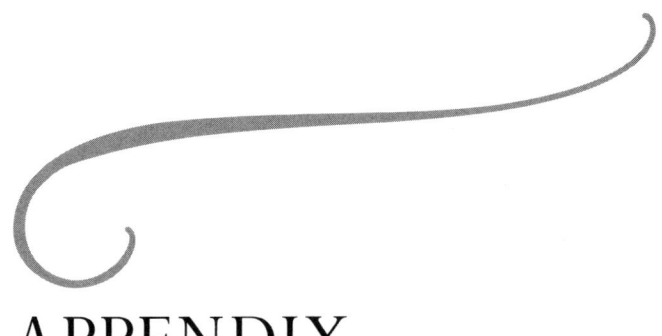

APPENDIX
True Male and Female Qualities versus Conditioned Distortions

Pages 164 and 165 present tables that list male and female qualities. The column on the left in each table lists the essential deep-seated qualities of man or woman. The column on the right lists the outcome or pattern when these intrinsic qualities become (unconsciously) distorted through sexual and societal conditioning. Because all human beings carry male and female poles within themselves, it can also happen that a man may sometimes demonstrate distorted female qualities, while at times a woman may display distorted male qualities. Approaching sex in a conscious, slow way leads to personal purification and healing of the body and psyche, promoting spontaneous inner balancing and integration.

TRUE MALE QUALITIES VERSUS CONDITIONED DISTORTIONS

TRUE QUALITIES	CONDITIONED DISTORTIONS
Pure consciousness	Unconsciousness
Power	Abuse of power, domination
Presence	Absence
Strength	Hardness, violence
Clarity	Judgment
Assuredness	Aggression
Directed action, dynamic	Activity, restless, doing
Creativity	Achievement, ambition
Will	Stubbornness
Courage	Compensation, arrogance
Leadership	Control, politics, law and order
Protector	Patriarch
Authority	Authoritarian
Wildness	Brutality
Clear mind	Arrogance
Charisma	Sexual manipulation
Sun, seed of creation	Sunburn, ecological destruction
Expression, articulation	Pomposity, uncouth behavior
Heartfelt, compassionate	Selfish, egoistic
Differentiation	Separation

TRUE FEMALE QUALITIES VERSUS CONDITIONED DISTORTIONS

TRUE QUALITIES	CONDITIONED DISTORTIONS
Unconditional love	Love with conditions
Pure energy	Hysterical
Electromagnetic field of attraction	Projects attractiveness
Appreciates inner beauty	Attached to outer appearance
Receptivity	Passivity
Loving	Jealous, manipulative, possessive
Softness	Weakness
Relaxed, nondoing	Inertia, laziness, collapse
Earth, manifesting creation, nurturing	Overbearing, interfering
Embracing	Overwhelming
Ability to surrender	Submissive, giving in, losing self
In contact with feelings	Emotional swings, sentimental, moody
Sensitive	Oversensitive, prickly, brittle
Nesting instinct	Obsessed with security
Intuitive, psychic	Suspicious, fearful
Enveloping	Sucking, taking
Sweetness	Hardness, stoniness
Silently strong	Masochistic, holding back energy
Connecting	Invasive
Trusting, allowing	Controlling, indecisive, lacking initiative
Connected to the universe	Spaced out, lacking personal boundaries

BOOKS AND RESOURCES

David, Marc. *The Slow Down Diet: Eating for Pleasure, Energy, and Weight Loss.* Rochester, Vt.: Healing Arts Press, 2005.

Honoré, Carl. *In Praise of Slowness: Challenging the Cult of Speed.* New York: HarperCollins, 2005.

Lloyd, J. William. *The Karezza Method or Magnetation: The Art of Connubial Love.* Charleston, S.C.: Forgotten Books, 2008. (Originally printed privately for the author in 1931.)

Richardson, Diana. *The Heart of Tantric Sex: A Unique Guide to Love and Sexual Fulfilment.* Alresford, Hants, United Kingdom: "O" Books, 2002. (Originally published in 1999 as *The Love Keys: The Art of Ecstatic Sex.*)

———. *Tantric Love Letters: A Collection of Experiences, Questions, and Answers.* Alresford, Hants, United Kingdom: "O" Books, 2011.

———. *Tantric Orgasm for Women.* Rochester, Vt.: Destiny Books, 2004.

Richardson, Diana, and Michael Richardson. *Making Love: What You Should Always Have Known About Sex.* DVD of a live talk. Voice tracks in English and German. Cologne, Germany: Innenwelt Verlag, 2011. Available at www.livingloveshop.com.

———. *MaLua Light Meditation for Women.* Guided breast meditation CD with music, available in English and German. Cologne, Germany: Innenwelt Verlag, 2009.

———. *Tantric Love: Feeling versus Emotion—Golden Rules to Make Love Easy.* Alresford, Hants, United Kingdom: "O" Books, 2010. (Originally published in German in 2006.)

———. *Tantric Sex for Men: Making Love a Meditation.* Rochester, Vt.: Destiny Books, 2010.

———. *Time for Touch: Massage Using Awareness and Relaxation.* Instructional DVD. Voice tracks in English and German. Cologne, Germany: Innenwelt Verlag, 2010. Available at www.livingloveshop.com.

Robinson, Marnia. *Cupid's Poisoned Arrow: From Habit to Harmony in Sexual Relationships.* New York: Random House, 2009.

Rosenberg, Marshall. *Nonviolent Communication: A Language of Life.* Encinitas, Calif.: Puddle Dancer Press, 2003.

Stockham, Alice Bunker. *Karezza: Ethics of Marriage.* Charleston, S.C.: Forgotten Books, 2008. (Originally published in 1903.)

Versluis, Arthur. *The Secret History of Western Sexual Mysticism: Sacred Practices and Spiritual Marriage.* Rochester, Vt.: Destiny Books, 2008.

"MAKING LOVE"
A Tantra Meditation Retreat for Couples

The author and her partner, Michael, offer weeklong retreats in Switzerland that guide couples into the art of slow, conscious sex. For more information about their work please visit their websites listed below.

www.livinglove.com
www.love4couples.com

You may contact Diana and Michael by e-mail at the following address.

info@livinglove.com

TANTRIC SEX
FOR MEN

TANTRIC SEX
FOR MEN

MAKING LOVE A MEDITATION

DIANA RICHARDSON
AND
MICHAEL RICHARDSON

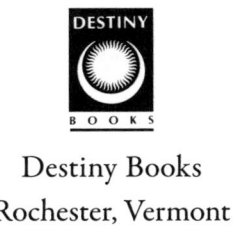

Destiny Books
Rochester, Vermont

Destiny Books
One Park Street
Rochester, Vermont 05767
www.DestinyBooks.com

Destiny Books is a division of Inner Traditions International

Text copyright © 2010 by Diana Richardson and Michael Richardson
Art copyright © 2004, 2010 by Diana Richardson

All rights reserved. No part of this book may be reproduced or utilized in any form or by any means, electronic or mechanical, including photocopying, recording, or by any information storage and retrieval system, without permission in writing from the publisher.

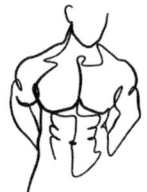

Volume II
of
Tantric Sex for Lovers
Boxed Set

Tantric Sex for Men

Printed and bound in India by Replika Press Pvt. Ltd.

10 9 8 7 6 5 4 3 2 1

Text design and layout by Virginia Scott Bowman
This book was typeset in Garamond Premier Pro with Weiss, Gill Sans, and Helvetica as display typefaces

All Osho quotes printed with permission of Osho International
Artwork prepared by Alfredo Hernando, Madrid, Spain
Author cover photographs by Shobha, Sicily, Italy

Dedicated to Mother Earth

Tantric Inspiration

Even after a lifetime of sexual experience we never reach anywhere near that supreme stage, near that divinity. Why? A man reaches a ripe old age, comes to the end of his life, but he is never free from his lust for sex, from his passion for intercourse. Why? It is because he has never understood nor been told about the art of sex, about the science of sex. He has never considered it; he has never discussed it with the enlightened ones.

OSHO, TRANSCRIBED TEACHINGS,
FROM SEX TO SUPERCONSCIOUSNESS

CONTENTS

	Preface by Michael Richardson	ix
	Introduction	1

1	Male Burden of Performance	7
2	Involuntary Ejaculation and Desensitization	15
3	Ejaculation Is Not Male Orgasm	25
4	The Equal and Opposite Force of the Female Environment	41
5	The Penis—A Potent Electromagnetic Instrument	53
6	Awareness, Movement, Penetration, and Erection	63
7	Dates, Foreplay, Kissing, and Positions	85
8	Sexual Healing and Male Authority	99
9	Mastering Love and Overcoming Emotions	119
10	Personal Experiences	139

APPENDIX	Exercises for Improving Your Awareness and Sensitivity	155
	Recommended Books and Resources	162
	About the Authors	165

Tantric Inspiration

When sex is just an unconscious, mechanical urge in you, it is wrong. Remember, sex is not wrong: just the mechanicalness of it is wrong. If you can bring some light of intelligence into your sexuality, that light will transform it. It will not be sexuality anymore—it will be something totally different, so different that you do not have a word for it.

In the East we have a word for it—Tantra. In the West you don't have a word for it. When sex becomes joined together, is yoked with intelligence, a totally new energy is created—that energy is called Tantra.

OSHO, TRANSCRIBED TEACHINGS,
PHILOSOPHIA PERENNIS

PREFACE

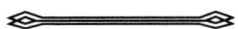

By Michael Richardson

Sex is not what it seems to be. We all have inherited preconceptions and ideas about sex, which are mostly false and form a screen, or barrier, that separates us from the real power of sex. When we look beyond the inherited screen of misunderstanding we discover that sex is completely different from what we generally think it is. Through sexual exploration I personally have discovered the true function of sex, which is to bring more love into the world. Each and every person can be a messenger of love by creating more love and contributing it to the world.

The screen of conditioning—our past experiences and ideas—limits our human sexual expression. After all, what does a man want when he makes love to a woman? What is the ultimate reason for making love? It is not to achieve ejaculation; it is to be loved by the woman.

Woman is the source of love, the mother of love, and I, as a man, am able to tap into that love. For me, love is what it is all about. Being in the here and now, I've discovered that in stillness, including inner stillness during movement, I can tap into or connect with the "garden of love" in woman. And there is nothing more satisfying and touching than seeing a woman radiating, blossoming in love.

I do have hope for humanity. The only hope is for man to find a way through his screen of conditioned sexuality, so that he may come to rest within his male authority. So that he can make peace with woman and make love to her body, heart, and soul.

INTRODUCTION

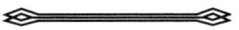

There are a great many books about sex offering a range of techniques best described as the "effort" or "doing" approach. Little is mentioned about the "relaxed" or "non-doing" approach in sex, which is why we decided to write a book from the man's perspective. The non-doing approach is not a technique, but the opportunity to change yourself through changing the ways you express yourself sexually. The orientation is one of sexual union as a meditation in which the intelligence is handed back to the genitals.

Tantric Sex for Men also complements the previously published *Tantric Orgasm for Women,* which many men say is actually a book for men. Nonetheless, to explore sex specifically from the male perspective is of immense value. Readers are also referred to *The Heart of Tantric Sex: A Unique Guide to Love and Sexual Fulfillment,* which offers the "Love Keys" and many specific details about lovemaking that do not necessarily appear in this book. Here our intention is to offer a completely new picture of sex, one that brings about a revolutionary and evolutionary shift in the way we *think* about sex, and therefore express ourselves in sex. Through a change of mindset we can intentionally allow the body to relax into its inner wisdom and express itself as nature intended.

Our body of knowledge is based on personal experience and has been confirmed by thousands of couples who have passed through our

Introduction

weeklong residential "Making Love" retreats over the past twenty years. During the retreats there is no nudity, no partner swapping, and each couple arrives committed to each other for the week. The atmosphere is respectful, supportive, and professional. We sometimes share with couples how fortunate we feel to have the best work in the world. Actually, it is pure pleasure and not work at all. We experience unlimited joy in seeing couples rise in love out of stagnation right in front of our eyes, in a handful of days. This is not only one couple, but twenty-five or more couples simultaneously. Everything proceeds easily, gently, naturally, and with virtually no effort on our part.

Although sex has been practiced in certain ways for thousands of years, we don't believe it has to continue in the same way forever. Over the years we have come to recognize that changing the way we make love changes and empowers our lives in loving, magical, mystical ways. However, this kind of transformation happens only through direct experience, and not by simply thinking that it sounds like a great idea. To gain access to insider knowledge, the experience has to be lived fully by the individual on a cellular level. Transforming our basic sex energy into its higher vibration of love, as described in the chapters ahead, raises the quality of love on personal, social, and cosmic levels of consciousness.

During our time working in the field of sexuality some couples who have attended our retreats have naturally separated and gone different ways. Our approach is not foolproof; rather, it depends on individual awareness, curiosity, and an interest in change. To our great astonishment, over the years we have witnessed a steady trickle of men returning to our retreats with a new lover. Actions are said to speak louder than words, and the return of so many men is their living endorsement of the immense value of changing the way one makes love. Once a man has been fortunate enough to have a taste of his male potency flowing into

Introduction

and through a woman, and being received by her, he naturally hopes to create similar experiences for himself in the future.

Sometimes women are more ready than men to change their sexual ways. If your woman is ready to embark on an adventure into the unknown, follow her lead and let her take you to new horizons. Give it a whirl; there is really nothing to lose. Quite possibly you will gain more love and insight than you can imagine.

Humans have progressed in countless amazing ways, yet sex, the dimension closest to home, remains unexplored territory. Perhaps now is the time to move beyond the familiar and take a step in human sexual evolution.

To those men and women who have already taken this step and have written to us about their profound personal experiences, we extend our deep gratitude to you for allowing us to use your words in encouraging others to explore their sexual potential.

Our spiritual master, Osho, formerly known as Bhagwan Shree Rajneesh, is the source of the tantric inspiration we now pass on to you. Osho's interpretation of the ancient Tantra scriptures addresses the search for harmony, wholeness, and love that is at the core of all religious and spiritual traditions, and that is also an integral aspect of the tantric relationship between two people. It is our privilege to include some excerpts of Osho's tantric inspiration throughout this book. His words, appearing in text form, were initially delivered as spontaneous oral discourses and later published in book form. The quotes included here are those that inspired us on our journey, and in no way represent the full range and extraordinary diversity of Osho's spiritual insight into the human condition.

We are both vitally aware that our lives have been shaped by Osho in ways that could not have been imagined at the outset, and for this honor we extend to him our eternal love and gratitude.

Osho Speaks on Sex

Osho's Spiritual Insight into the Human Condition

I have almost four hundred books in my name. Out of four hundred books there is only one book on sex, and that too is not really on sex; it is basically on how to transcend sex, how to bring the energy of sex to a sublimated state, because it is our basic energy. It can produce life. . . . It is only man who has the privilege to change the character and the quality of sexual energy. The name of the book is *From Sex to Superconsciousness*—but nobody talks about superconsciousness. The book is about superconsciousness; sex is only to be the beginning, where everybody is.

There are methods that can start the energy moving upwards, and in the East, for at least ten thousand years, there has developed a special science, Tantra. There is no parallel in the West of such a science. For ten thousand years people have experimented with how sexual energy can become your spirituality, how your sexuality can become your spirituality. It is proved beyond doubt—thousands of people have gone through the transformation. Tantra seems to be the science that is, sooner or later, going to be accepted in the whole world, because people are suffering from all kinds of perversions. That's why they go on talking about sex as if that is my work, as if twenty-four hours a day I am talking about sex. Their repressed sexuality is the problem. My whole effort has been how to make your sex a natural, accepted phenomenon, so there is no repression—and then you don't need any pornography; so that there is no repression—and then you don't dream of sex. Then the energy can be transformed.

There are valid methods available through which the same energy that brings life to the world can bring a new life to you. That was the whole theme of the book. But nobody bothered about the theme, nobody bothered about why I have spoken on it. Just the word sex was in the title, and that was enough.

The book is not for sex; it is the only book in the whole existence against sex, but strange. . . . The book says that there is a way to go beyond sex, you can transcend sex—that's the meaning of "from sex to superconsciousness." You are at the stage of sex while you should be at the stage of superconsciousness. And the route is simple: sex just has to be part of your religious life, it has to be something sacred. Sex has to be something not obscene, not pornographic, not condemned, not repressed but immensely respected, because we are born out of it. It is our very life source. And to condemn the life source is to condemn everything. Sex has to be raised higher and higher to its ultimate peak. And that ultimate peak is *samadhi*, superconsciousness.

OSHO, TRANSCRIBED TEACHINGS,
SEX MATTERS: FROM SEX TO SUPERCONSCIOUSNESS

Tantric Inspiration

And about sex also people are very, very worried. That very worry and that very effort to do something is the problem. Sex happens; it is not a thing that you have to do. So you have to learn the eastern attitude toward sex, the Tantra attitude. The Tantra attitude is that you be loving to a person. There is no need to plan, there is no need to rehearse in the mind. There is no need to do anything in particular: just be loving and available. Go on playing with each other's energy. And when you start making love there is no need to make it great. Otherwise you will be pretending and so will the other person. He will pretend that he is a great lover and you will pretend that you are a great lover . . . and both are unsatisfied. There is no need to pose anything. It is a very silent prayer. Making love is meditation. It is sacred, it is the holiest of holies. So while you are making love, go very slowly . . . with taste, taking in every flavor of it. And very slowly: there is no hurry, no need to hurry, enough time is there.

OSHO, TRANSCRIBED TEACHINGS,
THE OPEN SECRET

1
MALE BURDEN OF PERFORMANCE

Sex plays a central and crucial role in the life of a man from his early years onward, and remains significant regardless of whether a man is often having sex, seldom having sex, or not having sex at all. Since sex is pivotal to life, there are underlying aspects to the act that get hidden from sight, never brought into the light of day to be examined or questioned. Scratch the surface a little, however, and surprisingly soon men will start to express their feelings. Most men freely admit they would like to have sex more often, yet again and again they share with us in our seminars that as important as sex is, it is also experienced as a burden and a form of stress, which is sometimes subtle, other times not so subtle. The pressures implicit in sex can become a source of anxiety, which gives rise to a sense of insecurity and a lack of self-confidence.

When a man first gets together with a woman there is considerable pressure to be a good lover; perhaps he will even attempt to be the best lover this particular woman has ever had. There are many expectations, and the stakes are high. First, there has to be an erection, which is not guaranteed even in the most ideal situation, as we all know. Next, if and when the erection happens, it has to be maintained for as long as possible, which means that a certain level of stimulation and excitement is required. At the same time the man is praying that he doesn't ejaculate too quickly, at least not before the woman has her orgasm. And if everything works out just right, maybe it will even be possible to have an orgasm at the same time.

There are so many variables involved in the process that it is easy to get lost in the midst of monitoring and orchestrating the situation to best effect. At the beginning of a love affair a man's stress and performance anxiety are usually more obvious to him (but hopefully not to her), since he is more directly confronted by his wish to be successful. But after a while, as the relationship begins to unfold and assume a more day-to-day familiarity, his anxieties about performance temporarily bury themselves under a comfortable sexual routine. Even when a man is not consciously aware of his insecurity in sex, he nonetheless carries the emotional tension around with him each and every day of his life.

And in truth, the bottom line is that a woman can criticize a man about many things—being a lousy cook, a bad driver, unsuccessful at work, or even a miserable father. These criticisms are not easy to receive, but somehow they are manageable. But when a woman dares to criticize our sexual behavior, when she brings our performance into question, the words hit home and touch us at our most vulnerable place, rattling our male ego. To be not appreciated or valued as a lover can be very difficult for a man to digest.

RELAXING INSTEAD OF PERFORMING

Whether we are aware of it or not, much of our personality, identity, and self-perception is rooted in sex and in how we perceive ourselves as sexual beings. Sex also acts as a confirmation of our power and potency, thereby becoming connected—consciously or unconsciously—with pressure and performance in an attempt to prove our true value and worth.

Men who begin to experiment with a relaxed style of sex, as outlined in the chapters ahead, say it is an unbelievable relief to have the stress taken out of sex. All the big-time action that is unquestioningly accepted as part of sex simply falls away, because there is no longer a need for it. To relax in sex a man needs to be encouraged to abandon the idea that he, as the man, is 100 percent responsible for the quality of the shared sexual experience, whether it is very good, quite good, or unsatisfactory. In place of carrying the overall responsibility for the sexual interaction, which involves tremendous effort on his part, the man can discover how to simply *be* in sex—intensely present, in the here and now—and explore a more relaxing style of sex that does not include performance, effort, or tension.

Removing the Goal Removes the Pressure

In exploring a new style of sex, it is very helpful to shift our awareness from "doing" to "being." In order to alleviate performance pressure—the doing—the first step is to remove what we perceive as the goal. Generally the goal of sex is to have an orgasm. This goal of orgasm, which is the experience that usually makes people want to have sex in the first place, is what creates pressure. As we make love our deliberate intention and efforts are directed toward achieving that final end—a climax of heightened intense pleasure that lasts for a few short seconds.

There are significant disturbances that result from making orgasm the basic goal of sex. At the very outset, the focus on trying to get to the finish naturally causes us to get ahead of ourselves. This is true for men and women alike. If you pay attention you'll notice that your attention is more focused on the next penetration than the one happening right now in the present. Interest is generally in what lies ahead, what is coming next, and not what is occurring in the moment. The next penetration is more enticing because it brings us one step closer to the grand finale. We are unconsciously more focused on the future, so while the body remains engaged, there is little or no awareness of or in the present moment. We are following the mind with its specific ideas about how sex should go, and we are not tuning in and listening to the wisdom of the body.

Men often report wanting to have sex more frequently, but don't know how to make this happen. Many have lost confidence in reaching woman and have little clue as to how to get her more interested in sex. In our teaching we see how long-term issues like these begin dissolving in an extraordinarily short span of time—and only because of the non-goal-oriented, conscious style of sex we propose. During our retreats, we usually begin to see encouraging signs of response within individuals and between couples within two to five days. It is an honor to witness this miracle every time, like a shift from dark into light and from fear into love. All the barriers and problems that people arrived with begin to dissolve, and couples find a fresh sexual track leading to new dimensions, uncharted territory, and unlimited love. That it happens so easily is both astounding and reassuring.

Change Your Mind to Change Your Body
A shift of the kind experienced by our participants is possible *only* because the mind has reoriented to view sex and love from a diametrically opposite perspective. Without great effort you find you are indeed actually "making" love, and finally giving the expression its true meaning. When we stay present during lovemaking we naturally create love.

The solution appearing before us is quite simple—or so it seems! If we all change *our minds* about sex, we will possibly witness a dramatic reduction in the sex, love, and relationship problems to which people unhappily resign themselves.

HUMANS NEED MORE SEX

Sexual difficulties are experienced by both men and women, with the tragic outcome that human beings do not have enough sex. When sex finally happens the experience is short lived. Most partners do not have sex frequently enough for optimum mental, physical, and emotional health. Many do not make love for months and months on end, sometimes stretching into years. Sex satisfies our bodies, hearts, souls, intelligence, creativity, and most of all, our love—of self and of others. Sex is not the only way to access love, but if you are having or wanting sex, as most men are, then sex may as well be used to its highest potential.

When a U.K. satellite television channel recently conducted a survey on what people on their deathbeds regret most, seven out of ten British pensioners—both men and women—regretted not having "shagged around" (screwed around) more. As people were dying they were wishing they had had more sex in their lives. What an incredible revelation, that human beings are leaving this world sexually unfulfilled. Since it is becoming urgent and necessary for human beings to have more sex during their lifetimes, we need to develop a more evolved, sustainable style of sex that is manageable until our dying day. We need an approach that doesn't fizzle out when the newness is lost, disinterest or complacency sets in, or impotence or diminished hormones make sex more difficult.

EXPLORATION AND VULNERABILITY

To get more out of sex requires taking an adventurous step motivated by curiosity, intelligence, or both. The key is to make love frequently using the information and suggestions offered in the chapters ahead. If you follow where it leads and stay with what unfolds, you may soon notice a change in the quality of your life and a difference in how you feel about yourself as a man. You may even begin to perceive women differently.

As you begin to explore sex, old childhood wounds, memories, and insecurities may rise to the surface. It's better not to try to override or ignore any sexual difficulty or insecurity. Be open to yourself and allow your feelings to emerge, expressing any tears and vulnerability, not-knowing, insecurity, or confusion. Allowing yourself space to feel hidden aspects of your being is part of a healing and reintegrating process. Sexual exploration is a journey in self-discovery that not only leads to being a better lover with improved skills, but also can transform age-old restrictive patterns and generate more love and happiness. One thing is for certain—most women prefer a man's gentle, softer side to his hard, tougher side.

Rarely in the lifetime of the average human being are there altered states of orgasmic bliss, love, joy, and a peace that surpasses all understanding. The experience of being radiantly alive on a cellular level. Energized and aglow through merging with the body and its senses. Making love naturally presents us with an incredibly easy situation within which to "be present" and immerse ourselves in the body. Because of the absence of evolved sexual understanding, the human race suffers tremendous consequences. We are distorted by unconscious forces that affect our true nature, so that men are not truly men and women are not truly women. When we relate or connect through these distortions of our personalities and sexual identification, sooner or later the invariable result is tension and unhappiness.

SEXUAL CONDITIONING AND HOW IT SHAPES US

Each of us is unconsciously conditioned by society whether we like it or not, some more heavily than others. In conventional sexuality the majority of men tend to demonstrate the distorted versions of their true male qualities. Below you'll find a list of true male qualities in the first column, each of which is followed by a word or a few words describing the same quality after it has been distorted through false sexual conditioning. The 1960s-era saying, "Make love, not war," is actually a truth. A lack of sufficient fulfilling or nourishing sex often results in anger and aggression. Changing a man's understanding, and therefore his experience of sex, naturally calls forth his original, authentic male qualities.

TRUE MALE QUALITIES VERSUS CONDITIONED DISTORTIONS	
Power	Abuse, domination
Presence	Absence
Strength	Hardness
Clarity	Judgment
Assertiveness	Aggression
Creativity	Achievement, ambition
Meditation	Reclusiveness
Will	Stubbornness
Courage	Machismo, compensation
Leadership	Control, politics, law and order
Protector, authority	Authoritarian
Wildness	Brutality
Spontaneity	Performance
Wisdom	Arrogance
Charisma	Sexual manipulation
Sun, life giving	Sunburn, ecological destruction
Expression, articulation	Pomposity, boorishness
Action	Activity, bullishness
Independence	Isolation
Heartfelt, loving, compassionate	Selfish, egoistic

Tantric Inspiration

We live for sensations, we hanker for sensations. We go on seeking newer and newer sensations; our whole life is an effort to obtain new sensations. But what happens? The more you seek sensations, the less sensitive you become. Sensitivity is lost.

It looks paradoxical. In sensations, sensitivity is lost. Then you ask for more and more sensations and the "more" kills your sensitivity more. Then you ask for even more, and finally a moment comes when all your senses have become dull and dead. Man has never before been so dull and dead as he is today. He was always more alive before, because there were not so many possibilities to fulfill so many sensations. But now science, progress, civilization, education, have created so many opportunities to move further and further into the world of sensation. Ultimately, you turn into a dead person; your sensitivity is lost. Taste more foods—stronger tastes, stronger foods—and your taste will be lost. If you move around the world and go on seeing more and more beautiful things, you will become blind; the sensitivity of your eyes will be lost.

If you want the divine—the divine means the most alive, the ever-alive, ever-young, evergreen—if you want to meet the divine, you will have to be more alive. How to do it? Kill out all desire for sensation. Don't seek sensation, seek sensitivity, become more sensitive.

The two are different. If you ask for sensations you will ask for things; you will accumulate things. But if you ask for sensitivity, the whole work has to be done on your senses, not on things. You are not to accumulate things. You have to deepen your feelings, your heart, your eyes, your ears, your nose. Every sense should be deepened in such a way that it becomes capable of feeling the subtle.

OSHO, TRANSCRIBED TEACHINGS,
NEW ALCHEMY TO TURN YOU ON

2
INVOLUNTARY EJACULATION AND DESENSITIZATION

Perhaps the most common problem or issue faced by men is their lack of control over ejaculation, which results in an extremely high prevalence of premature ejaculation. And as we know, perhaps far too well, ejaculation usually marks the end of the sex act. As we come, we finish, at least for the present moment. Research has revealed that the universal average time of sexual engagement is between two and two-and-a-half minutes. Some men are able to extend the time to fifteen minutes, others to half an hour, or perhaps even forty-five minutes.

Enjoyable as these extra minutes definitely are, they are not really sufficient for a man to channel his vitality into a woman, and to have it received by her and returned to him. A man's ultimate fulfillment lies in being bathed in a woman's love, in overflowing radiant response to the love made in her. Man gives to woman who receives, and then woman gives to man who, in turn, receives. A reciprocal cycle of giving and receiving comes into play.

The truth is that if man wishes to make love for longer stretches of time and reap the true benefits of sex, then the level of excitement has to be drastically reduced and ejaculation consciously postponed.

EXCITEMENT CAUSES PREMATURE EJACULATION

Stimulation and excitement almost always end up in ejaculation. Yet at the same time it is a challenge to try to imagine sex without excitement. How would it look? What are you "doing" instead? Sex without excitement sounds like a contradiction in terms. Our impetus for wanting sex in the first place is precisely for sensation and intensity. After all, isn't that what sex is about?

Whether or not this is true for you, it is valuable to examine the role of excitement in conventional sex and perhaps come to the final conclusion that although excitement may be a great pleasure, too much of it can short-circuit the system. Facts are facts.

The basic problem doesn't lie with excitement per se, but rather with our sexual goals and the ways we manage the excitement. We begin sex with a strong intention, deliberately stimulate our bodies and genitals, and increase the level of intensity until there is a peak and overflow. These tactics basically produce too much heat, usually more than man can handle, so he boils over and discharges his life force, thereby unconsciously disempowering himself.

Sexual Fantasy Increases Excitement

Sexual fantasy is an accepted aspect of sex because it increases excitement. Fantasies in conventional sex are, in fact, a great help, but it is perhaps accurate to say that usually we are having sex with our minds, not with our bodies. We are unquestionably using our bodies, but we're not really understanding the way they are designed to function. Fantasy is a direct product of the mental powers of the imagination, and our bodies are forced to comply and satisfy the demands of our insatiable minds. As an example to show how sex and mind are connected, we remember a friend who told us that she had suffered an injury to her lower spine. This disturbance caused numbness and lack of sensitivity in the genitals over a period of several months. She couldn't feel a thing in her sexual organs. Nonetheless, she felt extreme desire for sex during this time. Finally she was forced to realize that the *source* of her sexuality lay in her mind, not in her body.

The mind is extremely powerful, but there are consequences to embracing fantasy as a sexual strategy. Fantasy is undeniably tied to excitement, which is tied to premature ejaculation; the three are linked together. Fantasy increases stimulation and excitement levels (as do all types of sexual aids), which in turn produce chronic premature ejaculation

Many people depend on fantasy and excitement for their sexual responses and in order to reach orgasm. The pornographic film industry is reportedly much larger than the mainstream film industry, and there are stripper bars in every major city in the world. Fantasy is an imagined situation; you are not with the person in the spirit of togetherness, sharing a mutual experience. You are mentally absent and not present, which results in the same consequence as focusing on the goal of orgasm; you are ahead of yourself or out of yourself. In both cases the mind, not the event itself, is the trigger. The mind wants orgasm and creates fantasy to satisfy its desire.

Staying Cool in Sex

If you want to avoid short-lived sex, it helps to heed an interesting folk aphorism: "A little is good, but more is not better." In the case of excitement this advice holds true; a little excitement is good, but more excitement is not better. Maybe more brings more pleasure and intensity, but if we wish to change, it's helpful to recognize the outcome of such behavior patterns.

In order to experience longer exchanges we need to cool down the sex act. A little excitement is fine, nothing is wrong in it, but then relax and take it easy. A retreat participant once shared his experience of having his thirty-year-old premature ejaculation problem vanish overnight, once he'd discovered the key of avoiding getting overexcited and remaining cool.

A style of sex that is cool and simple is more sustainable. It extends, expands, and increases the attraction between the bodies. The accepted cultural ideal is that sex should be as hot as possible, an approach that virtually guarantees premature ejaculation. Sooner or later excitement burns out, we take each other for granted, and boredom takes up residence. Boredom is natural; anything repeated again and again becomes a boring experience. Whenever the newness is lost, boredom takes its place. Excitement is triggered by the unknown, the newness of a situation, but the newness quickly wears off and the initial attraction burns up in the flames of excitement. Often couples report that after periods of heavy sex they experience a kind of physical repulsion and complete loss of interest in sex for a while.

SENSATION REDUCES SENSITIVITY

One significant by-product of excessive stimulation is that the penis becomes less and less sensitive. The more sensation to which the penis is subjected, the less sensitive it becomes. The same is true for the vagina. The repeated rubbing action of the penis within the vagina (or in the hand during masturbation) desensitizes both the penis and the vagina.

Repetitive in-and-out movements create friction between the tissues, which causes heat and a charge. After sex, a residue of tension remains in the body. This accumulates over time, and eventually the penis becomes subtly overcharged and tougher, and therefore less sensitive and less perceptive. Quite often the erect male penis feels unnaturally dense, hard, or even metallic to the touch. This rigidity reflects the tensions held in the tissue of the penis. Sensitivity is reduced, and a man loses the ability, capacity, and power to feel into the actual tissues of the penis. The penis itself loses inner vitality and consciousness, from its root all the way up to the radiant head. It forgets its slithering, supple, flexible nature that renders it capable of winding up and down inside the vagina exactly like a snake.

At the end of a retreat several years ago, a scientist who had participated told us that the loss of sensitivity in the face of intensity of stimulation had been scientifically proven in the second half of the nineteenth century by German physiologist Ernst Weber and physicist and psychologist Gustav Fechmer. Their research, formulated as the Weber-Fechmer law, is the theory of the relationship between stimulus and experience. Their research showed that the change in intensity of a sensation varies in increments proportional to the relative change of the stimulus. Today this is known to be true for every sensory channel within its range of dynamics. A simple example would be to light a match in the darkness. In this instance the light is like an explosion, but if you do the same in bright sunlight, it is barely perceptible. More sensation correlates to less sensitivity, and less sensation correlates to more sensitivity. Instead of endlessly seeking more and more sensation, we should begin to develop our senses so that we become capable of feeling the subtle yet vital life force moving through us at any moment of the day.

Mechanical Repetition and Loss of Sensitivity

To raise the intensity of sensation, we increase the tempo and frequency of our movements. We become mechanical, repeating the same thing again and again. Whenever there is an element of mechanical repetition in movement there is a corresponding lack of consciousness, and thereby loss of sensitivity, in each of the contributing individual movements. The steps that make up the journey are lost as we become climax machines, tense with the effort of getting where we want to go—orgasm!

Through being in a hurry we actually reduce the capacity to internally feel ourselves at a meaningful level. What is happening second by second in the body and genitals? Within the penis? Around the penis? Between the penis and vagina? If we are conscious in each moment, in each movement, the unfolding of sex can become a state of awe and wonder that lasts for hours. An experience of pure pleasure. A state of timelessness is entered wherein the moments emerge spontaneously from the body, unfolding naturally, one giving way to the next without fantasy or goals or mind being involved. The body is taken over by an innate force that intelligently guides it into loving expression. It is quite literally a mindless experience because we become utterly absorbed by our bodies in their state of heightened sesitivity. The more conscious and present a person is during sex, the greater his or her sensitivity will be.

Woman's Excitement Can Trigger Male Ejaculation
Most men have experienced coming very easily when the woman gets overexcited or too hot, especially as she strives to come to a climax. Ejaculation happens in a helpless enjoyable flash, and there is nothing to be done to avoid it. Many men confirm this experience, saying it is as if an ejaculation is virtually pulled from them, completely out of the blue. They are taken by surprise because they were nowhere near ready to ejaculate. Although the situation appears uncontrollable there is something that can be done, and that is to avoid making the woman too excited. If you'd like to make love last longer, maintain the sexual temperature at cool to gently simmering.

WOMEN'S SEXUAL RELUCTANCE

Let's face reality: men usually desire sex more often than their partners do. Ever wondered why? The truth is that for a woman the few minutes of sexual interaction are not really satisfying. There is hardly sufficient time for her body to warm up and celebrate the occasion. This sadly implies that women repeatedly return from sexual encounters feeling unfulfilled and at a loss—with the sense that the pleasures of sex are not worth the efforts of sex. Feelings such as these can get firmly embedded and cause many women to begin to avoid sex. Research reveals that 82 percent of women would rather kiss and cuddle than have sex; they find the exchange more nourishing. The choice to cuddle instead of having sex is a reflection of women's lack of true enjoyment when the penis is within the vagina.

Men can rest assured that the reluctant sexual response of a woman is not a mental or conscious response wherein she suddenly decides she does not want sex. (There are contraception issues that sometimes stand in the way of a woman's assent, mentioned in chapter 7.) The closing down of a woman's body is usually a slow, gradual process, unless she has suffered some trauma, in which case the closing down can be immediate. The withdrawal is physical yet very subtle, and something over which a woman does not have much conscious control. Many a woman feels she is alone in her unexpected and uninvited turnoff to sex, but it is a common and universal theme. Repeated lack of fulfillment plays a great part in why women experience loss of interest in sex. Women are definitely not frigid by nature, but their bodies start to freeze over when the sex is always hot, hard, and quick.

What's a man to do? Why precisely are women not enjoying sex? Why does your woman not want sex as much as you do? A recent *Redbook* survey shows that 52 percent of women regularly fake orgasms. According to a Durex Global Sex Survey, only 17 percent of women are likely to have an orgasm during sex. Forty-three percent of women report "some kind of sexual problem," such as the inability to achieve orgasm, boredom with sex, or total lack of interest in sex.

Basically women are not getting what they need sexually from men. At the root of the problems lies the male lack of understanding of the female body and man's loss of control over ejaculation. These facts are basic to female sexual withdrawal and difficulties in reaching orgasm. She doesn't enjoy sex because it doesn't feel good. How much sex would you want if you never even had an orgasm? If you want more sex from your woman, discover how to express yourself physically in a way that opens her, expands her body energy, and makes her ask for more. Once you figure that out, you won't have to ask. Trust us—she'll be asking you to make love to her. If you don't believe it, just try it.

There is an urgent need to discover how to extend the length of time of lovemaking, literally penis in vagina, for deeper sexual satisfaction of both the man and the woman. Their sexual experiences are inextricably intertwined, not separated into something one likes and the other does not. If a woman is not fully open to her partner, his sexual experience becomes one-dimensional, repetitive, and finally, boring. Then the need arises to introduce increasingly exciting and stimulating situations, porn movies, sex toys, party games, and the like to keep things rolling.

When woman is made love to consciously and at length, the man's experience is transformed; it becomes otherworldly, a multidimensional happening. When a man spends more clock time with his penis inside the woman he automatically thinks less about sex, because he is having it. Prolonged sexual experience in relaxation brings him a confidence and trust in himself, which in turn reduces presexual tension and excitement, and thereby postpones ejaculation.

Ejaculation can be postponed indefinitely once you discover the way to do so. Given that human beings do not make enough love, extending lovemaking by delaying, postponing, or even abandoning ejaculation sounds like the perfect remedy for bringing the situation into balance. There are always two opposing directions in which we can move with our sexual energy as human beings: emotional or mature, superficial or empowering, stimulating or relaxing, biological or spiritual, discharging or containing, reproductive or generative, unconscious or conscious.

PERSONAL SHARING
Enjoying Both Thrills and Silence

In the past six months of making love in silence without many outer movements, but with many more inner movements, it has become something that I had been seeking. It is the kind of making love that allows space for conscious encounters, deep love, unlimited variety, bubbling aliveness, powerful masculinity, and deep fulfillment. It is a wonderful path that leads me to who I truly am. At other times there is hot lovemaking with arousal. I experience excitement as something that pulls me in again and again. Sometimes it attracts me because I simply cannot let go of it, or it comes as a wave that overloads and overwhelms me. The experience is totally different from the silent lovemaking.

You taught us that, "Afterwards is your teacher." After the silent lovemaking I felt fulfilled and alive inside. After the love with excitement, in other words, after an orgasm, I felt tired and needed a break. In my personal experience there is another important difference. With the exciting love, I adhere to my partner energetically. In the silent love there is a space in which love can unfold between us. In regard to quality and sustainability, silent love is clearly leading for me, yet I'm not ready to say goodbye forever to lovemaking with excitement. I would be denying some parts in me that still long for that thrill, and I don't want to do that. I think further practice with tantra will lead the way. I allow myself to continue to be surprised as to where this path is taking me.

Tantric Inspiration

Ordinarily the energy is going outward and downward. You have to bring it backward, inward—and "inward" is synonymous with "upward." Once it starts coming back to you, and you become a circle of energy, you will be surprised: a new dimension has opened up; you start moving upward. Your life is no longer horizontal. It has taken a new route, the vertical.

OSHO, TRANSCRIBED TEACHINGS,
SECRET OF SECRETS

3
EJACULATION IS NOT MALE ORGASM

The general assumption is that male ejaculation is a man's version of an orgasm. However, some men have discovered that ejaculation is definitely not a true orgasm. They have experienced that nature designed the genitals for elevated, or evolved, sexual experiences. They agree that ejaculation is an intense pleasure, but these few seconds cannot compare with the timeless, blissful, relaxing experience of orgasmic fusion. You find your body empowered, rejuvenated, and your spirits lifted.

Physiologically it is possible for man to have an orgasm without ejaculating. However, a man can also ejaculate sometimes without experiencing any pleasurable sensations whatsoever. Orgasm and ejaculation can occur simultaneously, or they can be experienced independent of one another. For a man this means he is capable of a prolonged "valley" orgasm, or even multiple orgasms, without ejaculation.

LOSS OF ENERGY AFTER EJACULATION

It is well known that men usually, or perhaps always, experience loss of energy after ejaculation. Signs of energy loss occur as a negative type of relaxation that is the result of the unburdening of accumulated tensions from the system. Stimulation and movement are used to build up tension levels; the breath gets shorter and faster until the energy peaks into a climax. Accumulated tension is discharged downward and outward along with life-giving semen (in contrast to the energizing effects of orgasm without ejaculation, which keeps the energy in the body and sends it vertically up the spine).

There are a number of ways in which the loss of energy after ejaculation manifests: a sense of separation, emptiness, loss of interest in the partner, irritability, tiredness, wanting to switch off, or falling asleep. There has been a depletion of energy, inducing a negative type of relaxation. The by-product of true relaxation is increased vitality and aliveness.

A young man of twenty-five years attended our weeklong seminar for couples, during which he immediately started to avoid ejaculation and contain his energy. After several days of making love two or three times a day without ejaculation, he observed a distinctly different quality arising from his body and his being, as though he had entered a love paradise. He felt as high as a kite.

Then, on the second to last afternoon he decided to have an ejaculation just to check it out and see how it would feel. He told us that from one second to the next he felt himself falling from heaven into hell. There was an instant evaporation of the positive, uplifting, inspiring inner force he had felt building up within himself during the previous days.

Since that shattering experience he has been able to observe and identify certain emotional and physical states that accompany or follow his ejaculation. Here is the list he made:

An intense idleness spreads inside of me.

Contact with people becomes difficult for me. I do not feel like seeing people.

The front of my torso is extremely tense for the next two days.

My lower back is contracted.

My neck is tense.

My body is generally tense. There is no space in me, no mobility.

I am irritable.

I behave like a child that did not get enough sleep, even if I've slept a lot.

Even little things are often too much. If I have to do something, it often feels like an insurmountable obstacle.

My thoughts are racing

I doubt my profession, my relationship, my living space, and my life. Nothing seems as good as it is.

I lack serenity. I feel no joy. I am afraid that everything will get to be too much.

My eyes are blurred and my head feels foggy.

I do not want to look at my beloved any more, and I am hardly able to look at her. If I do it anyway, I do not see her clearly.

I feel restless.

In brief, nothing is fun.

I need two to three days (at least) in order to recover, unless I start watching movies endlessly and avoid contact with anyone.

The rest of this man's interesting observations appear at the end of chapter 9.

The Power of Containment

The containment of sexual energy is not a new idea by any means. Containment was advocated and practiced by ancient Taoists and Tantrikas thousands of years ago and was considered pivotal to enjoying a long, healthy, creative, happy life.

Today, the majority of men (and women) never question ejaculation. With the equation ejaculation equals orgasm never being challenged, ejaculation becomes the goal of sex. It's why we do it. Besides, we think sex without a buildup and climax can hardly amount to real sex, and so ejaculation is given a central place without consideration of the many possible negative effects. Enormous amounts of spiritual and physical energy are required to rebalance and revitalize the system—energy that would otherwise be put to better use in essential body maintenance, especially as a man gets older.

One tablespoon of semen is unbelievably potent. The fluid contains an immense amount of proteins, vitamins, minerals, and amino acids, as well as vital energies. Semen is like liquid gold. With each ejaculation a man releases around forty million sperm cells, which have the potential to reproduce that many human beings. What incredible power!

Man unwittingly and habitually depletes his essence each time he has sex because of the prevailing idea that sex is for the pleasure of ejaculation.

The Spiritual Aspect of Sex Energy Rises

The creation of a human being is a miracle, yet the reproductive potential of sex is its more superficial expression. The higher, spiritual aspect of sex lies beyond the biological aspect, and this is where man differs fundamentally from his animal friends. Animal reproduction is relatively infrequent, generally limited to brief seasons, and occurs when the male of a species is attracted to specific odors emanating from the female. Sexual behavior is rarely displayed in the phases between seasons.

However, human beings are able to make love all day, every day if it is their individual wish, so there must be more to sex than straightforward procreation. Man is able, through his consciousness, to raise his sexual expression to a higher level—one that is an evolutionary step. The containment of the life force through relaxation gives rise to stillness and a higher form of self-experience. Sexual experiences become uplifting, deeply moving, and nourishing. Further, the capacity to be relaxed in sex and avoid tension-filled climax-oriented sex gives rise to a quality of male authority and presence that is lacking today in the majority of men. (This aspect will be covered in chapter 8.)

A man's experience of the spiritual aspects of sex is limited because there is confusion about sex. Nature has an inherent commitment to reproduction (among all plant and animal species) and is not at all interested in states of ecstasy or fulfillment of orgasmic potential. Ejaculation, which serves nature perfectly well, also leads to a crash landing well before humans take off and start flying. The usual brevity of the sex act means that the majority of men are not experiencing the vagina as the true home and resting place of both man and penis. In a man's lifetime inestimable amounts of time and energy are locked up into sexual fantasy and longing, but the actual amount of time a man spends with his penis inside a vagina is minimal.

A style of superficial reproductive sex is basically not satisfying in the long term. Again and again the longing to repeat the same experience arises and can become a vicious cycle of desire and discharge. With repetition boredom easily sets in, so a man will change partners in order to keep his sex life alive.

When the ejaculation experience is truly fulfilling there is a sense of deep satisfaction and completion. Instead, most men, as already mentioned, feel depleted and devoid of creativity. Because the peak climax is not profound or deeply touching, the desire for sex continues almost as a compulsion or an obsession, and a man can find himself fully controlled by his sexual urges.

With the habit of building up and discharging energy the more subtle, delicate layer of sexual experience is bypassed. The life force is not given the opportunity to circulate within the body. Ejaculation interrupts the circle, and the higher potential of sex is lost. When a man learns to experience his higher orgasmic nature and finds deeper fulfillment through sex, there usually will be a corresponding decrease in his sexual obsession.

CONTAINING THE LIFE FORCE

For a man to shift gears and reach a higher octave in sex, he needs to prolong the sex act by cooling down and either avoiding ejaculation or postponing it until a moment of his choosing. The bodies of a man and a woman need to make love for an extended period of time for states of sexual ecstasy to arise. The human body is designed by nature to experience higher states, but this requires time, sensitivity, and awareness.

If a man understands that premature ejaculation happens through overexcitement, he can make ejaculation a conscious choice, rather than an accident or a habit, as mentioned in the previous chapter. Tantra masters also inform us that ejaculation is always preceded by the thought of ejaculation, that the origin of ejaculation is actually in the mind. Without the thought of ejaculation there is rarely an ejaculation (except when a woman gets overexcited and pulls an ejaculation from a man, as already mentioned).

Avoid the Tension of Ejaculation Control

Absence of ejaculation (nonejaculation) is not the same as ejaculation control. There is a significant difference between not ejaculating as a result of relaxation and controlling the ejaculation.

Osho says, "In sex, you are relaxing in it, not controlling it. If you are controlling it, there will be no relaxation. If you are controlling it, sooner or later you will be hurried to finish it because control is a strain. And every strain creates tension, and tension creates a necessity, a need, to release. It is not control; you are not resisting something. You are simply not in a hurry because sex is not happening in order to move somewhere. You are not going somewhere. It is just a play; there is no goal. Nothing is to be reached, so why hurry?"

This is different from sexual practices that suggest a man "dance on the verge" of ejaculation for a period of time without actually ever getting to the point of ejaculation. In other words, the man intentionally builds up the excitement and tension level, and then shortly before he feels he is about to reach the "point of no return," he relaxes his efforts, which represses the ejaculation. After a while the energy level is built up again, and then repressed again, and this process is continued with the effect that ejaculation is controlled for a prolonged period. (There are also specific techniques to repress ejaculation; for example, a man pushes finger pressure into his perineum/prostate area.) As the term *controlling ejaculation* indicates, by using such repressive techniques, the shift is from ejaculation to avoiding ejaculation—which means that the goal orientation remains the same.

Physical Pain after Hot Sex

Controlling ejaculation through repression as described above can have a short-term energizing effect on a man. However, the deliberate building up and pushing down of excitement will deposit tension in the prostate gland and genitals, which can later cause congestion. Because all repression is basically a type of tension, the practice of ejaculation control is not particularly healthy in the long term. When a man deliberately plays with excitement and controls his ejaculation, he should not be surprised if he experiences pain in the testicles or groin area afterward. The pain is usually a reflection of the tension produced through the buildup and repression of energy.

If, and when, a man does reach a point where he needs to ejaculate, it's suggested that he simply allow it to happen right then and there. Better not to interfere with the direction of the flow. Tell your woman out loud in words that you are coming, look into her eyes, remain present to the situation, and enjoy!

If you wish to postpone or avoid ejaculation, it's advisable to steer clear of too much stimulation and excitement right from the start of the lovemaking. Instead, become more slow and sensitive through relaxation and awareness. A cool approach can empower you to make love for hours.

Pain that Follows Relaxed Sex

After relaxed sex, surprisingly enough, there can also be pain in the penis, the testicles, the groin area, or the lower abdomen. When the sexual atmosphere has been one of relaxation, the pains are informing us that previously held accumulated tensions are leaving the tissues. These can be called "healing pains." If this should happen to you, accept the pain and do not be unduly concerned; the pain will pass in time. Movements such as gently shaking the body, including the pelvis, for ten minutes or more will help to disperse the emerging tensions. Often allowing simple tears of vulnerability will dissolve the pain. It is also recommended that masturbation not be used as a way to relieve the tension or pain. The body is healing and regenerating itself through the sexual relaxation. As layers of emotion and physical tensions rise to the surface and dissolve, body sensitivity and capacity for pleasure return.

Safety Concerns Regarding Nonejaculation

We have heard from a few men that they have been advised by their medical doctors to ejaculate regularly in order to "flush out the pipes," like a bit of do-it-yourself plumbing.

Personal experience has proved that it is possible to make love frequently for years on end without the need for ejaculation. It is not as though a man swells up into a balloon that eventually pops because of his unreleased semen! There is absolutely no physical danger for a man to go without ejaculation indefinitely. Sometimes there may be spontaneous emissions during the night, but these tend to happen more and more rarely as time passes. They occur frequently during puberty and adolescence, and the reason is thought to be sexual fantasies. These emissions have nothing to do with not having had an ejaculation for a long time or the body getting rid of old sperm.

Reserve Ejaculation for Conception

A man can, if he so wishes, reserve his ejaculation for procreation alone. There is no hard-and-fast rule, but a man should know that when he and his partner want to conceive, he can consciously decide to ejaculate at the time the woman is ovulating. (The time of ovulation can be determined through a number of different methods, such as changes in body temperature and vaginal mucus.) Conscious ejaculation will make conception an equally conscious event, rather than the hit-or-miss accident it often is. When a man ejaculates he can plant his seed along with an intention or vision for a conscious conception.

Women's Identification with Male Ejaculation

Men need to be aware that women often identify with their man's orgasm/ejaculation. In these few moments a woman feels that the man gives himself to her, and for woman this is somehow affirming. The irony is that she actually triggers the man into postejaculation syndromes, unwittingly disempowering him (and thereby herself) as the flow of intimacy and love gets interrupted or evaporates. Sometimes these breaks in the connection seem so normal that we would not immediately associate them with sex. We think this is who we are and how we are. However, a man who practices containment of energy will begin to experience himself as a completely different person in his daily life. Men report feelings of pleasure that rise to the heart with a lightness and glowing warmth that radiates throughout the entire body and being.

A man is equally identified with the woman's orgasm, because it confirms that he is a good lover, which supports the male ego. (However, many woman fake orgasm, so it is not necessarily reliable feedback.) The big disadvantage of making a woman come, as mentioned earlier, is that more often than not the man will ejaculate a few seconds too early due to the heightened level of excitement and tension, and so disempower himself.

BENEFITS OF COOLING DOWN

Many of the personality difficulties or relationship problems between partners disappear when there is a shift in the style of sex. An ambience of love surrounds the lovers, and radiant love shines from their eyes. Men's faces change completely when they are making love regularly in a relaxed, non-orgasm-focused way. The transformation is remarkable, certainly more effective than any facelift. Craggy, angular, mildly discontented grooves and folds transform into a widening and fullness of the face, as an infusion of *chi* or *prana,* the life force, enters into the facial tissues, energizing and rejuvenating the skin and leaving it rosy and radiant. The body is grounded as legs penetrate the earth; the heart is open, the eyes are shining.

Redirecting the Energy

In conventional sex the energy or vitality is normally forced downward and outward. To reach orgasmic states the energy has to be allowed to rise. It needs to be encouraged inward and upward, and this happens through relaxation in sex. An inner channel opens, and energy begins rising and expanding through the core, returning to its source in the brain. The ultimate source of the sexual energy lies in the brain. Roughly at the level of third eye lie the pineal and pituitary glands, known as the "master glands" of the endocrine (hormonal) system. Crucial substances and information are released and these filter downward through the system to eventually prepare us for sex. This cycle represents the reproductive, biological phase of sex mentioned earlier. When vitality is recirculated upward through inner channels and returns to its source in the brain it represents the spiritual or generative phase of sex. The inner design enables a man to reabsorb his vital energies and be empowered by them. Through relaxation a man can reach a vibrant and peaceful state, followed by the experience of feeling energized and rejuvenated.

It is an experience beyond and higher than the conventional reproductive expression, which is more "superficial." By allowing the life force to turn inward and upward, the man uses his intention to create the foundation for evolved experiences. He shifts from running mechanically after ejaculation to being conscious and present each moment, attentive to the subtle sensations unfolding within his body and being.

The Inner Rod of Magnetism

Perhaps you are wondering how these altered states transpire. What's going on? Both the male and female orgasmic experience can be explained most simply by comparing the human body to a magnet. Like a magnet, the body has two opposite poles—one in the heart and one in the genitals. Usually one pole is given a plus, or positive value, and the other a minus, or negative value. Whatever symbol or words you choose to use, the body's two equal and opposite poles create a difference in potential. This can give rise to an electromagnetic streaming in the core of the body and an amplification of the energy field surrounding the body. Tantra calls the experience of streaming in the core the awakening of the "inner rod of magnetism." And this is the true source of the human being's orgasmic experience. Through this miraculous inner design humans are able to experience ecstasy, alone or together.

Recent studies of chromosomes confirm the "magnetic" design of human beings. Science has proven that man is part woman, and woman is part man. Each human contains both parts, male and female. Both opposing poles are contained within each individual. We each have a male and a female pole, a heart pole and a genital pole. Each individual is, at a higher level and by design, an independent unit unto himself. Each person has the innate capacity to circulate energy and vitality within his or her self, which is ultimately the experience of "inner sex" and the most evolved form of human sexual expression.

PERSONAL SHARING
My First Full-Body Orgasm

I'm in India and it is 1993. I have been here more than a month, meditating every day, and suddenly I fall in love. It happens instantly, just by looking at her. We meet the first day of a meditative therapy that lasts three weeks, and after a couple of weeks of courting and wooing we meet at her home to make love. After long foreplay we get into the real act. Since I arrived in India I have not had any sexual contact with a woman, so even though I'm in ecstasy about making love with the woman I most desire in the whole world, I also have the classic male fear—some call it performance anxiety—that makes me think, "I hope I don't come immediately."

For me the first love encounter with a woman has always been like a testing ground: If the feeling is real, everything goes well and the experience is satisfactory for both partners; if it is not a real energetic feeling but the mind comes between us, then the experience is not satisfactory. On this night all best conditions are met—there is heart, our bodies like each other, and very importantly, we are both meditating regularly. I have always been a sensitive man, but tonight is pure magic. I can feel what she feels and I know exactly where, and how, and when to touch her. I really feel like I am one with her. The embrace really lasts a long time and every anxious thought is completely gone and I am totally relaxed.

The moment comes when she reaches orgasm and I, too, am captured by the escalation of pleasure that usually leads to a short, intense little squirt that we usually call "male orgasm." But this time it's different. In the beginning everything goes as usual, with the energy concentrating in my penis, ready to be scattered outside. This time, however, instead of going out, the energy goes up my entire body, shaking me in powerful waves. It could be described as a tremor, because the body can't be still, and there is heat, a kind of inner tingling, waves of pleasure everywhere, and maybe women can relate to this . . . these waves are not focused on the penis but wash through my whole body, all the way to my crown. Initially the interval between these long pleasure waves is a few seconds, and then they become less frequent, with longer intervals.

I feel the energy rushing through my body, flowing from me to her, *going through her body and coming back to mine through the contact between penis and vagina. I realize that if we keep a light contact with our tongues the waves pass more easily from my body to hers, creating a virtual circle that lasts long and eventually fades slowly, slowly . . . and it is beautiful to lie together, hugging, to watch the shaking of our bodies, the energy waves going up and down the spine, exchanging that state of ecstasy, indefinitely recharging each other. And when the waves calm and my ocean becomes still again I have the usual post-orgasm symptoms: my penis becomes soft again and my limbs are relaxed.*

Since that first time it has happened many times, but not always. This kind of orgasm, the valley orgasm, just happens of its own accord; I can't make it happen, I can only relax and allow it to happen. The biggest difference from a traditional orgasm is that after making love it takes less time for me to be ready again, because I've gained energy rather than wasting it, and the feeling of desire is untouched. After a night of these orgasms I need less sleep than usual, only a couple of hours, to be okay and get up perfectly refreshed. If I don't ejaculate I can go on making love for hours and hours. Of course I don't mean the boring "in and out" that we usually mean by making love. I mean following the energy, allowing the energy to guide me to move, to slow down, to stop . . . I wait, feeling what happens in my and her body, feeling the exchange of energy that goes through my penis.

The most important thing for me is to be relaxed. When I feel pleasure rising intensely, I have to remember to relax, rather than becoming tense as I normally would. It is particularly important to keep the muscles of the anus relaxed and soft, not tight and contracted. This expansion allows energy to go free, rather than being obstructed there: if the energy can't find the space to go up, it will be forced to go down into an ejaculation.

The other important thing is meditation. I've noticed that this type of orgasm is more likely to happen when I'm meditating regularly.

I don't think that technical knowledge about tantra is particularly important. That first time, in 1993, I was so completely ignorant about tantra that I was surprised and puzzled about what was happening to me, and thought I might be ill. I had to wait for years, till I met you both in 2000, to learn more about the circulation of energy in and between male and female bodies.

Tantric Inspiration

Tantra says do not try to escape; there is no escape possible. Rather, use nature itself to transcend. Don't fight—accept nature in order to transcend it. If this communion with your beloved or your lover is prolonged with no end in mind, then you can just remain in the beginning. Excitement is energy. You can lose it; you can come to a peak. Then the energy is lost and a depression will follow, a weakness will follow. You take it as relaxation, but it is negative.

Tantra gives you a dimension of higher relaxation, which is positive. Both partners melting with each other give vital energy to each other. They become a circle, and their energy begins to move in a circle. They are giving life to each other, renewing life. No energy is lost. Rather, more energy is gained because through the contact with the opposite sex your every cell is challenged, excited.

And if you can merge into that excitement without leading it to a peak, if you can remain in the beginning without becoming hot, just remaining warm, then those two warmths will meet and you can prolong the act for a very long time. With no ejaculation, with no throwing energy out, it becomes a meditation, and through it you become whole. Through it your split personality is no more split: it is bridged.

OSHO, TRANSCRIBED TEACHINGS,
VIGYAN BHAIRAV TANTRA

4
THE EQUAL AND OPPOSITE FORCE OF THE FEMALE ENVIRONMENT

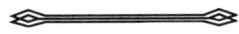

MEN AND WOMEN ARE NOT THE SAME

Much of the confusion and misunderstanding that occurs between men and women results from ignorance regarding our true differences. These deep-seated differences shape our respective roles during sexual communion. With insight into these differences we can begin to work together to reveal and unleash our sexual potential.

For deeper insight into our human potential we refer to information contained in the Tantras (the tantric scriptures), sacred knowledge from the ancients. These ancient sources contain compelling information that rightfully should be passed down from one generation to the next.

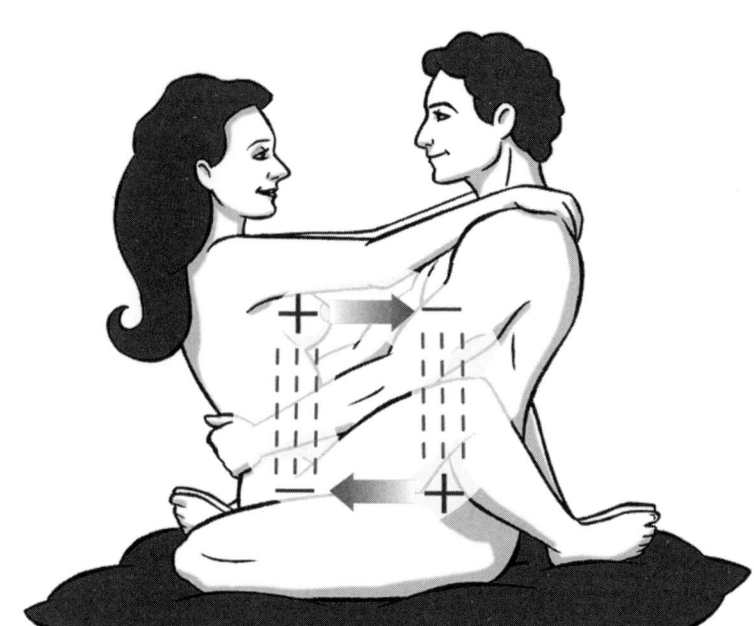

Fig. 4.1. Inner magnets of man and woman, showing poles, magnetic rods, and potential circular energy flow (in yab-yum position).

Male and Female Aspects within the Individual

The previous chapter explained the way in which each human being can be likened to a magnet, with a male and a female pole energetically linked by a rod of magnetism that, when awakened, gives rise to an inner electromagnetic streaming. This subtle internal by-product of the inner male and female forces at play within us represents our innate bisexual reality, and represents the very foundation of tantra and the biological basis of the orgasmic experience.

Of particular significance is that these two forces are equal. One is not more, one is not less; they are balanced, even. However, these poles simultaneously exist as opposite forces in relation to each other. The poles are equal forces, but opposite forces, not identical forces. Male represents an outgoing—"positive" or dynamic—force. Female represents a receptive—"negative" or passive—force.

The qualities of receptive and dynamic are diametrically opposite, and at the same time, they are equal and opposite and complement each other. They balance, correspond, and enhance each other, and one cannot exist without the other. Just as electricity requires two poles, positive and negative, no being or body can be without two poles, masculine and feminine, the universal forces of yin and yang.

Dynamic and Receptive Poles

In the male body the male, positive pole is represented in the genitals, the female, receptive pole in the chest/heart. The reverse is true for woman; the male, positive pole is in the breasts/nipples/heart, the female, receptive pole is in the genitals. When man and woman are in an upright, standing position, man can be visualized as a magnet standing on its head, with the positive (north) pole below and the negative (south) pole above. The woman is like a magnet standing upright: the positive (north) pole is above and the negative (south) pole is below.

Magnets Meet at Opposite Ends

When a man and a woman come together in an embrace, for instance, their bodies actually meet with energetically opposite ends aligned. The positives and negatives of each individual approach and meet simultaneously at the genital and heart levels. The inner rods of magnetism (as mentioned in the previous chapter as the source of the orgasmic state) flow in opposite directions to each other. When two magnets meet at opposite ends, there is an attractive force that pulls them together. And the same "magnetic" attraction can also be felt between male and female bodies. There is a perceptible drawing and pulling sensation as the equal and opposite forces influence each other. In addition, there is tremendous amplification of the magnetic or energy fields surrounding the two magnets/bodies.

The Dynamic Male Force

A man's body contains two poles, but the male dynamic aspect is the outer aspect, while the female (receptive) is his inner aspect. In a woman's body the reverse is true. The female receptive aspect is outer, and the male (dynamic) aspect is her inner aspect. One aspect is externalized, but both aspects are always present. Generally speaking, this implies that physically and energetically the man, predominantly male, is a dynamic force, while the woman, predominantly female, is a receptive force. Man does not have to take any direct action to connect with his feminine side, or his so-called inner woman. The more truly male man becomes through a relaxed, non-doing presence in sex, the more his opposite feminine quality of love will naturally and gradually open up. There will be a balancing within him. Similarly, a woman will access her "inner man" by relaxing increasingly into her feminine nature. The harmonizing inner opposite emerges and flowers as an alchemical process, as an outcome or a by-product.

Figure 4.1 shows the inner magnets of a man and woman with poles, magnetic rod, and potential circular energy flow while sitting in yab-yum position.

Genitals—Equal and Opposite Forces

The qualities of these forces, the intrinsically different polarities of man and woman, extend down to the level of the genital tissues. The shape of the male penis informs us that it is an instrument from which energy can flow or emanate. Likewise, the vagina is shaped as a canal or receptor with an innate capacity to receive, absorb, or draw out the opposite force.

The Equal and Opposite Force of the Female Environment

Energetically and physically our equal and opposite forces are complementary; they fit together to form a single unit. There is a completion in the joining of the penis and vagina, when a man's dynamic pole meets and penetrates a woman's receptive pole. When separate and apart, it can be said that the genitals exist as two incomplete halves. Tantra masters believe that everything that is incomplete is longing for completion and suggest that the search for sex, the longing for sex, represents a deep yearning for union, completion, and peace.

Through the understanding of polarity—the equal, opposite, and complementary forces—it becomes more apparent that man is not necessarily an independent unit unto himself. In order to invite the truly masculine qualities embodied in his penis, a man is dependent on the environment around him, namely, the vagina. The quality of receptivity determines or influences the dynamic qualities. A dynamic force can only be dynamic (experience its very self) through being received. In fact, the more receptive, the more dynamic; the two happenings are inextricably linked. Giving makes receiving possible, and receiving makes giving possible, which is why it is so important for a man to take into account his equal and opposite force and become aware of the vital role of receptivity.

The Significance of the Female Environment

To manifest the vitality of the penis and discover how best to call forth its dynamic male qualities (and essential function), the woman needs to be centrally placed in the sexual constellation. Man physically enters woman with his penis, so the environment surrounding the penis is to be given value and not underestimated. The polarity differences between men and women are best embraced and enhanced, not sidestepped, in order to make the most of the sexual situation. Acknowledging the woman's receptive nature allows the man to experience himself as a truly masculine force. He feels a deep sexual fulfillment when he experiences male energy flowing through him and being received by the woman.

Man is inextricably dependant on woman for his higher experiences, and her environment needs some preparation to be able to warmly receive the guest. Man basically can be ready for sex at any given moment if he so wishes, which is probably the by-product of being a positive, dynamic force. Woman's lack of instant readiness is a by-product of her nature as a receptive, passive force. Any reluctance or unwillingness in sex is not a mental hang-up or frigidity, but rather a reflection of the intelligence of the body.

Woman's Body Needs Clock Time to Open

Usually man prefers to penetrate woman as soon as possible. Getting inside her becomes his primary focus, often from fear of losing his initial erection response. When a man has to hang around on the fringes waiting for the woman, he easily loses his erection and may have to wait some time for another. In reality, a leisurely, extended time frame, even an hour or three, will normally suit woman very nicely. She is able to tune into her body and relax into herself. If the man takes the time to "be" with the woman, perhaps to lovingly and softly (as a feather) caress her body into an energetically expanded state *before* entering her, he will be amazed by what an awesome experience it is. To consciously enter and be received by an inviting and absorbing channel changes the entire experience, which in turn transforms man.

When woman is entered too early, without feeling truly ready to receive, without the feeling of a total yearning "yes," her body may begin gradually to close down, interest in sex may dwindle, and reluctance to have sex may increase. During the initial phases of lovers' meeting, the woman's heart is wide open, so receiving man totally and at any time is not an issue. But sooner or later a woman will require acknowledgment of her differences if she is to continue enjoying sex well into her later years. The same is true for man. On an encouraging note, once a man of eighty years attended a couple's workshop with his wife of seventy-six; four years later they continue to have genital union as a daily practice. Their motivation in attending was to have one more adventure in life, and they both report a vastly improved quality of life; each day is a joy and filled with love.

When man enters a woman before her body is "open," it is similar to butting his head against a closed door. You can get only so far, but no further. However, when you have the keys to the door, you will find it opens easily and often. When man accepts the fact that woman is basically slower than he and her system requires preparation, then his sexual experiences will begin to transform into empowering acts of love.

Energy flows from positive to negative. This is the direction of movement, penis into vagina. A doorway opens, energy moves. When woman is vibrantly receptive, the direct connection between penis and vagina forms one vital unit. There is a flow and exhange of energy, potency, and life force.

The Diminished Role of the Clitoris in Tantric Sex

The vagina naturally has greater significance (for both men and women) than the clitoris because it is understood to be the receptacle for man's dynamic force. Normally the clitoris is considered to be the saving grace, the sun around which everything revolves, because clitoral stimulation can easily, but not necessarily, bring woman to orgasm. Clitoral stimulation will intensify excitement, which can, in fact, have a subtly disturbing effect on the cellular receptivity of the vagina. This tension in turn disturbs the capacity of woman to accept and receive the dynamic force into her. Clitoral stimulation elicits sexual desire but causes tension and confusion in the vaginal vibration, and the potential of the penetration is reduced.

Basic to experiencing higher states is maintaining a lower level of excitement, as introduced in chapter 2. A cool, nonstimulating approach allows the vagina to remain free of tension, able to maintain a relaxed, receptive atmosphere. If a woman is able to monitor her own excitement, to relax into her body rather than work at building up the intensity, she is less likely to inadvertently trigger man's ejaculation. Likewise, if man does not attempt to excite his woman, ejaculation can be postponed and lovemaking can be extended for hours.

A woman can get a bit fixated on her clitoris because of the pleasure and intensity experienced though these nerve endings. Sometimes it can be challenging to let go of things we know and have enjoyed. All the same, an elevation of sexual experience requires curiosity and intelligence by both partners and a willingness to explore the unknown. (See chapter 8 for more about the clitoris.)

Female Sexual Energy Is Raised in the Breasts

The big question is now how to knock on heaven's door. The true way to expand female sexual energy is to initially shift the emphasis away from the vagina and clitoris toward the breasts, which signifies *a shift from negative pole to positive pole in woman.* The breasts are the positive, dynamic pole from which energy is awakened, the key to accessing the female body. Energy can only be raised from a positive, dynamic pole and not from a passive, receptive pole. First the breasts need to become energized and filled with awareness (and this takes time), and then as a result the vagina will respond and become an invitation. Through merging with her breasts a woman is capable of experiencing the most profound orgasmic states. The vagina/clitoris,

The Equal and Opposite Force of the Female Environment

which is the usual starting point in conventional sex, is—energetically speaking—the passive, receptive pole in the female body. In truth, the vagina can only become fully alive and energized via the positive and dynamic pole of the breasts.

When man knows that the breasts are the doorway, the access to woman, his approach can be simpler and more informed, with less guessing or fiddling around to find the clitoris and get it just right. Instead, loving attention can be given to the breasts, which doesn't even require much effort on man's part. It is more a matter of "being" in your hands, without any intention or agenda lying behind the touch. A warm hand that gently embraces and lovingly molds to the breasts is absolutely perfect. There is no need to stimulate the nipples directly, but only indirectly through simple hand contact or a feather-light brush once or twice. Some women have hypersensitive nipples, so it's best to find out what suits your woman. (See more on breasts and foreplay in chapter 7.)

Ancient tantric wisdom makes it possible to initiate a thrilling journey of self-discovery, the outcome of which is the true experience of masculinity. This requires a revolutionary reevaluation of sex and the discovery that the "how" of sex plays a profound role in maintaining an active sex life and a loving, joyful relationship. The key is to treat woman as complementary and not the same. Any limitation in the sexual experience of woman inevitably limits the sexual experience of man. If woman is adversely affected through a lack of orgasmic experiences, then so is man, even if he is not aware of this.

SHIFT FROM SENSATION TO SENSITIVITY

There is a general requirement to shift away from sensation and excitement toward sensitivity and nature's subtle energetic connection.

Lovemaking must be reconceived as an interplay of dynamic and receptive forces that give rise to extraordinary energetic experiences. A shift away from sensation toward sensitivity imbues man with true male attributes and the ability to be present to his penis. To give value to, and opportunity for, the male-female connection within the vagina, where the vagina becomes an embracing sheath that elicits the essential qualities imbued in the penis, supporting man's experience of himself as authentic man. A natural biological ecstasy is possible, an exchange that satisfies every cell in the body and lies beyond the pleasure of ejaculation and fantasy.

The penis has a definite intelligence and innate sensitivity. When the female environment is open, warm, and loving, the penis responds positively to the intrinsic force-flow. When the female environment is closed, tight, or unwelcoming, the penis can easily shrink and withdraw as it loses cellular interest. For a man it is a profoundly moving and touching experience to feel deeply welcomed into the vagina by a woman.

Awakening Polarity

You and your partner can make yourselves more aware of your complementary polarities before you start lovemaking—as a kind of foreplay. Or at any other time.

Sit opposite each other on the floor on cushions situated a little distance apart so that your knees or hands aren't touching. Close your eyes and tune into your positive poles: for you that would be at the root of your penis (the perineum), and for your partner, her breasts and nipples. Take a few minutes for this. After a while when you feel you have managed to pull your attention into your penis and testicles, imagine the penis radiating energy, light, and warmth toward your woman's vagina. She should imagine herself receiving the love and light into her vagina and at the same time radiating warmth, light, and love out through her breasts to you. Imagine receiving all this beautiful energy and absorb it into your chest and heart.

You can use the breath to support the experience if you wish (but should you feel more relaxed without any special attention on the breath, this choice is fine too). As you breathe out, radiate love and light from the penis. As you breathe in, absorb the love and light coming from her breasts. Breathe in together and then out together for a while. Or as one breathes out, the other breathes in, then vice versa. When you feel ready, open your eyes in a gentle, receptive way, and sustain an inviting, gentle eye contact.

If you feel a physical attraction arising between you, woman can move across the space, and you can assist her to wrap her legs around your waist while sitting in your lap (yab yum position); cushions can be used to support her if necessary. This position brings the genitals into closer proximity and the breasts and chest into correspondence. This means the inner magnets are meeting at opposite ends. Embrace lightly and feel the inner sensations, or use the imagination to circle the energies.

If you wish, you can also change the breathing pattern—as you breathe in, woman breathes out; as woman breathes in, you breathe out. This practice will intensify the feeling of the energy and aliveness circling between your bodies. After a time you probably will begin to feel subtle sensations of the energy circulating. If yab-yum is not comfortable to sustain, you can move into a standing position, or you can do the entire exercise standing. Experiencing this circling energy may lead to a mutual desire for union, but if not, slowly separate your bodies so that you don't suddenly break the energetic connection. Sit with closed eyes and settle your attention inside your own body for few minutes.

Tantric Inspiration

And this merger should not become unconscious, otherwise you miss the point. Then it is a beautiful sex act, but not transformation. It is beautiful, nothing is wrong in it, but it is not transformation. And if it is unconscious then you will always be moving in a rut. Again and again you will want to have this experience. The experience is beautiful as far as it goes, but it will become a routine. And each time you have it, again more desire is created. The more you have it, the more you desire it, and you move in a vicious circle. You don't grow, you just rotate.

Rotation is bad because then growth is not happening. The energy is simply wasted. Even if the experience is good, the energy is wasted, because much more was possible. And it was just at the corner, just a turn, and much more was possible. With the same energy the divine could have been achieved. With the same energy the ultimate ecstasy is possible, and you are wasting that energy in momentary experiences. And by and by those experiences will become boring, because repeated again and again, everything becomes boring. When the newness is lost, boredom is created.

If you remain alert you will see: first, changes of energy in the body; second, dropping of thoughts from the mind; and third, dropping of the ego from the heart. And when this third thing has happened, that energy, your sex energy, has transformed into meditative energy.

OSHO, TRANSCRIBED TEACHINGS,
MY WAY: THE WAY OF THE WHITE CLOUDS

5
THE PENIS—A POTENT ELECTROMAGNETIC INSTRUMENT

A man who experiences his penis as a divine instrument of love and ecstasy develops a profound trust in his manhood, which rests easily and gently at the center of his being. He has the capacity to listen to his body, loves and respects his penis, and knows how to be male in relation to female. He understands the source of his erection and is in control of his ejaculation, and not vice versa. He becomes able to prolong the sex act at will and capable of holding a relaxed, timeless space that supports woman (and thereby himself) as an equal and opposite force in experiencing orgasmic fulfillment.

When man and woman are rooted in nature—man as dynamic force, woman as receptive force—there is an intrinsic movement as a by-product of the meeting of opposite polarities. Spontaneous, inherent circles of giving and receiving come into play. Man gives to woman, she receives from man; woman gives to man, he receives from woman. Many men have probably experienced, however briefly, no greater blessing than being the recipient of woman's love; there is nothing more gratifying or significant in the life of a man. When he receives a shower of female essence, divine feminine nectar, the pure sweetness of it is a magically empowering experience for a man. It is the love that is awakened in her through the power of a loving penis. Such enchanting experiences are the true outcome of sexual union, but happen much too seldom. Normally at the outset of a relationship, when the situation is fresh and new, magical experiences naturally occur. The knack is to keep re-creating the newness and not fall into habit or take each other for granted.

SEXUAL CONDITIONING INFLUENCES SEXUAL BEHAVIOR

Very few men have conscious control over themselves or their penises in sex, which puts them at a disadvantage in creating love. Lack of control exists because there is a complete absence of constructive information. Instead, unconscious impressions about sex from earliest childhood accumulate and shape the individual, gradually forming a sexual conditioning that distorts the individual's natural sexual responses or expression.

Although clarification about sex, or useful sex education, is virtually nonexistent in our culture, sex continues to be a driving and distracting force. But at the same time this powerful force is kept under wraps, like a secret. Most people are involved in sex in some way, but nobody acknowledges it, shares information, or even talks about it. Sex shifts away from the body and becomes an aspect of the mind as expressed in thoughts, fantasies, dreams, and voyeurism, and this is true even in self-pleasuring. Sex leaves the realm of the humanly sensitive flesh to become something you think about a zillion times more than you actually do.

When a man finally gets together with a woman, he operates on his accumulated past experiences and guesswork, and hopes for the best. Beneath multiple layers of bravado and performance frequently lies a sexual insecurity that gnaws away at the depths of his being. Such tension will exacerbate any other presexual tension, causing the man to perhaps feel out of control, especially concerning ejaculation.

Correspondence between the Penis and the Vagina

To shift to a higher realm of sexual experience a man has to reevaluate his penis and the way he uses it inside the vagina. He must use his penis with intelligence, maturity, and vision.

Nature intended the penis to operate as a highly sensitive, perceptive magnetic instrument. Although the penis and vagina are physical organs, they are designed to communicate on a refined energy level. The entire penis is a channel, a conduit through which life force moves from man into woman. Woman receives this force and draws it into herself. The response or communication between the genitals can first be felt as a vibrant sensation of aliveness on a fine cellular level. When we are caught up in sexual doing, there is no opportunity to relax and simply be in the body and experience this subtle vitality. When mechanical movements cease, we can begin to tune in to a finer level of sensitivity and delicate sensation.

The vagina and penis as equal and opposite forces are designed by nature for a "happening." When one fits into the other, man can begin to experience emanations from his penis, like electromagnetic streamings, that become increasingly ecstatic as they spread throughout the body. By developing an inner listening to—and with—his penis and genital region, his overall approach to making love will become more sensitive and conscious.

DEVELOPING SENSITIVITY THROUGH BEING CONSCIOUS

When a man begins to make love with awareness and experiment with stillness, he may be surprised to notice a relative absence of sensitivity in his penis. Without the familiar stimulation and intensity, it's not so easy for him to find a real inner connection to his genital area. Such lack of sensitivity is to be expected after many years of tense, goal-oriented sex. The good news is that sensitivity will quickly return to the penis through a relaxed style of lovemaking.

On the eighth and final day of our workshops we usually ask the men, "Does your penis now feel more sensitive?" Virtually all raise their hands to confirm a dramatic increase in sensitivity. By reducing the friction movements—the doing—they are able to redirect their attention to an inner awareness of the penis and its vitality. Even men who have used the penis in another way for forty or fifty years notice a change in sensitivity and aliveness within just a few days. The body's regenerative power under conducive conditions is extraordinary. There exists an intrinsic drive toward purity and wholeness when the intelligence of the body is embraced.

Using the Imagination

If you lack sensitivity in the penis when there is no movement or stimulation, your creative imagination can help your body to cooperate with your inner reality. Imagination can be a powerful tool for awakening an inner, cellular experience. You can take your attention into the penis and visualize it as a channel for potency, warmth, love, light, gold, or whatever encourages an inner perception and flow. Energy follows imagination, so by leading the way with visualization, you can actually begin to experience vitality and sensation.

We know how well the imagination works in sexual fantasy, but in that situation we are imagining something that doesn't exist, so we are completely absent and disconnected from what is happening in the here and now. When imagination is directed toward something that actually exists in the energetic realm, it has the power to elevate the experience and gradually open man to the inner experience of his radiant penis.

Bringing Attention from the Head to the Perineum
Generally speaking a man will tend to have most of his attention on the head of the penis, naturally, because this is where he experiences the most intense pleasure. To begin to shift attention away from the head of the penis, visualize your penis as a channel for potency, warmth, and love. Imagine that it is a fountain of light and liquid gold energy, circulating its dynamic force back into your body. Envision your penis as a channel or conduit, and refocus your attention on the base of your penis, in the area of the perineum. The perineum, a small, coin-sized area of knotty muscle lying directly in front of the anus, is virtually the root of the penis and is its energetic source. It is where the muscles and tissues that form the penis initially emerge from the floor of your pelvis.

When you begin to make love and feel the sexual heat rising, bring your attention to the perineum. Consciously relax the entire pelvic floor area, including the anus and testicles. When you notice your attention start to drift—there are, after all, abundant distractions—you may notice that in your absence the pelvic floor area once again contracts and tightens. Relaxing the anus frequently and maintaining awareness of the base of the penis will give you an inner feeling of your penis as a complete unit, rather than a disembodied tool for thrusting. It becomes a divine instrument capable of channeling subtle energies that flow or stream from the root upward to the radiant head, and beyond into your receptive partner. Be aware of your breathing and of the subtle sensations deep within your physical core as your inner rod of magnetism awakens. Notice how the life force rises to caress your heart into vibrant aliveness. (See the appendix at the back of the book for specific ways to increase sensitivity.)

A HIGHLY SENSITIVE MAGNET

The silky, slippery, smooth, sensitive head of the penis bears testament to its powerful magnetic properties. The head radiates life force, energy, and potency, which correspond directly with the receptive, relaxed, inviting vaginal environment. The head of the penis also acts as a catalyst with profoundly healing properties (see chapter 8 on sexual healing and male authority). When the head of the penis corresponds to its equal and opposite pole, the connection is able to generate states of ecstasy. Tantra master Barry Long, from Australia, says that a man should attempt to "become" his penis while making love. Through awareness and presence a man can gradually learn to merge with his penis, and be his penis.

There is a ruthless emphasis in our culture on the size of a man's penis when erect, and even when it is flaccid. Sometimes the two don't even correlate, since it's impossible to estimate the erect size of a penis based on its flaccid state. Convention insists that bigger is better, so a man may have feelings of shame or insecurity because of his size, which affects his capacity to trust, love, and value his own penis.

In the tantric approach, sensitivity and capacity of presence are more important than size and performance. It is true that a bigger penis is able to cause more friction in the vagina, but a penis that is big and hard can also be numb and insensitive in itself, as well as cause discomfort to a woman. However, when there is a shift in our thinking about sex, we can begin to give value to our subtle energy exchanges, which means that any size is perfect. Many men discover that their optimally perceptive sensitive state is when the penis is only half erect. How you do something is much more meaningful than what you do, or the size or rigidity of your sex organ. The penis is innately intelligent, and if man is able to relax back into himself, nature will express itself through him.

PERSONAL SHARING
Focusing on the Inner Body

During the lovemaking retreat we repeated one exercise several times, which involved closing my eyes and focusing just on the inner body (the home in my body) in order to feel a connection with my pelvis. It was always a beautiful experience for me.

When I felt connected with myself, I slowly opened my eyes, still focusing on the inside, and slowly turned to my partner, who had just done the same exercise. While slowly coming together in this manner, I was full of joy and love. I realized that my penis stiffened and I wanted to share this pleasant feeling with my partner and rub my penis against her, as I used to in the past.

However, this time I tried something new. I stayed with my feeling, sensed my penis from inside, and experienced a strange energy filling my body and rising to my heart. This wonderful connection, this streaming of energy from my penis to my heart, was very fulfilling for me and left a deep impression. All this happened just because I was alert and contained my feeling, and did not automatically project my feeling out of my own body.

PERSONAL SHARING

Swaying in a Tantric Dance

One sensation that came up again and again was of a kind of dance happening between penis and vagina. When I was inside my wife, I perceived a soft motion between us—like leaves swaying gently in a warm breeze, or as if my penis were surrounded by soft, warm liquid. Although seen from an outside perspective our bodies did not move, my motions were, in fact, in harmony with her motions, and I felt deeply connected to my beloved in what felt like a dance between the female and the male. As I remember this event, I wonder again about the untapped potential of our sexual organs. Tantra is a true adventure to me. My perceptions during lovemaking have become more refined, diversified, and intense. This makes lovemaking more touching, colorful, and deeply conscious for me, both physically and energetically.

I have a beautiful experience to share: One morning when we were making love and were inside of each other, I felt as if my penis were surrounded by warm liquid honey. My wife's vagina was soft and receptive, I was very present and focused, and a common space formed between us, a healing space in which my masculinity encountered the femininity of my beloved. Energetically there was just this one space, within which we could love each other in total freedom. After some time we changed position, and my wife suddenly got aroused and had an orgasm. After that her vagina felt tense and tight, and the space between us had disappeared.

PERSONAL SHARING
One with Myself and with My Lover

I've begun to notice the ability of my penis to stay erect without my being aroused. Previously erectness was inextricably connected with arousal. I happen to see a sexy woman, and poing—my penis gets stiff. My wife touches my penis—poing. But now the poing happens without any arousal, but only if we are inside of each other and I am present, focused, and relaxed. There are two factors that make it extra easy: If my lover is also present and if I am deeply in her vagina. Most of those times I feel a strong energy flow within myself and between us. Everything around us becomes unimportant, and I am one with myself and my lover. I feel held, loved, and simply at home in myself and in everything that is.

Tantric Inspiration

Remain with the beginning; do not move to the end. How to remain in the beginning? Many things are to be remembered. First, don't take the sex act as a way of going anywhere. Don't take it as a means: it is the end in itself. There is no end to it; it is not a means. Secondly, do not think of the future; remain with the present. And if you cannot remain in the present in the beginning part of the sex act, then you can never remain in the present—because the very nature of the act is such that you are thrown into the present.

Remain in the present. Enjoy the meeting of two bodies, two souls, and merge into each other, melt into each other. Forget that you are going anywhere. Remain in the moment going nowhere, and melt. Warmth, love, should be made a situation for two persons to melt into each other. That is why, if there is no love, the sex act is a hurried act. You are using the other; the other is just a means. And the other is using you. You are exploiting each other, not merging into each other. With love you can merge. This merging in the beginning will give you many new insights.

If you are not in a hurry to finish the act, the act, by and by, becomes less and less sexual and more and more spiritual. Sex organs also melt into each other. A deep silent communion happens between two body energies, and then you can remain for hours together. This togetherness moves deeper and deeper as time passes. But don't think. Remain with the moment deeply merged. It becomes an ecstasy, a *samadhi,* cosmic consciousness. And if you can know this, if you can feel and realize this, your sexual mind will become nonsexual.

OSHO, TRANSCRIBED TEACHINGS,
VIGYAN BHAIRAV TANTRA

6
AWARENESS, MOVEMENT, PENETRATION, AND ERECTION

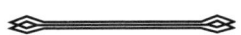

AWARENESS

The expression "It's not what you do, but how you do it" is more deeply understood through these simple yet profound words of Osho: "Tantra is the transformation of sex into love through awareness." These few words encapsulate the essence of tantra, which is about awareness—nothing more, nothing less. If we are aware and conscious during sex, sex transforms into love. Awareness changes the whole quality of sex, and the fragrance and climate of love is naturally generated through awareness. Woman's heart and body respond vibrantly to man rooted in the present through his awareness.

Staying Present within the Body
The elusive present moment is created through bringing awareness to the body, holding the attention in the body, millisecond by millisecond.

Being aware of body position, movements, and breath and relaxing habitual tensions are basic tools to accessing and staying in the present. The body always exists in the present; it is the mind that roams around in past and future thoughts. Before a man can understand how to remain present while making love with a woman, he must first establish a relationship with his own body. He can literally embody his own body by taking his attention inside the body and away from thoughts and fantasies. As one retreat participant a few years ago reported, "It's incredible, I am a fifty-four-year-old man, and nobody has ever told me to feel inside my body. And it is paradise in there!"

Another encouraging example was this: less than twenty-four hours into the retreat a man raised his hand and complained, "It's all very well for you to say, 'Feel all the subtle pleasant inner sensations.' You've been doing it for more than twenty years. I can feel absolutely nothing." We assured him that he needed to give himself more time and that practice makes perfect. The week continued without any further comment from him, so on the final day we asked how he was feeling in his body. He looked at us, eyes and face radiant with love, and said just one word: "Unbelievable!"

See the appendix for specific exercises to bring attention into your body.

Relax and Breathe

There is a tendency for us to tighten various muscles or clench muscle groups unconsciously, without really realizing it. Such tensions have become a habit and a way of life to the extent that as we are falling asleep, we may realize we are unconsciously holding ourselves up on the bed. We are not letting go and allowing even our place of comfort and repose to fully receive us. Physical tensions compress the energy system and restrict the expansion of vitality through the body. So it is enormously helpful to become aware of these tensions and release them, or breathe into them, while you are making love. Physical relaxation and conscious breathing will also reduce the pressure to ejaculate. (See the appendix for particular ways to scan the body and check for tension.)

Eye Contact and Communication

Generally speaking people make love in the dark, with closed eyes and without much meeting of the eyes. Although it might feel a little awkward in the beginning, connecting eye to eye immediately creates a feeling of intimacy and brings you in touch with the present. The eye contact is not a fixed stare, but an introverted, soft, receptive gaze that invites your partner into you. As you enter woman, or as you change positions, allow the eyes to meet and engage. And at the same time, feel how your genitals engage. Maintaining eye contact is not a rule but a suggestion, a tool to increase awareness and presence. Closing the eyes and taking awareness into your own body, in order to strengthen your inner connection and sensitivity, will also be necessary from time to time. It's a good thing to tell your partner why you are closing your eyes, so the person doesn't feel abandoned or excluded.

To amplify the experience of the present moment, you will be surprised how much sharing what is happening to you on an inner body level—communicating out loud—helps to intensify the inner experience. Acknowledging your inner sensitivities and sensations verbally has the effect of intensifying them, and you'll find your body unexpectedly rewarding you for having noticed the existence of its cellular subtleties and vitality. Only a few words are needed to convey what you feel within yourself on a body-heart-soul level, as if you are giving an inner weather report. Your partner does not have to respond directly, unless she wants to communicate what she feels within herself. These kinds of body reports are a great key to tracking your way to the present and can be done either before as a kind of foreplay or while actually making love. It will also eliminate any need for the clichéd, "Was it good for you?" because you will know during the process.

Consideration of the Receptive Force

As we now can appreciate, there is a distinct advantage to the female partner being in a state of receptivity in order to allow the male force through her. Like man, woman also needs the opportunity to enter her own body and become alive to her inner world. Since you know it will take longer for woman's body to warm up, wait until your woman says she is ready to take you in. Wait for a "yes," an invitation. Women tend to yield to pressure because they have not yet learned to trust and honor their feminine systems. They get messages from their bodies, but there is a tendency for woman to override her inner wisdom; frequently she feels compelled to let man into her before she is truly ready. Part of woman's sexual conditioning is to please man, usually because she is afraid of losing him or losing his love. When man is aware of the pleasing tendency of woman, he can begin to understand it as the female counterpart to the male pressure to perform.

When you wait, create space, and support woman to relax into herself and connect with her internal world, she opens with ease and enthusiasm. Man creates the potential to be inside woman endlessly and tap her higher orgasmic energies. When a "yes" comes from woman in her totality, it is as if she's plugged into a circuit from which she finds it difficult to disconnect. She is neither frigid nor rigid, but vital and receptive. For man to be a channel or conduit for his true male energy, the equal and opposite force must also be available, so man needs to be constantly aware of the receptacle that is receiving the flow of his life force.

MOVEMENT

There is a common misconception that tantra means no movement during sex. We heartily endorse movement, not for the sake of movement itself, but because it creates more aliveness and presence.

Movements should also seek to enhance the correspondent dynamic-receptive potential of the genital contact. Stillness is an option, and something that you may develop an appreciation for over time, but initially most people usually enjoy alternating phases of movement with phases of stillness.

Awareness and Tempo

Any movement done consciously, which means you feel yourself as you do it, changes the quality of the experience dramatically. Done with awareness, all movements naturally become slower, and the body becomes more sensual and sensitive; you become totally engaged in the unfolding present. Be alert and aware as you approach each other, embrace, kiss, move, change position, move the penis within the vagina—be aware in whatever you do. There is a natural slowing down when any action is done with awareness. You are not slowing down to follow a rule, but instead discovering that when you are aware, you do in fact move more slowly. And you can feel more; your sensitivity increases. Slowness is an outcome, a by-product of being more conscious. Out of curiosity or for fun, you can ask yourself, "How slow is slow?" And get into an inquiry.

Come together in an unhurried way, while staying in awareness. Remain alert, attentive, and conscious in the body. Let there be a flow; allow it to happen, rather than forcing or pushing it in certain directions. Allow an easy, innocent, playful, spontaneous unfolding without knowing what will happen next.

Goal-oriented Movement Becomes Mechanical

Movements that have the goal of building up to a climax will have an intrinsic pressure powering them, whereas movements that do not have a goal can arise fluidly from the requirements of bodies in the moment. There is nothing wrong with movement per se; movement is life, but at the same time we need to remain aware and steer clear of the tendency to be mechanical in the sex act. The usual movement of the penis in the vagina is forward and backward thrusts, a linear movement. But movements can also be made in a more expansive three-dimensional way, reaching into different angles of the vaginal canal (as described later, in chapter 8 within the context of sexual healing and male empowerment).

Movements made with the intention of creating pleasure and excitement will tend to become mechanical, and when we become like machines, we lose awareness and sensitivity. With the focus on stimulation, our awareness of what is taking place in the body on a more subtle level tends to diminish. Our attention or focus is more on building up intensity, rather than on taking delight in each of the individual movements taking place.

Usually, a woman will push her genitals forward (using her pelvis) at the very same moment the man thrusts or moves into her. Physically speaking, just from the mechanics of the musculature, the vagina becomes narrower and tighter during a forward push. This tightening results in the vagina being less receptive in this phase of the movement. As a consequence, woman is not truly available to the dynamic force entering her body.

Another option is to let man do the moving, while woman holds still. Instead of woman pushing forward to meet man's movement, she tilts her pelvis upward at an angle and remains still. In this nonmoving position a woman is able to put all her attention into her vagina—into the receiving, absorbing, and welcoming of the penis into her body. A pillow can be placed beneath the buttocks in order to raise the level of the pelvis, if so desired. Man will perceive his conscious movement in woman far more deeply if she is able to fulfill her part of the design, which is to act as receptor for the dynamic force.

The Difference between Lust and Passion

When the dynamic and receptive forces in our bodies are honored, we become more present and naturally more passionate. Passion is pure presence, aliveness, and spontaneity. In passion there can also be strong movements that might look the same as the movements of conventional sex from the outside, but the inner experience is vastly different. The movements contain an inner stillness because they belong to the domain of the here and now; there is no direction, no goal, and no agenda. Nothing is planned or expected. Instead, each individual is engaged, with full awareness merged into the unfolding of each and every millimeter of movement. Each millisecond of any movement is a completion in itself.

In contrast, when movement contains lust, there is a tendency to be ahead of oneself, slightly mechanical, with the movements being focused on building up to a crescendo. The individual movements are not independent or complete in themselves. When lust drives the lovemaking, frustration and disappointment are likely to follow a sudden interruption because something desired was not reached or achieved. The act is incomplete because the goal was not fulfilled. By contrast, when passion is unexpectedly interrupted, everything is simply perfect as it is. Each second has been utterly complete in itself, so there is simply no sense of any loss at all. In fact, passionate sex can be resumed at any moment, while in lustful sex there will usually be a sense of deflation and loss of interest because the heat and excitement will have gone out of the situation.

THE ART OF CONSCIOUS PENETRATION

When erection is present it is recommended that the very first movement into the vagina be exceptionally conscious. The first move sets the stage for what is to follow. The penis should enter the vagina slowly, millimeter by millimeter. A number of positions are possible, the most direct and easy being the missionary position, with woman lying on her back and man kneeling between her legs. The head of the penis can enter the vagina and gradually open it along its entire length, gently probing slowly but surely up the canal. Resting from time to time allows you to take in the view, which means feeling in and down into your body and especially into your penis. A single movement can easily be extended to many minutes, or an entire lovemaking session of several hours can be one divine immersion in woman's body. These experiences can change your life and your whole view of sex.

The problem with an entry by the penis that is fast or aggressive and lacking in awareness is that woman (unconsciously or consciously) closes her vagina to protect herself from possible intense pain. The upper vagina tightens to prevent the penis from thrusting into the very delicate and sensitive cervix—the entrance to the womb. When woman is hit here it really hurts. Such naturally defensive contractions, both physical and psychological, definitely influence woman's receptivity and capacity to absorb, which means she is no longer feminine in relation to man. With conscious, slow penetration, woman has the chance to invite, welcome, and caress each millimeter of the probing penis.

There is a distinction between being careful and being conscious. One is not being "careful" in relation to woman; carefulness implies a certain tension, a holding back, a fear of hurting the other, which is more an attitude lacking in self-awareness. With carefulness, one's attention is externally focused on the other and not on the self. We are up and out, and have left home, so to speak. When one is conscious, one is self-aware and automatically acts with care as a by-product of that awareness, rather than as an intention to "be careful." When a man is conscious, he also becomes more confident.

Awareness, Slowness, and Sensitivity

The greatest advantage of awareness, of being conscious during penetration, is that you can feel "into" the penis on a cellular level. Finally you have the time and there is nowhere to go (toward ejaculation), so you can instead focus your attention inside the penis itself. Listening to the

Awareness, Movement, Penetration, and Erection

penis and becoming aware of its gradual movement greatly increases its sensitivity and allows the perception of inner, fine, cellular, delicate, delightful sensations that expand throughout the body. An unhurried, aimless, no goals approach is vital to making this possible.

Ecstatic, thrilling, touching experiences occur through a correspondence of opposites. In fitting snugly together with sustained contact, penis and vagina respond to each other according to an innate intelligence. The penis is a powerful instrument able to generate divine states of ecstasy when arriving in its truly complementary environment.

Deep, Sustained Penetration

As a general orientation, when there is erection and the possibility of gradual, sensitive penetration, the penetration should be sustained in the depths of the vagina. (This subject is also dealt with in chapter 8 on sexual healing and male authority. Both chapters should be read in order to grasp the full implications of remaining deep inside woman.) This means that when you eventually arrive (after the minutes given to the first journey down the canal), you remain with the penis inside, resting in the depths, and do not immediately withdraw in order to repeat the movement. Instead, take the time to intentionally bring your entire awareness into the penis and "be" your penis, attempting to sense the tissues from within, to merge and melt with them. You do not force your penis into woman, but you force your awareness, your point of attention, into your penis, remaining at the same time relaxed and observing. These are two very different experiences for both parties involved.

At the end of the vagina lies the extremely sensitive cervix; and as already mentioned, it can be indescribably painful if the penis head aggressively hits this spot, so it is important to arrive here with sensitivity. When you arrive at the end of the canal or as far as you can go or whenever you have the feeling that the penis head is pushing into the walls with pressure anywhere along the way, it's very important to drop back a hairsbreadth or two. This minute fraction of space removes any pressure and intention, and creates "breathing room" for the "porous" contact that is required for an energy exchange. When the push is purely physical and hard, the vaginal cells withdraw and close in response. When the contact is subtle, gentle, easy, and spacious, the cells are able to relax and open. Sometimes during penetration the penis will encounter pains held in the vagina, a topic that will be covered specifically in chapter 8 on sexual healing, along with diagrams of suitable positions for deep, sustained penetration.

Lubrication—the Secret of Sensual Penetration

A slippery, smooth, silky, slow, sensual penetration simply has to be one of life's greatest joys, for both man and woman. Use lubricant without hesitation and with pleasure, and use it every time. Oil the penis, the vaginal lips, and the entrance. It's a great part of foreplay, especially when woman does the oiling. Oil was used by Taoists thousands of years ago and is said to reduce bacteria levels in the vagina. Use thin, fragrance-free vegetable oil, such as almond oil. It is also suggested that woman hold her lips/labia open when man is about to enter her. Using both hands, she clears the entrance from any obstructing skin folds and holds her hands in position for a while. This assistance guarantees a smooth, pleasurable journey.

Vaginal Dryness

Without high levels of stimulation woman is less likely to become "wet," which is quite normal. Also, when women approach menopause and suffer from dryness, penetration can become difficult, painful, or impossible. With a slow, conscious, oily penis, miracles are possible. Women who have not been able to make love for years are able to get back into it with ease. Gradually, in time, the vaginal tissues relax, regenerate, and naturally become more moist.

Condoms

Condoms are sometimes necessary for contraception or health reasons, and are without doubt a layer between man and his sensitivity. However, according to people who have used them and our own personal experience, man is capable of feeling the delicate, subtle, electromagnetic exchange through condoms. The basic sensitivity is not seriously affected or compromised.

If condoms are used, don't use oil as a lubricant; oil destroys rubber and compromises contraception. Use only water-based gels, which can be obtained from a pharmacy. This is a good moment to stress the importance of genital hygiene and daily cleansing of the penis, particularly underneath the foreskin.

While on the subject of contraception, it is important to acknowledge here that a woman responds to sexual invitations much more readily if there is no fear of pregnancy. Such fear can definitely contribute to a woman's reluctance or lack of availability during her fertile years. If man is willing to take responsibility for contraception, either in taking care of himself or supporting his woman to take the appropriate care in the moment and not in theory, he is helping himself enormously. Some men choose the option of a vasectomy as a solution for contraception, and from time to time we receive queries asking if vasectomy disturbs male potency. We can say with confidence that vasectomy does not appear to affect male potency and may even increase potency, in that it allows woman to be more free with herself. Relieved of concerns about conception, she can be more spontaneous and may also wish to make love with greater frequency.

Soft Penetration—Entry without Erection

Soft entry is a pure and simple alternative when there is no erection. It completely eliminates the pressure of having to have an erection in order to have sex. Given the general lack of stimulation, not having an erection is quite normal and nothing to be concerned about. Soft entry actually bypasses many erection concerns and issues, and gives us a humble, human way to get our bodies together. The advantage of a soft start is that both man and woman begin at zero, so to speak, allowing their temperatures to warm up together. Soft entry is very easy and, with practice, can happen in the flash of a second. There are two possibilities: man puts his penis inside woman, or woman puts the penis inside her. We recommend the second option.

Man Initiates Soft Penetration
Man kneels between woman's open legs, as seen in figure 6.1. Woman can place a flat, firm cushion underneath her buttocks. The lifted position raises the level of the pelvis and brings the vagina closer to the penis. Woman holds her labia open, as described earlier, and man introduces the head of the penis into the entrance of the vagina using his fingers. Push the head in a little bit (be sure your fingernails are trimmed), move the fingers back a few centimeters, and insert the penis a little further into the vagina. Step by step, wiggle and walk the penis inside the entrance.

When the penis is in the vagina as far as you can manage (even the head is a good start), remain kneeling and bring the pelvises together. Or lower yourself down on top of your partner, holding yourself up with your arms. Or lie forward on your partner and then roll onto your sides, man remaining between woman's legs.

Woman Initiates Soft Entry
The easiest and most comfortable position for soft penetration is the side position called scissors, because of the scissor-like interlacing of the legs. The advantage of the scissors position is that nobody is on top and nobody is underneath, which is indeed very relaxing. Man is on his side, while woman is lying on her back with her legs inserted, scissors fashion, between man's legs. You can stay in this position for several hours quite easily. From scissors position any number of other positions can be reached, which will be elaborated on in chapter 7.

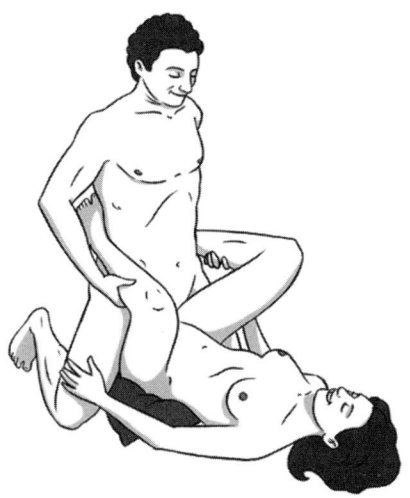

Fig. 6.1. This figure shows man in the middle position suitable for soft entry

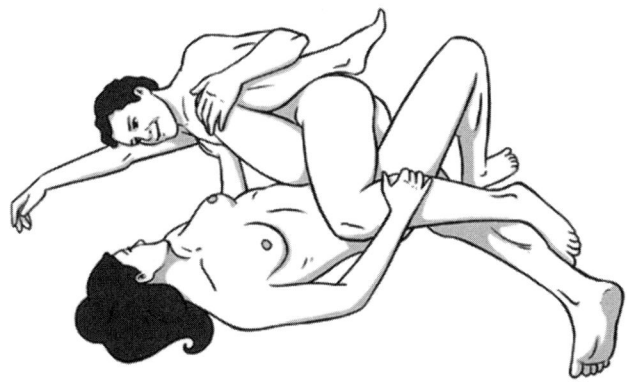

Fig. 6.2. The scissors position for soft penetration

Bring your legs together, as shown in figure 6.2. The scissors position can be assumed from either man's left side or his right side, and it's a good idea to change sides regularly to avoid getting habituated (and therefore less alert) to one side only. Woman opens her legs, opens her labia, and then reaches for the penis, which has been oiled in advance. By now it's probably not so soft, so the entering is made even easier.

The first two fingers of one hand (short nails so as not to scratch the vagina) are put behind the head of the penis and squeezed firmly to get a grip (see fig. 6.3). The same two fingers on the other hand can stabilize the penis at the base. Woman pulls the head toward the vagina and inserts it in the entrance. Fingers are moved back a few centimeters, then gradually walked step-by-step into the vagina. At first the head may be as far as it gets, but with practice, it does get perfect. Woman must avoid looking between her legs during this delicate operation because the tightening of her abdominal muscles (needed to lift up the head to look) will also tighten the vagina and make penetration difficult, if not impossible. Looking is fine as you get set up, but then lie back and relax before you initiate the insertion.

Then move the pelvises together, joining firmly in connection. If by any chance man rolls back slightly—which pulls the penis out—wedge a flat pillow from behind, under his pelvis/buttocks. The pillow wedge tilts man's body forward slightly and stabilizes the position. Pillows can be used for support wherever needed, for instance, under the calf/knee of man's upper leg. This also reduces the weight on woman's body, as well as giving man a floating feeling. Be sure to get yourselves as comfortable as possible so that your systems can relax. Small discomforts can be distractions, and instead of delighting in your inner pleasures, you tune in to your lack of comfort.

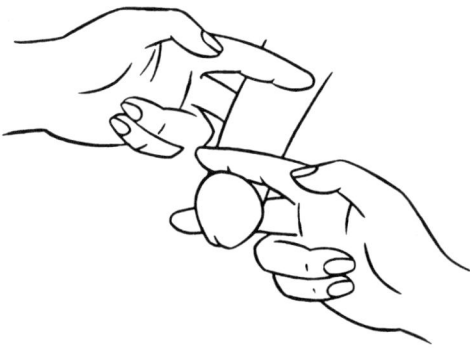

Fig. 6.3. Woman's finger position behind penis head

SPONTANEOUS ERECTION AND IMPOTENCE

Spontaneous erection within the vagina is not something that can be expected or demanded of the body. It is a by-product of a special constellation of factors, among which are awareness, presence, relaxation, and love.

Erection Responsibility Is Shared

Until now, whether he likes it or not, erection has been considered man's job, which has been a big part of his performance pressure. Conventionally, erection usually depends on stimulation and excitement, and many anxieties or fears about erection can cause a disturbance in the psyche, perhaps becoming expressed in distorted ways.

As a partnership continues, a man can easily experience a lack of erection because of a lack of excitement. The woman is known, the situation is known, and the routine is known, so there is nothing to get him really excited. However, with a new vision of sex we realize that excitement is not necessarily a basic ingredient of the sexual experience.

Erection is definitely possible without stimulation and excitement when a man begins to trust his penis. A true erection is an electromagnetic response to the equal and opposite force exerted by the vagina. From a soft state, the penis can slowly rise as a direct response to the vagina surrounding it. The female force plays an equal role; through receptivity it starts to "draw" and effectively pulls the penis into an erection, millimeter by millimeter. The penis unfolds like a slow snake winding upward in a circular spiraling motion. Erection without stimulation or excitement can also happen when in close proximity to a woman. The female force exerts an influence on the male force without your actually being inside her. Men say that it is as if the penis awakens in the atmosphere of love created through presence and awareness.

A spontaneous erection is one that arises out of the moment, due to the polarity between dynamic and receptive forces and the presence two people bring into the situation. Erections that arise spontaneously do not require stimulation or fantasy to keep them going; they simply need presence and awareness. The instant one person's attention wavers, the penis starts to wind back down, coiling like a snake. Quickly retrieving one's presence and releasing distracting thoughts will cause the erection to grow again. The penis is capable of performing a snake dance within woman—a miraculous experience for any man.

Lack of Sensitivity

The first few times soft penetration is tried, most men will find that they do not "feel" much in their penises (as mentioned earlier). This is very common and will change as soon as the penis adjusts to a new way of being used and perceived by man. This insensitivity is due to a long history of stimulation, so for it to be a little numb is not really surprising. The way to retrieve sensitivity is to relax into woman, spend as much time inside her as possible, and take full consciousness down into your penis. Begin to "be" inside the penis, treat it with love, and gradually sensitivity will return.

Usually the woman is able to feel your penis, even if you cannot perceive it. She is usually very content with soft penetration and the experience of subtle, ecstatic emanations from the penis. It is a great support to the man if a woman can communicate what she feels within herself (her inner sensitivity) out loud in words while making love, particularly in the situation where a man discovers he is not (yet) able to feel the power residing within his own penis. At the very least, it's relaxing to know that woman can feel man, even if he cannot feel himself. And she, as container, is bound to be more perceptive initially.

Impotence Issues

Impotence—lack of erection—is a deep-seated fear in most men, provoking anxiety at an almost primal level. Excitement leads to a certain type of erection that is very fragile and requires stimulation to keep it going. Impotence is no longer an issue when soft entry used. And—surprise, surprise—erection may take place on its own. The best cure for impotence is to keep putting yourself in the situation and continue making love with no erection. In time things are highly likely to change as sensitivity returns.

Several years ago a man with an inherited erectile dysfunction came to our group with his wife. He had been using penis implants up until this point and was wondering whether to drop the implant and instead try the way we had been explaining during the group. His success has been incredible. He does not have full erections now, but enough that it is no longer a problem. He describes his experience below.

PERSONAL SHARING
From Impotence to Daily Lovemaking

First of all, we bought your new book, Tantric Love—Feeling versus Emotion: Golden Rules to Make Love Easy *(the German edition). My wife read it within three hours. I took more time, but also read it quite quickly. We can confirm all that you have been saying. Emotions and feelings are too often mixed up, and very few people are aware of this important difference. (See chapter 9 for more on the distinction between feelings and emotions.)*

Last December we attended a workshop for Vipassana meditation. The theme was arrogance; the solution is humility. The insight and the teaching was: Our minds are constantly using our senses to compare all our perceptions and assess them as positive/good (I want more), negative/harmful (I want to get rid of it), or equal/good (which is not really satisfactory either). As long as we constantly compare, we are never relaxed in life and are unable to enjoy a love relationship with awareness and equanimity.

It lines up perfectly with your explanation of why there is so much incomprehension and jealousy between couples. In any event, we learned that making love your way takes away so much of the pressure that many reasons for comparison vanish, and disappointment (emotions) within yourself and against your partner just doesn't manifest. For us making love has become a kind of meditation, combining intimacy with spirituality, which we consider the whipped cream on the cake.

But let us tell you what happened to us since we attended the course with you a second time. After the first course with you a few years ago we practiced love within my almost nonexistent erection capability (owing to my medical condition). In the beginning we made love two to three times a week, and slowly cut back to making love once a week, keeping this frequency stable. We noted that regardless of the unhurried and relaxed way of making love, there was often the feeling that after almost an entire week it was about time to have sex together, and this created increasingly unpleasant pressure to perform.

After the first course, my wife started paying a lot of attention to my penis, massaging me and holding my penis in her hand every night when we went to bed, falling asleep this way. My penis got so much attention that it started to react to her contact, not with an erection, but with a kind of aliveness. It swells up just enough that I can introduce it into her vagina without great effort, and is also firm enough to go for an ejaculation, if I so desire. Even if my penis extends less than four inches, it is good enough to have the real feeling of having sex. Since my wife has never had an orgasm by penetration, but only by stimulation of her clitoris, this "handicap" of my shortened penis is not really bothering us. Sometimes I feel that I'm not a "real man with a hard one," but the sexual satisfaction I experience with my wife vastly exceeds the short event of conventional sex and ejaculation.

After our second course with you we both had the impulse to say, "Why don't we decide to have sex every day to get rid of the pressure of having to do it after a number of days? Let's create an atmosphere in which making love daily is as normal as eating meals." We decided to connect our genitals every morning at daybreak. We set the clock one hour earlier in the morning and start with twenty minutes of cuddling and caressing each other. Then my wife celebrates the oil ceremony, oiling her vagina and giving a short oil massage to my penis—just enough for it to be gently hard and easily introduced into her vagina. We remain connected for another twenty minutes, and then either turn and change position or share some moments of in and out movements. About once a week one of us—or both—feels like going for an orgasm, and we celebrate it without restriction. Finally we have another twenty minutes of cuddling—relaxing, drowsing, caressing, and so on. After an hour we get up, my wife takes a shower, and I sit down for Vipassana meditation till she is ready to leave the house for work. Often our genitals radiate pleasant vibrations and pulsate throughout our entire bodies for the whole day. It is just gorgeous.

We started this a few months ago, and since then have hardly missed a day of making love. It has become so natural and uncomplicated that we actually long for it if we have to miss one day. Our entire relationship has reached another level because we can behave so freely and openly, which I never before thought possible.

Sometimes we look back and ask ourselves what triggered our starting to insist on making love every day. We don't know, really, it just clicked and we knew we wanted to try it. During our second course with you we heard from a couple resolutely doing a fifteen-minute tantric get together every morning who seemed to be happy and united, so maybe this was the final kick for us to start.

We are very thankful for having met you and having been able to learn this method of making love from you. In my special situation with a medical condition, I often wonder what I would have done after conventional sex was no longer possible for me. I don't even want to imagine.

PERSONAL SHARING
Viagra Is No Longer Necessary

Since puberty, erection has been of great importance for me. The first time I had sex with a woman it happened in a very small compact car, and

I had no idea where to put my long legs. Due to the excitement, I did not find my way into her vagina and had a premature ejaculation. Ever since, ejaculation and penetration were stressful for me. Each time I met a new woman, I immediately had a fear of failure and thus, difficulty with the erection. It wasn't until my first longer partnership that this theme began to lose its importance.

My penultimate partnership was very much affected by wild sex and strong emotions. It was sex that glued us together and helped us to come together again and again, but in the end, even sex did not work any more. This resulted in new emotions, mutual hurt, and finally, in separation. Since I was nearing the end of my fifties at that time I presumed that sex was over for me, until I found out about the remedy for erections: Cialis (Viagra). I was very relieved to be able to have sexual contact with new women, and realized that I retained my capacity for erection even beyond the action time of the remedy. This also showed me the psychological aspect of the erection deficit. When I met my new wife, we had a weekend relationship for the first two years. I got used to taking Cialis each time before we met, because it gave me a sense of security. When we took a two-week vacation, one pill at the beginning of the holiday was enough.

After we read your book, The Heart of Tantric Sex, my wife didn't want me to take the remedy any more, so I promised to take it only after having talked to her. At home, where we were already comfortable with the relaxed way of lovemaking, I found taking it less and less necessary.

Before the lovemaking retreat we had not seen each other for three weeks. During the first three days of the seminar, I again experienced some pressure with the issues, and had trouble keeping my sense of humor about erection and penetration. I feared that since I was sixty-three years old, my virility was definitely over, so I told her that I would like to take Viagra again. When she declined my request, we had a talk with the two of you and somehow I relaxed after having talked about it so openly. The loving support of my partner, and the length of time that we took for lovemaking, has resulted ever since in much heartfelt and relaxed sex. I learned that even with a weak erection at the beginning, lovemaking lasted longer, and was heartfelt and deep. Our love grew and I was able to relax more and more deeply. Since then our love and our sexuality have reached a new dimension. For me it has been a gift. Being able to let go of goal-oriented male sexuality as my erection was getting weaker has caused our love to grow. Thank you both for this wonderful experience.

PERSONAL SHARING
My Body Keeps Me Honest

During lovemaking, my body lets me know if I am touching from my heart. I became aware of it when I was lying in bed with my wife in a close embrace one morning. With my right hand I was touching her skin, which felt warm and soft, and in contrast I experienced my hand as stiff, wooden, and lifeless. All of a sudden it came into my consciousness: "You are not touching your woman with your heart." That's why my hand felt so dull. When I thought about why this was so, I realized I felt trapped in my old pattern of not getting enough. The root of this pattern is not love, openness, and trust, which explains why my hand did not feel loving, trusting, and open. I decided to watch my hand as I shifted my attention away from the pattern to a deep and relaxed presence toward myself. Very swiftly my sensation of my hand changed. My hand softened, became alive, and was gently tingling. Immediately the breath was flowing through my hand and became one with my whole body. My hand was reconnected, and I was again able to touch from the heart. I was aware of the whole and no longer focused on my pattern. This experience taught me what is most important when touching my wife: relaxed, loving presence toward myself. So every touch is a delight and a touch of my heart.

Tantric Inspiration

If you can go on growing in this intimacy, which is no more excitement, then the joy will arise: first excitement, then love, then joy. Joy is the ultimate product, the fulfillment. Excitement is just a beginning, a triggering; it is not the end. And those who finish at excitement will never know what love is, will never know the mystery of love, will never know the joy of love. They will know sensations, excitement, passionate fever, but they will never know the grace that is love. They will never know how beautiful it is to be with a person with no excitement but with silence, with no words, with no effort to do anything. Just being together, sharing one space, one being, sharing each other, not thinking of what to do, what to say, where to go, how to enjoy; all those things are gone. The storm is over and there is silence.

And it is not that you will not make love but it will not be a making really; it will be a love happening. It will happen out of grace, out of silence, out of rhythm; it will arise from your depths, it will not be bodily really. There is a sex which is spiritual, which has nothing to do with the body. Although the body partakes in it, participates in it, it is not the source of it. Then sex takes on the color of Tantra, only then.

Osho, transcribed teachings,
Let Go!: A Darshan Diary

7
DATES, FOREPLAY, KISSING, AND POSITIONS

MAKE LOVE DATES

Knowing you are going to have sex can really be a big turn-on. Nothing beats looking at your diary and seeing that from 6 to 9 p.m. tonight you have an appointment with your partner—to make love! You know that *today*, for sure, it's going to happen, which is not generally guaranteed under ordinary circumstances. How many times does your woman brush you aside before she lets you be close? Several years ago there was a story about the famous musician, Sting, and although we don't know whether or not it's true, it makes the point about women's general lack of availability in a humorous way. According to the story, Sting made a comment to the press about his sex life, making himself almost as famous for this as for his music. His claim that he had made love for six hours or so caused an international stir. Some weeks later, or so the story goes, he clarified his statement by explaining that five of the six hours had consisted of begging.

Initially, setting a fixed time for sex may seem somewhat strange, because we have the idea that sex ought to be spontaneous—without preparation or premeditation. In fact, sex is rarely truly spontaneous, but happens more on an accidental or habitual basis. Sexual thoughts accompany man throughout his every day, but although he makes endless appointments for other things, no time or space is consciously set aside for the actual act of sex. Real sex (as opposed to virtual sex, which is increasing at an alarming rate since the advent of the Internet) appears to be low on a man's list of priorities. After work, socializing, putting the kids to bed, and watching TV, then perhaps (if he's not too tired) sex will happen. Hopefully, but not necessarily.

Attunement and Relaxation
With guaranteed sex on the horizon, you will perhaps observe yourself feeling more positive, present, and enthusiastic about being alive. You'll feel more at ease knowing that sex will happen, that your partner has actually agreed to meet you and make love. The knowing allows you to settle into yourself in advance, bringing awareness to your body, your legs, perineum, and breath. Inwardly preparing for sex is an effective form of foreplay.

Set aside three or more hours for lovemaking, if possible. It probably sounds like a lot right now, but after a bit of experimentation, three hours may turn out to be a bit on the short side. If three-hour slots are difficult to carve out for yourselves, then settle for one or two hours. Sometimes give yourself an entire day in bed, with breaks for meals and so on. When lovemaking transpires several times on the same day, bodily ease deepens to the extent that bodies enter a state of spontaneous letting-go, undulating, moving, and dancing of their own accord in a divine choreography. In states such as these, the bodies are unable to stop, so you find yourself making love for hours, totally absorbed, present to each split second, unaware of the passage of time.

The Tantric Quickie

The tantric quickie is also highly recommended. Soft penetration for ten, fifteen, or twenty minutes is a perfect way to start off the day. It brings you back home to yourself before you leave home and allows you to relax into the center of your being, which transforms the quality of the day ahead. Last thing at night is also perfect for a tantric quickie, or during an afternoon nap on the weekend. Soft union without erection is so simple and easy; just slip it in, no big performance needed, no great expenditure of energy. You just connect the genitals, relax into the moment, and become present in your body.

Quite possibly the experience of jumping into sex at a fixed time every day feels clinical and unromantic. Also, putting the unerect penis into the vagina (as described in chapter 6) may feel somewhat cold-blooded and technical. You may even feel shy and self-conscious because you are used to making love in the dark or being more concealed. Don't give concerns such as these too much attention, because first impressions fade quickly. Conscious meetings in broad daylight where everything is natural and out in the open are a dream come true for many of us. How easy is this? How sane and sensible is this? Both people are present, willing, and committed. It is ordinary, yet extraordinary. Any initial feelings of awkwardness will soon be replaced by the joy of simplicity and ordinariness, in which you can connect with yourself and your partner in a relaxed and relaxing way.

FOREPLAY

The majority of women, when pressed, will admit that the usual ways men touch and stimulate them actually turn them off. This is sobering news, but relaxing, too, because it means there is less fumbling and guesswork required. A perfect guideline for foreplay: "It's not *what* you do, but *how* you do it."

Presence and Awareness, the Greatest Aphrodisiac

Osho says, "Tantra denies nothing, but transforms everything," which means that awareness changes the situation; any action carried out with awareness is transformed through awareness itself. This basically means that almost anything goes when we are aware, consenting parties. Best is to keep everything simple, innocent, and exploratory, not following any program or putting yourselves under any pressure. Get into your body and enjoy being in it. Touch, stroke, kiss, embrace, and stay in the awareness. Stay present in each and every movement or gesture, with nowhere special to go, being innocent in the simplicity of the situation.

Any kind of touch should bring about an expansion of the other person's energy field, not a contraction. Foreplay becomes simple with the realization that there is no need to excite your partner to make her horny. Excitement will often cause a contraction of the energy field, and any hard or pressuring physical touch will do the same. Try feather-light touches instead.

What women respond to is man's presence and awareness, and awareness is basically effortless when compared to all the usual action in sex. Of course it initially takes effort to maintain presence, but it becomes increasingly familiar and effortless with practice. Presence is easily accessed through the body, and it takes time for an individual to relax into a cellular experience of self, which naturally captures or holds one in the present.

Patience

Foreplay is not so significant for men, because the male positive pole is more or less ever ready, but women definitely appreciate being given time to warm up to love. A woman requires space to relax into her body, her senses, and her receptivity. As an equal and opposite force, this prerequisite is a basic need for her, as explained in chapter 4. Patience and a selfless approach will pay off for the man in the long term. Patience is not some kind of obligation, but simply realizing, accepting, and appreciating that woman (whom you wish to enter physically) is different from you and needs time to open internally before the marvelous experience of entering and joining with her can be of any true value.

Barry Long said that for man, "Patience is the beginning of stillness." Stillness is a quieting of the system and the lessening of thoughts, staying present in the body and inwardly "holding the space." It is simply being in the here and now, resting in your body and being, present to woman. It is not turning her on, but opening and accessing her, supporting her to relax and melt into herself, giving her the feeling of being at home and at ease. If the initial pace is easy, relaxed, and slow, lovemaking is more likely to be filled with timeless delight and pleasure.

Losing Your Erection

Waiting for, or being with, a woman as her body opens means that most probably you will lose your initial erection, if you have one. Don't worry if this happens! An erection can easily return in an atmosphere of loving presence and awareness. And if not, who cares? You always have the five-star option of soft entry without erection.

Remember, true erection is a by-product of consciousness, love, and presence. It is a magical electromagnetic response to a unique set of circumstances, as explained in chapter 6, which deals with erection in more detail.

The Role of Women's Breasts in Male Erection

The wisest place to give a woman loving attention is her breasts. Woman experience their deepest orgasmic experiences through melting into their breasts. As mentioned earlier, in chapter 4, breasts are the positive dynamic poles of the female body, from which sexual energy is awakened. After some time of relaxing into her breasts (and being supported by her man), a woman will usually feel an overflow, experience a vibrant response, in her vagina. Woman's body then becomes filled with a deep yearning for penetration, and her body and being give an unconditional "yes." When a woman has a strong inner connection to her breasts, the spontaneous erection response is likely to happen more easily (as described in chapter 6).

Woman needs to feel her own breasts for herself, from within. You cannot do the internal feeling for her, but you can definitely create the situation that helps her to feel into, and sense, her breasts from the inside. You can touch both breasts at the same time if you are in a position that allows for a two-hand hold. Otherwise, touching just one breast is also fine, and the woman may wish to touch her other breast herself.

How to Hold the Breasts

With open hands, cup the breasts while lifting upward from underneath them. Let the hand contact be "porous," not compressing or squashing the sensitive breast tissue. Then take your attention into your hands; relax your hands, arms, and shoulders; and simply be present and melt into your hands and into her breasts. Mold your hands to fit the contours. Send love, light, warmth, energy, and good vibrations through your hands into the woman's breasts.

There is no need to stimulate the nipples directly, especially the favored radio-tuner style. Some women become hypersensitive to direct touch of the nipples. For other women, nipple stimulation raises the level of excitement and sometimes triggers orgasm (for both), so they choose to keep things cool. Talk about what kind of touch or hold feels good and helps your woman gain an inner connection to her breasts. Reaching around her body to hold her breasts while you embrace her from behind (right hand—right breast, left hand—left breast) can be a beautifully opening and healing experience for a woman. Right hand on the left breast, left hand on the right breast is also a possibility, where man's arms cross over in front of woman's body. But be careful when crossing the arms. Doing so can make the embrace too tight, which squashes the woman, effectively compressing her energy field and her capacity for relaxation and expansion. She may want to escape your hold instead.

In the situation where a woman has had surgical removal of her breast or breasts, the deeper energy centers remain unaffected. Women will continue to feel the expansion of energy in the breasts even in the absence of the physical breast.

Basically with women there are no general rules to be made. What works one day may not necessarily work the next day. Women are very sensitive to any signs of male intention. Woman can feel immediately if a man has intention behind his touch, and this very often closes down her body. Drop your agendas and programming when you are with a woman. Just be present in yourself and in your heart, sharing your being, touching, and caressing with love. Finding a touch without intention is a subtle art.

In the past it may have appeared that a woman functions counter to the man, in that she demands this, needs that, and has many preconditions to be satisfied before she opens sexually. But we now realize that the obstacle is due to a misunderstanding about her body, and not some kind of mental resistance, personality difference, or lack of interest in sex. Sadly, during the lifetime of a woman the female sexual energy is not often awakened sufficiently for her to have deep orgasmic experiences.

By beginning with her breasts instead of stimulating her clitoris, you will access a woman's sexual energy on a profound inner level. The more a man is able to simply wait for his woman's sexual temperature to rise, to meet and equal his own sexual temperature, the more satisfying the sexual experience is likely to be. Man's deepest longing is to bring woman to orgasmic fulfillment and feel her love flowing toward him.

Oral Sex and Masturbation

Oral sex and mutual masturbation are given a great deal of emphasis in the conventional style of sex because of their stimulating and exciting effects. When we start to create a more relaxed and sensitive environment, the need for stimulation is reduced. So it is possible that in time some things that you previously enjoyed or gave a value to slip out of significance because they no longer serve you. Many men have told us that they reduced their masturbation habit when they experienced how it was having a desensitizing effect on the tissues of the penis.

You may also find another way to do the same thing, remembering that "tantra denies nothing but transforms everything." Touch yourself or the other with love and awareness. Bring their or your body to life, a state of being awake and alert. Get into your senses and sensuality. Expand the pleasure through relaxation. Explore the valleys long before you think of heading for the peak, or perhaps you don't even bother to go there this time. Experiment with how it feels to retain your vital juices.

TANTRIC KISSING

Learning to kiss tantric style has great value. You begin to really enjoy kissing and become incredibly kissable at the same time. Some women say they experience kissing as more intimate than sexual union.

Anyone can be an excellent kisser. Just relax your lips with your mouth lightly closed, bring your full attention into your lips, and become present in them. Tantric kissing is done with full, sustained lip contact. This means you don't stop; you stay connected. You remain joined at the lips, which are fused in a relaxed, sensual fashion. You get together and stay together, so a tantric lip kiss can easily last a few hours. Each person enters the lips with presence and awareness, becoming their lips.

The tongue is usually not used in tantric-style kissing; or if it is, only a little, and delicately. Perhaps the tip of your tongue gently caresses the lips. The famous French tongue kiss can cause a sharp rise in the level of man's excitement and encourage early ejaculation, which means the tongue ought to be used with caution.

Like most things, kissing takes practice, so do not abandon the tantric kiss before you "get it." Suddenly one day it will click. There is nothing obvious to be seen from the outside (except that you do not stop)—a kiss is a kiss—but from within, the experience can be electrifying.

POSITIONS DURING SEX

Positions are relatively unimportant. One position is as good as the next if you enjoy it and it works for you. What is most important is to be present in a position and for the position to enhance the correspondence of penis and vagina, so that it encourages and supports the flow of life force. In general, the actual physical fitting together is maintained as much as possible in any given situation.

Changing Positions through Rotating Moves

Changing position increases awareness and enhances presence. Positions can be changed regularly in order to renew and refresh the environment of the penis and vagina. Positions can be changed when there is a need to move, the pull to sleep, or the urge to stretch.

The sequences of what we call rotating positions are shown in figures 7.1 and 7.2. These are changes of position using circular, dimensional movements, rotating around a focal point—penis inside the vagina. As the bodies move, they endeavor to maintain the connection between penis and vagina. If the penis slips out, just quickly slip it in again. Man can do it, woman can do it—whatever is easiest. Nothing is lost if this happens, but a sense of humor helps.

The starting point of the sequences in figures 7.1 and 7.2 is the scissors position used for soft penetration as described in chapter 6. Scissors is a good beginning position—man on his side, woman on her back, relaxed and easy for both. Scissors position is equally wonderful for slow penetration with erection and is a comfortable position for a short sleep.

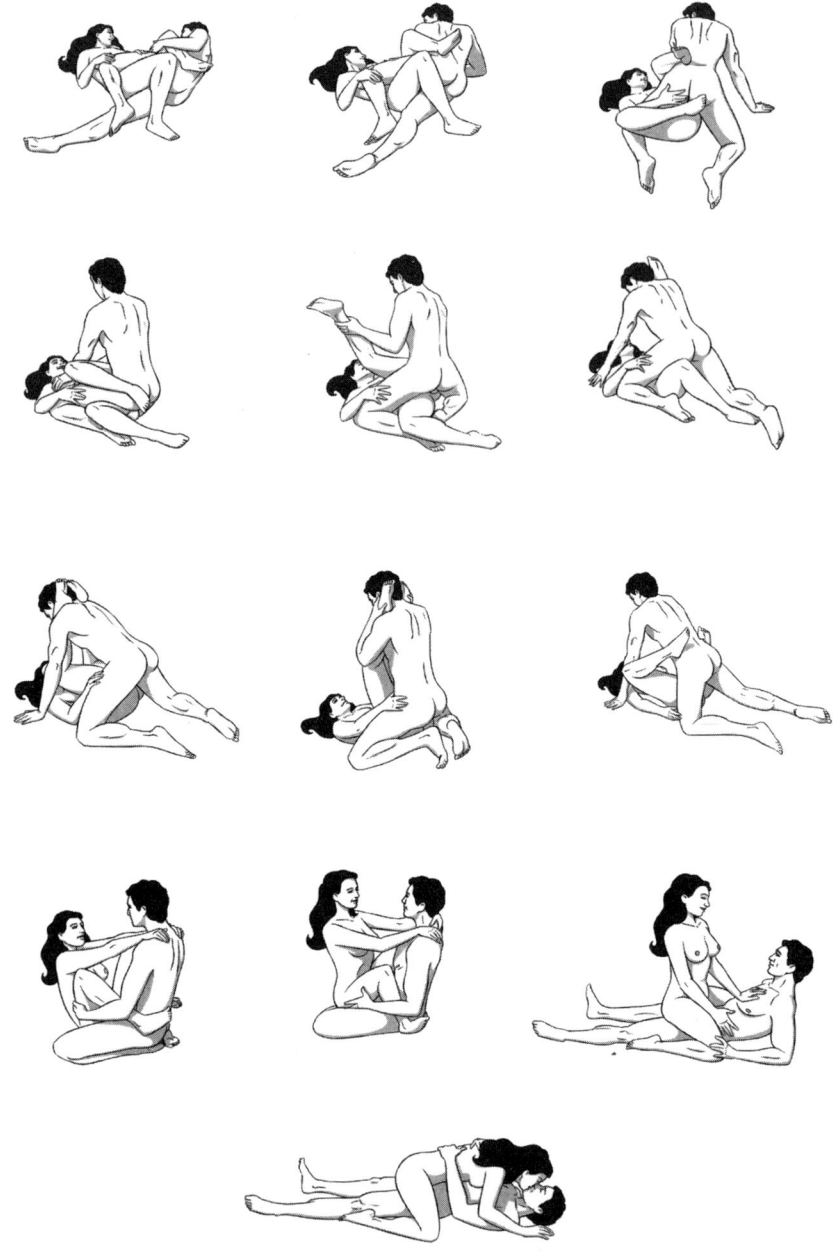

Fig. 7.1. Sequence of rotating positions through front approach

Dates, Foreplay, Kissing, and Positions

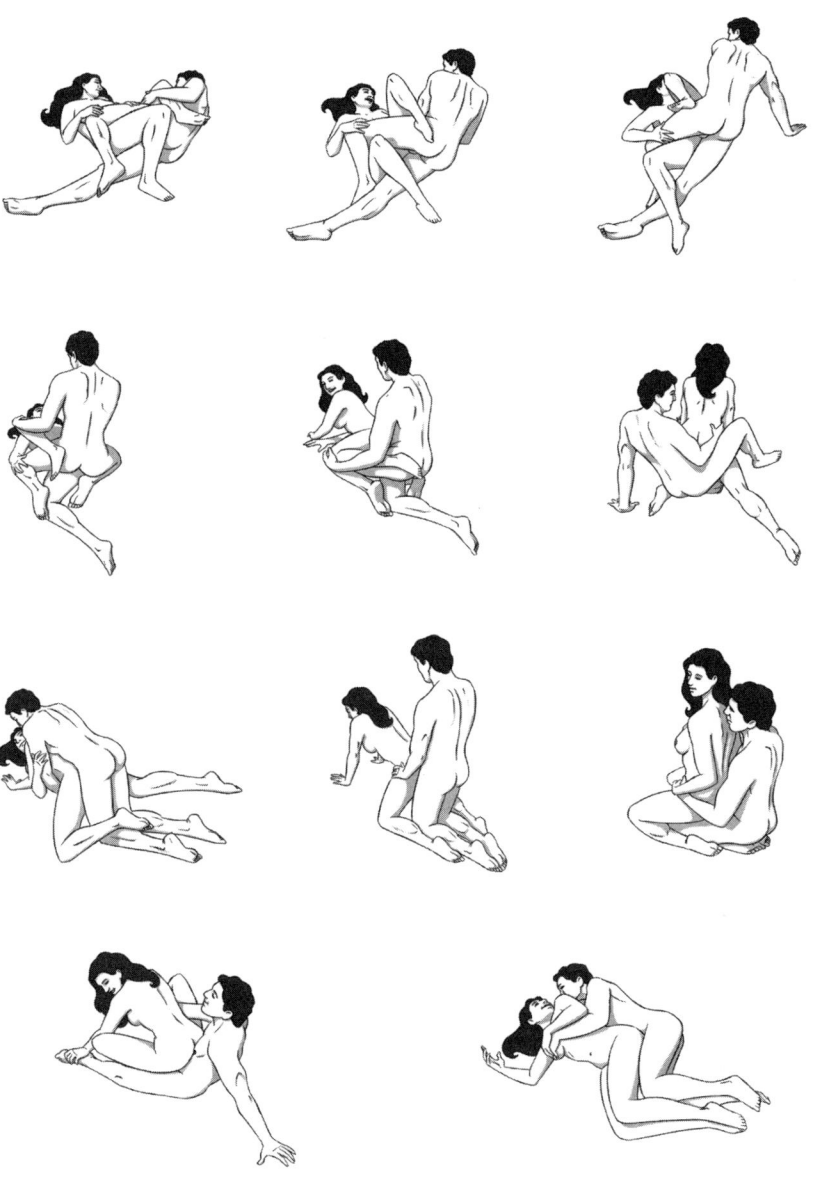

Fig. 7.2. Sequence of rotating positions through rear approach

After five, fifteen, or fifty minutes the position can be changed, as often as necessary, as often as desired. Shifts in position can be done slowly, all movements in a deliberate, step-by-step, unhurried, unfolding and rearranging of bodies.

> **Tantric Inspiration**
>
> And while making love, forget about orgasm. Rather, be in a relaxed state, relax into each other. The Western mind is continuously thinking about when it is coming and how to make it fast and great and this and that. The thinking does not allow the body energies to function. It does not allow the body to have its own way; the mind goes on interfering . . .
>
> Relax . . . If nothing happens there is no need for anything to happen. If nothing happens then that is what is happening . . . and that too is beautiful! Orgasm is not such a thing that it has to happen every day. Sex should be just being together, just dissolving into each other. Then one can keep making love for half an hour, for one hour, just relaxing into each other. Then you will be of utter mindlessness, because there is no need for the mind. Love is the only thing where the mind is not needed; and that is where the West is wrong: it brings in the mind even there.
>
> OSHO, TRANSCRIBED TEACHINGS,
> *THE OPEN SECRET*

PERSONAL SHARING
Finally Getting Enough

My biggest source of stress has been not getting enough sex. Two factors have helped to considerably diminishing this source of stress. First: I have learned to plan sex. Planned sex! Only a short time ago this would have sounded terrible to me. I thought sex had to be spontaneous, there had to be butterflies in the stomach, and I had to be horny, otherwise it wouldn't work. This has changed totally. Nowadays I am planning sex with my wife. On Mondays at 8 p.m., for at least an hour or two, we make time for love. Week by week we have a second look as to when we want to schedule time for sex. This doesn't eliminate spontaneity. Spontaneous love encounters often happen when we're on vacation, but during the normal workweek, it happens rather seldom. With this schedule we make time for something that is very important for both of us. For me this is a great relaxation from the tension of not getting enough. I know that at least once, and maybe twice, per week I will have sex. Wonderful, isn't it? The reason planned sex is nearly always possible is because of tantra. I learned to meet my wife without focusing on sexual desire and excitement. Nowadays I seldom use the word sex; I talk about making love. When we make love, we first tune in, in the form of a common meditation. Each time it is a treat to encounter myself, to open up, to go into my own male power before engaging with my wife. For some time we had put aside meditation preceding lovemaking. Then we often got caught up in discussions, the energy didn't flow, or just about nothing else happened. Generally the lovemaking gets easier, more loving, and more intense if I meditate beforehand.

Secondly: Through tantra, our love is lifted into a totally new dimension. It is fulfilling, sustaining, and very alive. The knack is (and this is really true) to be aware of myself during the lovemaking. This is the opposite of my previous belief that I should do anything possible to make the sex act enjoyable for my wife, and my expectation that she would lead me to a great orgasm as soon as possible.

Tantric Inspiration

In meditation, if two meditators share their energies, love is a constant phenomenon. It does not change. It takes on the quality of eternity. It becomes divine. The meeting of love and meditation is the greatest experience in life, and only then does duality between man and woman disappear.

OSHO, TRANSCRIBED TEACHINGS,
THE REBELLIOUS SPIRIT

8
SEXUAL HEALING AND MALE AUTHORITY

Every fifth woman a man meets in the Western world is likely to have been sexually abused, according to official statistics, and this number does not include women who prefer not to disclose their histories. Perhaps we can even say that every woman has been inadvertently abused or misused to a certain extent, due to the relatively aggressive and hard (unconscious) conventional style of sex. Culturally there is deep misunderstanding about the female body and the way it opens and responds to male energy (see chapter 4). Likewise, because of lack of awareness and information, the way men generally use their bodies in sex is actually abusive to their intrinsic male energy and creates a kind of "overcharge" or disturbance in their systems.

Many men feel a heartfelt concern and unease about the pain and suffering women have been subjected to through sex. At the same time, men feel quite helpless and powerless, and unable to extend support or healing to women on such a sensitive level. Sexual abuse has long-lasting, injurious effects on the life of a woman. The memories in her body and the scars in her psyche can fundamentally affect her capacity to love and enjoy her body and sex. At times in a relationship, abuse issues from the past can reappear out of the blue, become reactivated in the present, and turn into a source of conflict and unhappiness. A man may even carry a lurking guilt about sex in general, in view of the sexual injustices a woman may have experienced in her past. Following the guidelines below will give man a positive alternative and direction for his energy, which is just as beneficial and healing for him as it is for a woman.

This chapter is dedicated to sexual healing and male authority and completes the generative or meditative sexual orientation that we give our retreat participants toward the end of the weeklong retreat. A few threads from themes of earlier chapters will be picked up and drawn together here into a single frame. There will be glancing references to aspects previously addressed in more detail.

VAGINA, NOT CLITORIS

Here we will explain in concrete terms how to deepen our sensitivity so that man and woman become more sensitized in relation to each other. We first need to examine the role of the clitoris and how this has affected woman's capacity to receive. In conventional sex, the clitoris is generally considered by both women and men to be central to female sexuality and orgasm. This leads to a tendency to focus on the clitoral area, which actually lies well outside of the vagina. In addition, within the first few inches of the vagina are some muscular rings that constrict the penis, stimulating it slightly with pleasurable sensations. Because of these considerations, the movement of the penis usually consists of short, repeated, frictionlike thrusts that enter only the first part of the vagina.

These two factors have also caused an external focus in woman, so that her awareness is drawn downward, toward the front of the vaginal/

clitoral area, and away from the deeper regions of the vagina, where, in fact, she is most receptive. Often during hard sex women deliberately have to contract the vagina to close and protect the sensitive cervix (as mentioned before) because it can be painful. Sometimes the deeper area will also contract and "close down" due to the tension of old memories buried deep in the vaginal tissues. These stored memories might include overstepped boundaries, aggressive sex, abusive sex, rape, abortion, gynecological visits, or even anxiety learned from parents or church.

Female Receptivity and Stored Tension

Anxiety, memories, and the external focus on the clitoris result in the deeper regions of the vagina moving out of woman's awareness and thereby becoming a bit inaccessible. There will usually be a corresponding lack of awareness and vitality higher in the vagina. At the same time, most women recognize the significance of this deeper place in their bodies and would like their man to stay deep within what we call the "garden of love" that lies at the entrance to the uterus—the cervix. Even if a woman has had her garden of love area (or the entire uterus) surgically removed for medical reasons, the energy center remains intact and will continue to be a place where woman longs to be touched. But in the normal course of events, man usually reverses out again before woman has a chance to say a word. The place where she is most receptive, most feminine, and best able to experience divine feminine nectar is not available to her, and thereby not available to her man. When an area is closed down there is a lack of inner perception or sensitivity, which can affect a woman's receptivity and sexual experience.

For example, if a woman has a history of sexual abuse, therapy can help to release the trauma, but memory fragments usually remain stored on a cellular level in the tissues, disturbing female receptivity. Fortunately, by the grace of nature, we have been given one magical instrument that can remove these memories and tensions from a woman and awaken her receptivity and femininity—the penis. There are other methods of internal vaginal massage that release tensions by using a finger. However, compared to the magnetic, silky head of the penis, the tip of the finger is almost as rough and crude as sandpaper. Further, there is no real energetic connection between fingers and vagina when compared to the inherent electromagnetic potential between penis and vagina.

THE PENIS AS HEALING CATALYST

The head of the penis is like a highly sensitive magnet with the capacity to draw out disturbing tension. It purifies vaginal tissues, purifying itself in the process, so that there is a reciprocal cycle of purification. Men have their own accumulated traumas and memories from the way we have used and abused our penises. And many men have also been victims of childhood sexual abuse, and carry memories and tensions relating to the experience.

It's important to realize that the penis is not like a vacuum cleaner that sucks up all the woman's tension, leaving you stuck with a full bag. It is more like a catalyst that precipitates the release of tension. The penis causes tension to be released from the system. Through this process man's tensions soften, his male energy gets refined, and the penis loses its overcharge and becomes more supple, pliable, sensitive, and relaxed.

This is very good news, because while an unconscious penis can cause a lot of damage, a conscious penis can create tremendous healing. One of the reasons why the world is suffering from so much war and so many natural disasters is that male and female forces are out of balance. Over the centuries woman (and the feminine energy) has not been treated at all nicely, and while it's perhaps less obvious in Western society, the way woman is still treated today in some cultures is shocking. Man has used and abused woman for his own selfish reasons and when she was no longer interesting, thrown her away and taken another woman. Frequently woman is also used by man to discharge his inner tensions and emotions (see chapter 9). Even if this is not your personal history as a man, the collective human memories over centuries are probably stored in every woman.

Conscious Love Can Heal the Past

By entering woman consciously, in love and presence, man can have an impact on the larger planetary imbalance. It's as if woman is burdened with this collective past that she cannot shake off, but which can be "displaced" and released by a conscious, loving penis—freeing woman and bringing her back to her essential self, which is love. And in purifying woman of her tensions, man is also purified. There is an innate circle of reciprocity; man heals and balances woman, who in turn heals and balances man. By welcoming man in at this level, woman brings him into a state of purity, relaxation, and love (as opposed to fostering the insecure, defensive, and aggressive stance that leads to war). Nature is truly remarkable.

There is a beautiful talk by Barry Long called "Love Brings All to Life," in which he recounts the Greek myth of Pygmalion (see Recommended Books and Resources). Pygmalion was a sculptor who carved a life-sized statue of what he considered to be the perfect woman—the woman of his dreams. He worked passionately, and when he was finally finished, he fell in love with her. He caressed and admired his idealized woman in stone with so much tenderness, so much love and longing that the statue came to life.

Long perceived contemporary women as being in a similar situation. Woman comes into this world already a bit hard, a bit stoney and protective, and for very good reason. She has been abused and misused for much too long, so she is often born with defenses and not truly open to love. Long said that like Pygmalion, man must use the power of his love to soften and melt woman so that she can give up her hardness and protection and return to being pure love.

Female versus Male Essence

Woman in her essence is pure, unconditional love. Man in his essence is pure presence, pure meditation. There are two ways, or polarities, on the spiritual path: one is of love and devotion, and the other is of meditation, presence, and being here now. Osho says these are the two highest polarities in existence; love is female, and presence is male. As woman relaxes in love, meditation or presence grows by itself. As man relaxes into meditation and being present, unconditional and pure love grows by itself.

Through cellular purification woman can once again experience her birthright as pure love. Likewise, man learns to relax into his essence rooted in the present and, very specifically, present in woman in his penis. This is what a woman most wants from a man, that he be present to her. She is not so interested in a great performance as a lover, but that man be present to her while he is inside her. Some men may question this, because often women ask for hard and aggressive sex, but this is more a reflection of her sexual conditioning whereby she has become slightly male herself. It is up to woman to examine this response pattern in herself.

STAYING PRESENT

The capacity to be present really defines what it means to be a man, particularly in light of our cultural confusion. Men are looking for some kind of male authority, but what does it actually mean to be a man? It is nothing less or more than the capacity to be present.

If man can be present in woman—not enter her with a hungry or demanding penis (an emotional penis, see chapter 9), but with a penis that is loving in the here and now—then the penis can begin to "catalyze" what has accumulated in the female body and allow her to relax and transform into pure love—the true quality of woman. For a man there is nothing more gratifying than to see transformation happening before your eyes. Far from being a burden or a job, it feels more like a noble task, an honor to be in woman in a conscious way. To be a chosen one. It gives me (Michael) a certain trust in myself—a male authority. Many men confide at the end of the retreat that they finally have a constructive vision of manhood, and that it is a life-changing experience. And yes, when you cooperate with your sexual nature you do mature and emerge as more of a man. You are more present, relaxed, and connected to your being; you are a more loving human being.

Altering History

Man can do tremendous damage to woman because she represents the container, the space, the environment. Man can leave all his tensions there for selfish reasons, but by putting himself in a larger frame of mind, he actually has the power to change the course of history. That which has been out of balance for thousands of years can start to change today.

There are no mass solutions for the world's problems. There is only one solution, and it starts with this man and this woman. If you can bring the balance back, here in this couple create harmony between man and woman, you do true peace work for the world. And really, there is no other way. You will see that when balance is created here, in the relationship, it radiates out to the world in a palpable way. So sometimes perhaps we feel, "Oh, this is boring . . . not so exciting." Always put yourself into a bigger frame of mind, remembering that we are connected to a much greater energy field encompassing all of us.

DEEP, SUSTAINED PENETRATION

How do we go about deepening polarity, purification, and healing on a practical level? When erection is present you enter the vagina very slowly (see chapter 6), and you look for places that feel painful, strange, weird, or numb—and you stay exactly on that spot. Sensitive, painful spots can be anywhere—just inside the entrance of the vagina, along the walls, or in the upper regions, the "garden of love." Woman will help you to identify these places. We suggest you maintain soft eye contact as described in chapter 7. Open eyes help to keep you present and available, and subtle reactions and responses expressed in her eyes can sometimes give you information about what is happening internally.

Usually pain is something we avoid; we do not like to touch sensitive areas, naturally, because doing so is painful. But now we are intentionally looking for them. Pain or lack of sensitivity (deadness) indicates held tension and memories in the vaginal tissues. By going in there very consciously, with great awareness, it's possible to contact these areas with the penis. Woman will usually allow this because you do not push into the pain, you just want to gently contact the pain. You make a "porous" contact with the area. You don't want to push hard against the vaginal walls, because that would reinforce woman's protective instinct. You find a sensitive area, and then you pull back a hairsbreadth—more like a withdrawal of intention. This creates space for an interaction of energies, so that things can shift. You just stay there without moving; you sustain the contact in the depths. Your woman can use simple words to communicate what is happening, and you can do the same. This begins a journey of discovery over a period of time, touching all sides of the vagina, the entire canal, seeking out those areas we usually avoid.

If a woman has pain at the very entrance of the vagina, you can just place the head of your penis there and let it rest. Often penetration becomes very painful when women go through menopause, and this approach relaxes the tension. If the movement of the penis in the vagina has a burning sensation for a woman, it can mean that the entry is too fast. Ask your woman if she feels any burning. If she does, stop, withdraw half an inch or so, and wait for a little while to enable the vaginal tissues to soften and relax. Then move again, very slowly, and stop as soon as your woman again reports burning sensations. At times an additional, generous application of oil to the head of the penis and to the vaginal lips and opening will counteract any burning sensations.

Some women experience painful penetration throughout their sexual lives. Recently a woman in our group had a pain-free penetration for the very first time in her life, after forty years of every sexual experience being painful. Just the head of the penis can do so much healing, so try this healing approach any time you wish. Let it be a new orientation. Pain is interesting; it is a doorway, and there is usually treasure hidden behind that pain.

Loss of Erection

When you find painful areas and stay in contact with them, you might suddenly start to lose your erection. Usually when this happens we will try to get the erection back as fast as possible, but now in this new situation we understand that this is the way the penis does the job. When the penis has done its job, it is going to be relaxed, naturally. Like everything in life, there is an active phase and a passive phase, but in sex we want an active erection all the time, 100 percent.

If you accept this relaxation of the penis from time to time and do not interfere with its withdrawal, you allow your penis the opportunity to regenerate. Often, just as the penis is about to slip out of the vagina entirely, it will again begin reaching out, spiraling upward and erecting in the vagina (see chapter 6). Soon you may get the feeling that the genitals themselves are making love and that actually they know how to do it better. It is almost like handing the intelligence back to the body, and it is such a remarkable experience that you can almost lean back and watch the show.

Trust Your Penis

The experience of my penis responding of its own accord gives me a trust in myself, because basically we men do not trust our penises; they are not completely reliable. But when I know that this is going to be the process, then I can trust my penis, and that gives me trust in myself as a man. I no longer feel I need to be strong or ambitious, need to prove this and that. My definition of man has changed. The only thing that is required from me, as man, is to be present, to develop the capacity to be here now. Then miracles are possible.

When there is erection, you enter as far as you can go and sustain the penetration; you stay where you are. We call this deepening polarity through deep, sustained penetration, because as the woman gets more receptive, man gets more dynamic, and the potential between male and female poles increases. In general in your life, as a style of lovemaking, you begin to "hang out" deep in the vagina, allowing the dynamic and receptive forces to start to play with each other. Here woman is "minus" while man is "plus," and any obstructions (tensions) lying in the way of this moving magnetic force are displaced so that healing, purification, and regeneration can take place.

The effects of deep, sustained penetration also work with and through condoms; the energy exchange is relatively unaffected (see more about condoms in chapter 6).

Effectiveness and Penis Length

Some men worry that the penis may not be long enough to reach all the way up to the "garden of love." Both women and men have reported to us that the cervix also seems to be drawn downward as it reaches for the head of the penis. Always remind yourself that these are energetic phenomena, not purely physical, and the energy exchange works in any case. Even with a soft, relaxed penis that remains still within the first couple of inches of the vagina, purification and healing is taking place.

Unexpected Ejaculation

During deep, sustained penetration, at times a woman's buried tensions are suddenly discharged down the vagina, almost like a rush or wave of excitement. This can easily cause a man to ejaculate instantly, without any warning. Should it happen, do not feel something went wrong—it's a natural part of the purification process.

ALLOW OLD FEELINGS TO SURFACE

As you make love and pay attention to places in the vagina that are painful or numb, it is likely that for your partner tears, sadness, or anger may come to the surface. You yourself might experience similar feelings. This is all good. These feelings are trapped and held in the body, and the old must come out to create space for the new. Expressing previously unexpressed feelings (see chapter 9) cleanses our poles, our genitals, and our bodies become more sensitive and sensitized. One becomes increasingly receptive, the other increasingly dynamic.

Don't try to figure out what's happening when old, buried feelings or emotions emerge. Thinking about what is going on distances you from the experience, so just stay with the feelings and allow them to flow. Sometimes spontaneous understanding will occur, an insight into the source of the pain, but not necessarily. Healing takes place in any event.

If uncomfortable feelings start to arise, be aware that it is not the fault of your partner. Your partner is simply a trigger to help you to retrieve the past. Old feelings stored in the cells are going to rise to the surface, offering the opportunity to finally express feelings you may have been storing since childhood. So if suddenly a lot of tears come up, don't think, "Oh, now I have to be alone to deal with my old feelings" (see "golden rules" in chapter 9). No, it is the genital connection that is triggering the release of old feelings, so just stay together inside each other. Or if suddenly anger pops up, which can easily happen, you can simply explain, "I'm just really angry, I have to move this energy." Then you disconnect and quickly do something physical, like jumping up and down, to burn up the anger. As soon as you feel the wave of anger has passed, climb back into bed and continue making love. Through a polarity exchange, purification is happening on both sides, and it changes your whole experience and sense of yourselves as man and woman.

Self-healing

We talk more frequently about the abuse of women, because they do suffer more abuse, but many men, too, are carrying a history of pain, insecurity, and self- or other-inflicted abuse in their bodies, so it is important to understand that sexual healing is not only for woman. It really is a self-healing that happens through awareness and channeling and directing energy in a constructive way. After a time any pains will usually disappear.

Sometimes you might lie in bed and just cry and cry, perhaps not only for yourself, but for all of humanity. If you allow yourself to be washed through, you will experience how much it empowers you to feel the pain of humanity flowing through you. So avoid trying to understand what's going on; just accept it with gratitude.

When we first met we spent days and days, three weeks crying. I (Michael) don't know what or why, except that it was just wonderful. It felt like very old pain, and at the same time was exquisitely beautiful.

Communicate, Share, Express

As you make love in this way you communicate all of what's happening—strange feelings, numbness, beautiful sensations—in simple words. Do not try to explain anything; just acknowledging is enough. Sometimes when tension is released there is laughter. So whether it is tears, laughter, shivering, shaking, or sweating, simply allow it and be with it. These are all signs of the body purifying and detoxifying the cells of past memories.

POSITIONS SUITABLE FOR DEEP, SUSTAINED PENETRATION

Since the painful places can be anywhere in the entire vagina and cervix area, there is quite a lot of room to explore, and many angles can be used. A variety of positions are suitable, as suggested in the diagrams (see figures 8.1–8.7). However, even subtle shifts of the penis in the vagina, moving one centimeter and staying there, represent a shift in position. You do not have to always move your entire body, but instead reach to different parts of the vagina through subtle shifts in the angle of the pelvis. Positions are covered in more depth in chapter 7, where the basic guideline is that positions per se are not as significant as the level of awareness that a person brings to them. Any position is perfect when it feels right.

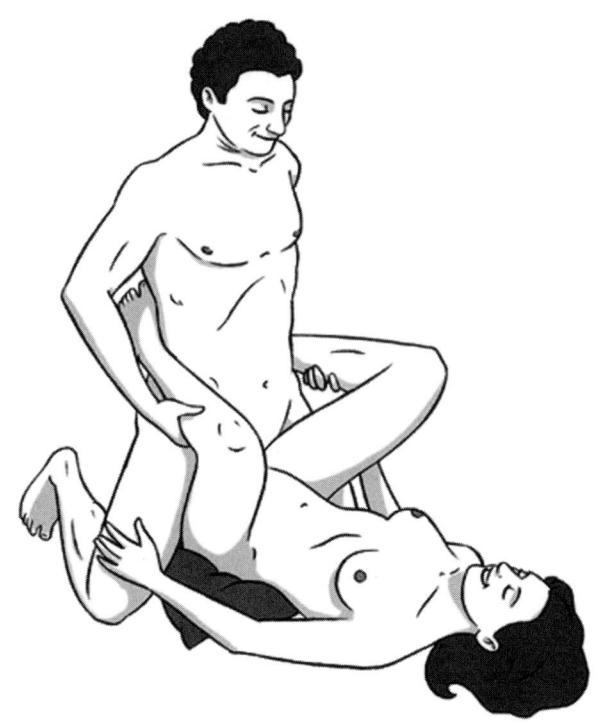

Fig. 8.1. Middle position, man kneeling
(with pillow to raise woman's pelvis)

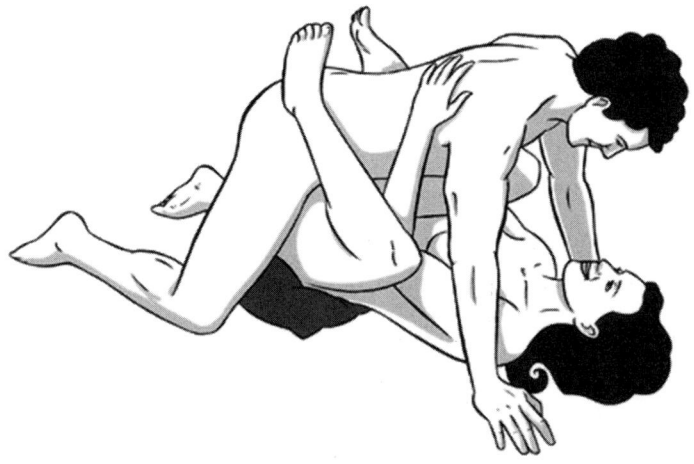

Fig. 8.2. Middle position, man on hands and knees
(with pillow to raise woman's pelvis)

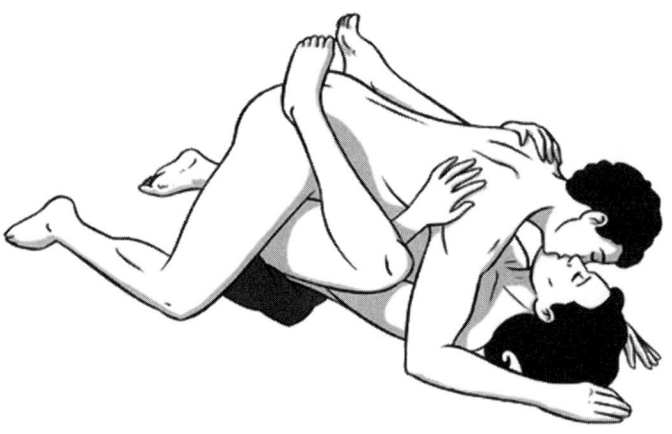

Fig. 8.3. Middle position, man lying forward, half kneeling (with pillow to raise woman's pelvis)

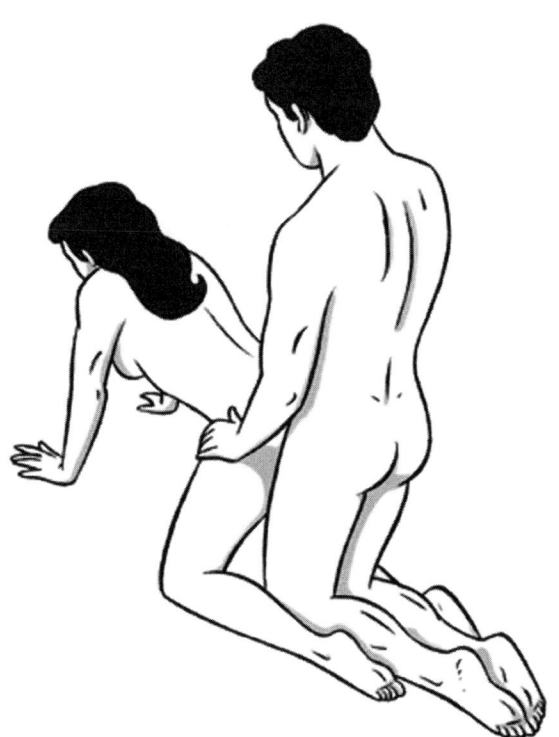

Fig. 8.4. Rear position with man kneeling

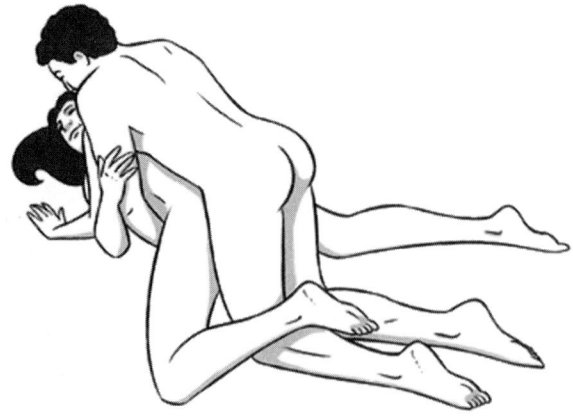

Fig. 8.5. Rear position with man lying on top of woman

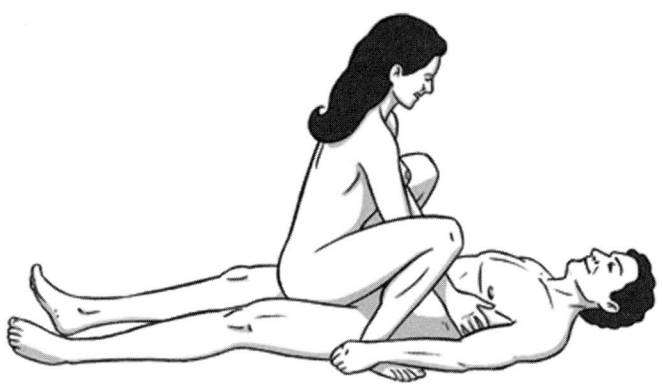

Fig. 8.6. Woman sitting on top

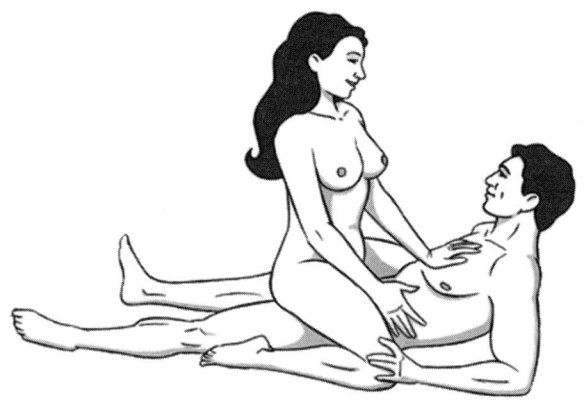

Fig. 8.7. Woman kneeling on top

PARTNERING WITH WOMEN

If woman has the garden of love, then we men are the "gardeners of love." We have to take care, remove the weeds, and plant roses. When man becomes rooted in his penis as a positive force, he experiences true male authority with the capacity to heal woman of her past. Sex can be lived as a spiritual, loving meditative force, becoming the roots of powerful self-healing and transformation.

On the surface it may appear as if man has to tune into woman and do it her way, or that tantra is for women and not for men, but the issue extends to deeper levels. In making love from the inner dimension, man will discover his true male authority. He will certainly feel a new authority or competence when he is able to open the heart of woman with his penis. Allowing woman to be the guide may be unexpectedly fulfilling. Yes, after thousands of years it does seem intelligent to make a change, and to realize that it is for male empowerment in the long term. If we want to have more love in our lives, make love to women, and have women want to make love to us, we have to allow women to help us to find our true inner man.

Easy, Natural Orgasms

Often woman say, "I don't really feel that I lose energy with the conventional orgasm. How does this fit into the picture?" The approach to take regarding orgasm is not to take an approach. You don't want to go looking for orgasm, hunting or pushing for it. But when an orgasm happens easily and naturally, with no effort, then it is beautiful. So first a woman really has to observe and ask herself, "Am I relaxing into the moment or am I pursuing—even a little bit—orgasm?" In general, if woman allows the clitoris to be more passive and fade into the background, she will find it easier to take her awareness higher up into the vagina where her divine energies are accessed.

Woman's Healing Contribution

Basically women, as the receptive element, are very vulnerable; their one and only defense is to deny man entry. Women's no to sex can be a reflection of a painful personal or collective history, but in either case it's a by-product of our cultural lack of sexual information. So what a woman can do for this healing process is to start to say yes to man when he is committed to being conscious inside her. Woman can begin to allow him in so that healing can begin. She can step beyond sexual politics and invite the male force inside of her. Through this a tremendous amount of healing is possible for both woman and man.

Over the centuries sex and love have become two separate things entirely. Much too often sex has nothing to do with love, but when a woman allows man to enter and be present in her in consciousness, aspects that have been separated for centuries can reunite. Sex (the lower vibration) and love (the higher vibration) of the same life force become one expression. When we understand how bodies cooperate, we can completely change our inherited sexual patterns.

PERSONAL SHARING
The Joy of Feeling Welcome

Tantra helps me to tap in to the unexplored aspects of my being. Even without pursuing the goal of becoming more conscious of deep-rooted patterns, primal fears come up from time to time while practicing tantra. And at the same time, it leads me into dimensions, takes me toward energies I would not have reached and felt without tantra and without my wife. The following situation brings up the most significant sensations: Whenever my penis is softly lying in the vagina of my wife, its mere presence creates a deep connection between the male and the female pole. I have the sense that I am pulled in by her vagina, yet I also feel that by my penis stiffening, my male energy is growing into my woman. The sensation of being pulled in to her vagina is one of the most beautiful feelings that I know. It tells me on a very deep level: "You are welcome." One of my deepest fears is that I might not be welcome, so to experience this welcome again and again relaxes me in the depths of my soul. This fear is a basic fear of all manhood. Many men have confirmed this by sharing with me that they personally have this primal fear. When I first had this experience of being pulled in to a woman (during the tantra course) I was simply overwhelmed. I had never expected to experience being so deeply welcomed, ever in my life. I just cried with joy, but also because such a deep pain started to be released. Today I can honestly say that the fear of not being welcome, not getting enough and being rejected, has largely been healed.

PERSONAL SHARING
Penis Tension Resolved

Besides the changes on the spiritual-energetic level, I also feel changes on the physical plane. Previously, when I touched the top of my penis, the sensation was always partly unpleasant. It made me back off inside and become tense. I experienced that as a defensive tension in the tissue. As far as I can remember, it had always been like that. Four months after the tantra course, this unpleasant part dissolved and has not returned. I am surprised by this experience, but it teaches me that my body becomes soft, vulnerable, and receptive through tantra.

The most important experience with tantra is that each time it is different; nothing happens twice in the exact same way. It's like life itself—every day brings something new. Therefore, I experience tantra as a precious teacher for my whole life.

Tantric Inspiration

What is love? Love is the fragrance, the radiance of knowing oneself, of being oneself. . . . Love is overflowing joy. Love is when you have seen who you are; and then there is nothing left except to share your being with others. Love is when you have seen that you are not separate from existence. Love is when you have felt an organic orgasmic unity with all that is. Love is not a relationship. Love is a state of being. It has nothing to do with anybody else. One is not in love; one is love. And of course, when one is love, one is in love—but that is an outcome, a by-product, that is not the source. The source is that one is love.

OSHO, TRANSCRIBED TEACHINGS,
THE GUEST

9
MASTERING LOVE AND OVERCOMING EMOTIONS

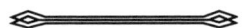

Tantra sees human energy in terms of polarity: feminine energy as "being" and masculine energy as "doing." Within woman, the inner masculine is active, logical, and result oriented; and in man, the inner feminine is receptive, intuitive, and process oriented. Tantra takes a step further to say that the highest spiritual polarity in existence is love and meditation, that woman embodies love and man embodies meditation. This implies that woman's inner man is meditative and man's inner woman is loving.

To be whole human beings, operating with wisdom, passion, authenticity, and spontaneity, we need to master both energies: masculine and feminine, meditation and love. Woman becomes more meditative the more she loves, and man becomes more loving the more he meditates. In more precise sexual language, to love in woman means to welcome the penis in and surrender to its power, and to meditate in man means to merge with, and become fully present in, his penis, inside woman, in stillness.

DISTINGUISHING BETWEEN EMOTIONS AND FEELINGS

Deep personal and societal wounding prevents many of us from balancing our energies in a way that serves us. We repress the memories of our hurts, suppress our real feelings and energies, and then unconsciously begin to control or manipulate others, or fail to channel our energies in a wise or creative direction. As we change the way we make love, we initiate an alchemical process of awakening the inner, opposite polarity, which will, in time, enable us to use both energies powerfully and productively. This, in turn, helps us to dissolve emotional patterns that have caused us pain in the past and enables us to create the life and love we long for in the present.

To create the life of sustained, loving harmony that so many of us wish for, an important step is to keep emotion out of love. As Osho says, "Love is a state of being," and "One is not in love, one is love . . . it has nothing to do with anybody else." With the new input about harnessing polarity and our orgasmic potential, we might be able to conceive of days of "being love" as a sustained state that is not associated with the highs and lows of relationships. But what about these highs and the painfully difficult, emotion-laden lows, when love becomes scrambled up with irreconcilable feelings and fears? Despair or resignation can set in when a couple can see no way out of the cycle of conflicts.

Regaining our power in love is dependent on knowing the difference between feelings and emotions, knowing that "love has to be separated from this category of emotions." (See the tantric inspiration at the end of this chapter.) It is crucial to understand that emotion comes from the past, while love and true feelings arise in the present. When too much "emotional baggage" from the past gets dragged into everyday life, love is quick to wane; love flourishes in the delicacy of the now. That doesn't mean emotion is some kind of demon. Emotion is understandable, but it's important to be aware that you are emotional and to know what is happening, when it is happening. The recognition of emotionality causes a big shift in the maturity of an individual and a couple.

Symptoms of Emotion

Until now we have had no frame of reference to understand what is truly going on in the split second in which emotions surface—the instant when, seemingly out of the blue, the love boat begins to rock dangerously. What we need is self-awareness. The immediate physical symptoms of emotion can be described variously as "suddenly feeling paralyzed" or as if "a wall suddenly comes down." You may experience a jumble of feelings you can't put into words, find it impossible to look the other in the eyes, or have the awkward sensation of feeling disconnected from everything, utterly separate, lonely, totally misunderstood, and physically collapsed. Often we find ourselves feeling vengeful and wanting to hurt back. We start blaming our partner for the situation, using the accusing words, "You never . . ." or "You always . . ." When a breakdown like this takes place, we must recognize that emotion is in play. It takes some practice to recognize emotion, but after a while, it does become obvious.

This inner acknowledgement immediately puts things into better perspective. Emotion is the resurfacing of old or repressed feelings that we were unable to show or express at the time the feeling was actually taking place. This is why emotional reactions are often quite disproportionate to the slight comment or mild action that triggers them. The trigger itself does not usually warrant the huge upset that follows in its wake. It's those old, unexpressed feelings that begin to resonate and bubble to the surface and create confusion. When you acknowledge these old feelings for what they are and work their negative effects out of your system, emotional reactions will begin to diminish. In a few years your partner will be able to say precisely the same words to you, and the comment will slip by you like water off a duck's back.

The Solar Plexus and Emotion

In addition to emotional alarm signals like suddenly feeling paralyzed or disconnected, you can learn to recognize states of emotionality through your solar plexus. Consider this area as a sensor, because here the tensions of emotions can gather and create a lot of discomfort. These tensions try to seek discharge in various ways—through irritation, complaining, nagging, or passing on your frustration to family members or colleagues. When you develop awareness of the solar plexus, the moment someone says something that strikes an uncomfortable chord in you, you will probably notice a response in that part of your body: the sensation of tension or congestion, like having a stone in your stomach, or a hollow, empty, nervous feeling in the stomach. These kinds of body responses let you know that you are emotional and that something unresolved is being triggered. If the solar plexus is free of tension, it allows for unobstructed flow of sexual energy between the genitals and heart. There may be slight feelings of nausea when first relaxing into lovemaking (perhaps more common in woman), but this is nothing to be concerned about. It is a sure sign of the surfacing of old tensions seeking release. Nausea is usually a by-product of the sexual energy expanding, displacing, and cleansing the restricting tensions from the body.

OVERCOMING FEARS CREATED BY LACK OF LOVE

Many people begin experiencing feelings of being separate, wrong, unworthy, or not good enough very early in life, already as young children. We become separate from ourselves, from each other, and from the whole of existence. As we cut off from our pure energy, we also cut off from our love source, and as fear replaces security and joy, a false self gradually develops around us. The fear is due to imprints made by an absence of love in the immediate surroundings (family and parents). It provokes a child into behaving differently in order to try to get approval (or disapproval, through rebellion, where at least some attention is gained) and secure the love so necessary for survival. And so our parents begin to write the script for who we are and how we should behave, and we gradually lose our authenticity.

Emotionality is an unconscious, automatic reaction to a situation or circumstance, like when a switch is flicked off, and light turns to dark. It can even be a learned habit: some people learned to be emotional as young children by mimicking their parents' behavior. As the years go by, we begin to define ourselves according to our emotions, thinking our emotional part is who we really are. It is as if we are in a movie, and the situation is not actually real. Only the past makes it real. (If we were to wake up one morning without our memory, with no past, what then?) But in spirit and essence we are all interested in love, and to keep love alive, love has to be separated from the unconscious backlog of stored emotions. As we begin to release these old feelings consciously (whenever we notice them arising), pieces of the past get healed.

Toxic Emotions and Conventional Sex

Emotions are extremely toxic and will poison the atmosphere by striking deadly blows at the person we most love. This is a big problem; we unconsciously put all our unresolved feelings onto the person we most love and thereby contaminate the love. We say the most awful things to our partner in an attempt to unburden ourselves of our emotions. Emotional statements stick like glue in the mind and revolve endlessly in the thoughts, long after the fight is over. Did she really mean that? Am I really like that? And then the mind will create more emotions from endlessly rethinking the past. In truth, love cannot withstand too much emotion; it is a delicate and fragile flower that requires awareness to keep it blooming. Love will slowly slip through our fingers when we let emotion have the upper hand.

A big source of emotionality lies hidden in sex. When energy moves downward, as it does in conventional sex with its usual discharge, tension and anxiety are by-products. This is why arguments and dissatisfactions easily follow. Sexual tensions eventually create a subtle overpositive charge in man and a subtle false-positive charge in woman. These falsely acquired charges make woman slightly male and distort her essential female qualities. Man's essential qualities are also distorted as he becomes a "tough guy." These accumulating tensions have to be discharged in some fashion, and they are often released through arguing, finding fault with each other, or complaining. When emotions are in the air they easily spawn excitement, which gives rise to the famous fucking-after-a-fight syndrome to heal the rift. But trying to repair the damage through sex and ejaculation/orgasm is a vicious cycle, because through that very same fuck we acquire more charge, which can flare up into emotion at any moment. This explains why, even in the absence of an argument, after a so-called good fuck, a fight can start so easily.

Recent brain research has revealed that chemicals released during a conventional peak orgasm have a separating effect that causes withdrawal and disconnection (see Marnia Robinson's book *Cupid's Poisoned Arrow* in Recommended Books). Previously we mentioned a tendency for men and women to withdraw and feel separate after peak orgasms. Now we know that behavior is actually controlled by a chemical event in the brain. Conventional sex ultimately causes separation, not union.

False Female Emotionality

The false charge built up through a misunderstanding about how genitals relate to each other is a big factor in the emotions for which women have become famous. The overcharge, tensions, and stresses present in the system seek release in order to keep the system in some kind of balance. One way they manifest is in the form of overwhelming emotions. Women seem so sensitive, get upset easily and cry, have dramas, and start blaming. This is man's nightmare! These emotional reactions affect a woman's equilibrium and her capacity to love and be loved. The tensions can also be reflected in women as various menstrual syndromes or genital disturbances.

Man unknowingly contributes to this. When man has hot sex and ejaculates, he frequently (but not always) deposits some of his sexual/emotional tension in woman's body, which she later has to process in some way or other. Woman is unconsciously accumulating stress and tension on a few fronts, which affects her behavior and self-perception, and men's perception of women.

The Emotion of Jealousy

Jealousy is perhaps the most debilitating and excruciating of emotions. Jealousy is about having the desire to possess and control another person; it is not an expression of love for that person. Jealousy has its roots in comparison, and we are taught to compare ourselves in all kinds of ways, particularly in the sexual sphere. Comparison is a useless activity because each individual is unique and incomparable, and once you truly understand this, jealousy can evaporate. Sex certainly creates jealousy, but jealousy is a secondary thing, so it is not a question of how to get rid of jealousy. It is more a question of loving without conditions. Love that does not control or posses but honors the other's freedom to live their own life.

GOLDEN RULES FOR GETTING RID OF EMOTION

There are some "golden rules" (elaborated on in *Tantric Love: Feelings versus Emotions;* see Recommended Books and Resources) to help in processing emotion. The very moment you recognize that you are emotional—through the solar plexus, the experience of disconnection, or in whatever other way you recognize your emotion—the first step is to acknowledge it and say aloud to your partner, "I am emotional." This verbalization instantly brings a touch of relaxation, because at least now your partner knows that you know that you are emotional, which takes the other out of the picture and no longer makes that person responsible for your unhappiness. It is a difficult and challenging step to take (at first), to admit you are emotional by actually saying so, because the ego will be justifying and fighting like crazy, trying to blame the other. But until you take yourself back to yourself and acknowledge the unexpressed past within you, your love life will remain a series of good times followed by bad times.

In such circumstances, having said the three golden words, "I am emotional," to your partner as gracefully as possible, physically leave the room, adding the words, "I need some time to myself and will return soon." Close the door gently and go outside or to another room in the house and take some time alone. (Do not drive off and feign that you are abandoning the relationship in that moment—accidents happen.) Now is not switch-off time, but the time to switch on and release, to get in touch with old feelings residing in your system by moving your body. In fact, when emotions get activated the toxins of feelings gone sour move through a layer of connective tissue in the body, called fascia. This explains why sometimes at the onset of an emotional attack you will feel the event in your body very clearly, almost as if a substance with density is swirling through you. (Indeed, fascia does weave dimensionally through the body and from head to toe about five times, connecting the superficial layers with the deepest physical layers.)

To get rid of these emotions, you need to use physical movement to help them move out of the body. Be active in some way, and do whatever you do purposefully; for example, beat a pillow for twenty minutes, bang on a drum, go for a jog, chop some wood, or dig in the garden. Talking gibberish (nonsensical words) also helps to clear emotion. It's important to be physically active and do what you do with intention and not give in to any inclination to contract and collapse. Surprisingly, when you return to your partner after a bout of physical release you are likely to experience that the feeling of disconnection has diminished, you can make eye contact again, and the distancing "wall" is slowly crumbling to the ground.

If this is not the case, if you feel you are still looking over a half wall, that there's still some sense of separation, you likely need an additional round of body movement. This sounds almost too simple, but it works. If you need two or three hours, or days, to get over the attack of emotion, then take the time required. As you begin to operate in this way with your emotions, soon the whole process gets faster—the recognition, the acknowledgment, and the burning up of the past.

Being creative in this way certainly beats the alternative option of dragging the emotions around for a few days, miserably wondering what has become of love, until eventually, sleepless nights later, one side breaks down into tears, gives up the fight, and starts to express the feelings lurking behind the emotions. You have experienced this yourself many times, for sure; the very instant one side gives up and starts to express inner feelings, the fight is over. We pick up the remaining threads of love and start again.

You may wonder why it is necessary to separate physically in order to deal with emotions. One of the telltale traits of emotion is that it enjoys discussion and argument, each one trying to convince the other why he or she is right. Emotion is full of ego. If you do stay in each other's presence when emotionally activated, it is really best if you can speak only about yourself and say, "I feel . . ." This is the most direct way to step out of emotion, by expressing and releasing your deep, hidden feelings. Bring the congestion of emotions from the solar plexus—where it is likely to have formed a knot—up to the heart, and get into your inner feelings for real. Do not make your partner responsible for creating unhappiness in you. Reach behind the emotion and find what is truly happening inside of you, the old buried hurts that have nothing to do with this individual in front of you. She has only been a trigger.

Even if this person is in some way responsible for some of the hurts you carry from the past, the fact that you repressed your deeper feelings at that time and did not express them is really the issue in the present. If feelings had been authentically released at the time, they would not keep bubbling up inside of you. You would have felt a great deal better for having expressed the feelings, even if a particular issue remained unresolved between you. Through expression you release emotions you've been dragging around and accumulating year by year. You keep yourself free from the past.

THE ROLE OF EMOTIONS IN SEX

Because of our emotional patterns, as couples we tend to get a bit high on emotions and begin to believe that this intensity is a part of love, and that a good hurling of china is an expression of our love. We once heard Barry Long say that all anger is, in reality, the result of sexual frustration. This certainly gives food for thought, especially in light of all the wars going on around us and how little satisfying sex is being enjoyed on Earth. Men and women have pressures and frustrations associated with conventional orgasm, so they are quite likely to have anger about this as well. Many women feel deep rage toward men for their abusive behavior, a rage that extends beyond the personal to the collective level.

Discharging Emotions through Sex

Very often men use sex to discharge their emotional tension. Since they generally express their real feelings much less readily than women, men often have an overload of unexpressed feelings, along with their accompanying tensions. These cause an "itch" in the system, and a man can start to feel horny and want quick sex, excitement, and discharge in order to balance the system. This type of sex has nothing to do with man's basic sexual system and how he is designed to operate as the male principle on Earth. Barry Long referred to the hot excitement/ejaculation style of sex as "emotional sex," and a demanding or hungry or aggressive penis as an "emotional penis."

For man to discover his true male qualities he is advised to refrain from using the sexual channel to release emotional tensions. Ejaculation is certainly an extremely pleasurable way to release them, but there are consequences to such discharges. Men need to find alternative ways to release the tensions they accumulate through life in general, which often involves high levels of stress and anxiety, including survival anxiety. Men will benefit enormously from using their legs in regular daily exercise—for example, jogging, gym workouts, ta'i chi, dance, squats, and any kind of stretching—as well as receiving regular deep-tissue massage in order to relax and free tension in the musculature of the legs and feet.

Tantric Sex Reduces Emotionality

When love is made consciously and emotional or hot sex is avoided (or reduced), there is soon a visible shift in the emotional state of woman. She becomes more radiant, open, and content. Nagging stops, and she begins to flower. Women in our couple's workshops experience a shift within two or three days of making love regularly without forcing a peak orgasm. Men also notice a big change in their own emotional state, as they become calm and centered, grounded in the body, more present and aware, more relaxed, and more loving. Sounds perfect! Men also notice that anger is not provoked so easily. Anger and frustration levels reduce dramatically when hot sex and ejaculation are avoided or reduced.

How we make love profoundly affects who we are and how we conduct ourselves as human beings. It is of eternal value to explore evolved sexual approaches and observe how these experiences begin to shape who you are, how you feel on an inner level, and your perception of each other and the world around you.

EXPRESSING FEELINGS IN THE PRESENT

In addition to keeping the past in the past by recognizing when emotion steps in, and experimenting with relaxing into sex to avoid adding emotions to those you already have, the art now becomes one of staying in touch with your feelings so that you can begin to feel what you are feeling. To keep love fresh and free of emotion it becomes essential to express feelings as they arise. Do not hang on to your feelings for an instant, unless you are in a hopelessly inappropriate situation. Move with the rising feeling and don't let your mind talk you out of it. Allow tears to flow, laughter to erupt, and roars to unleash. Jump up and down, do something fast, and above all, do not repress feelings and in so doing form fresh emotions, which happens very quickly. Equally quickly, any sadness, pain, anger, or frustration, if fully lived as it is happening, will have a life span of about eight intense seconds, after which it is all over.

When you practice consciously expressing anger there are a few hard-and-fast golden rules that come with it, and these are not to be broken under any circumstances. If you feel anger, do not direct it onto your partner, even if your emotions are convincing you that she is at fault. Do not touch her or do anything to hurt her physically; do not even face her. Turn to face in the opposite direction, showing her your back; then let a deep roar emerge from your belly.

PERSONAL SHARING
Releasing the Roar

The first time I consciously allowed my anger to flow was unforgettable. In the very instant that I felt the rising anger for being blamed for something I did not do, I contacted a deep, roaring sound in my belly that was so powerful it shot me up into the air to virtually touch the ceiling, and this one was higher than most ceilings. By the time gravity pulled me back to terra firma a second or two later, it was all over. I felt no anger, no emotion, no resentment—nothing. I stepped back into the moment without hesitation, ready to continue relating, I felt liberated and refreshed.

When anger arises, welcome it, knowing that it is old tension within you that can be transformed. By expressing it you are released from its restrictive grip. Contacting feelings is a cleansing experience; energy that was locked up suddenly becomes available. When you express a feeling or transform an emotion into a feeling you feel lighter, expanded, and fresh; you're more connected to your partner, open and soft, clear and radiant, even loving. Emotions bring the experience of quite opposite qualities: darkness and gloom, despair and collapse. The whole range of positive uplifting experiences arise when you share your feelings. (Learn more in *Nonviolent Communication: A Language of Life*; see Recommended Books and Resources.)

HUMANS NEED LOVEMAKING FOR CONTINUED WELL-BEING

Relaxing into sex brings you into a state of being that is quite apart from the whole range of emotions. Through relaxation we reach a rare state in which our energy is regenerated, and we become suffused with peacefulness as opposed to frustration. As life force moves upward through the energy centers (chakras), it cleanses and purifies them and makes the inner-body experience increasingly dynamic and alive.

Contemporary women suffer from a mass of issues: extreme menstrual syndromes with hormonal ups and downs, poor self-esteem, fears of aging, menopausal anxieties, disappointment, and often disinterest in sex. At a certain point sex is considered by many women to be too much hard work with very little reward, and for this reason they abandon it.

For men the situation is equally dire. Until given the chance to enjoy the expansion of his sexual energy through direct experience, man cannot begin to imagine it. And since excitement and ejaculation are the only experiences he knows, it is not so easy to consider doing something differently. A man's inability to channel his real life force can result in frustration, aggression, anger, restlessness, obsessive fantasizing about sex (both alone and during the act), and all types of sexual perversions.

When the life force circulates freely through man he finally feels himself as more of a man. At the end of a recent workshop a man said, "This is the first time in my life of fifty-four years that I have been given any insight or guidance on what it means to be a man." And that was not the first time we've heard this. When a man knows how to use his sexual energy correctly, allowing it to expand throughout his body, the sense of self changes. Sex becomes less to do with the other or with getting something, and becomes more a way of valuing and loving oneself, of being with oneself. And in this frame woman is likely to be more interested in making love. With insight into our body mechanisms we are able to direct the sexual energy and be more in command of love and life. Man will be in wonder, even a bit awestruck to learn how the same elements—the penis and the vagina—can produce two such vastly different experiences.

MALE AUTHORITY THROUGH TAKING RESPONSIBLE ACTION

Many a man is interested in producing a peak orgasm for a woman because he believes it validates him as a lover, but this attitude has grave consequences for both men and women. Until a man can manage to fully satisfy one woman, he will never feel himself to be a true man, in spite of any other achievements and successes. The need for man to feel himself as masculine, for woman to feel herself as feminine, and for both to have orgasmic experiences through each other is a burning need for humanity today. Without the generative, spiritual, sexual expression, the human race will slowly die from love starvation.

Eliminating or reducing the usual orgasm-driven sex may sound like a loss, but this is truly responsible action on the part of a man. With responsibility you gain freedom, higher sexual experiences, and greater sexual fulfillment, and you transform from an emotional human into a loving human. You lift yourself out of the cycles of unconsciousness that have been going on between people for generations. Life changes its whole quality when the genitals are reserved to serve love, which is their higher purpose. Reproduction is the lower purpose of the sexual interaction. Through understanding the genitals anew and using them according to the inherent polarities embodied in male and female, it is possible to create love in the here and now, with the person you are with today. You learn to contain the energy, embrace it, expand with it, and melt into it.

When physical love reaches a refined level of exchange through polarity, love is generated as a tangible reality between a man and a woman. In being profoundly touched, woman connects with the source of her own love and showers man with her love, thereby completing the circuit of love and joy. Remember again and again: any level of awareness brought into sex will begin to create love; it is the awareness itself that transforms sex into love. Once again, it is not what we do but how we do it. Woman is love, this is the quintessence of her very soul; thus, love to her is as essential as food. She requires the opportunity to relax into her feminine nature and receive the contentment and regeneration of ecstatic experiences to sustain her life. The sincerity and willingness of both parties is clearly a contributing factor, but the responsibility also lies in the individual's hands. Through cooperation in sex we can regain power and balance as male and female forces.

Tantric Inspiration

There is certainly something very similar in very different emotions: the overwhelmingness. It may be love, it may be hate, it may be anger—it can be anything. If it is too much then it gives you a sense of being overwhelmed by something. Even pain and suffering can create the same experience, but overwhelmingness has no value in itself. It simply shows you are an emotional being. This is typically the indication of an emotional personality. When it is anger, it is all anger. And when it is love, it is all love. It almost becomes drunk with the emotion, blind. And whatever action comes out of it is wrong. Even if it is overwhelming love, the action that will come out of it is not going to be right.

Reduced to its base, whenever you are overwhelmed by any emotion you lose all reason, you lose all sensitivity, you lose your heart in it. It becomes almost like a dark cloud in which you are lost. Then whatever you do is going to be wrong. Love is not to be a part of your emotions. Ordinarily that's what people think and experience, but anything overwhelming is very unstable. It comes like a wind and passes by, leaving you behind, empty, shattered, in sadness and in sorrow.

According to those who know man's whole being—his mind, his heart, and his being—love has to be an expression of your being, not an emotion. Emotion is very fragile, very changing. One moment it seems that is all. Another moment, you are simply empty. So the first thing to do is take love out of this crowd of overwhelming emotions.

Love is not overwhelming. On the contrary, love is a tremendous insight, clarity, sensitivity, awareness. But that kind of love rarely exists, because very few people ever reach to their being.

OSHO, TRANSCRIBED TEACHINGS,
OM SHANTIH SHANTIH SHANTIH

PERSONAL SHARING

Tantric Sex Completely Changed My Life

It is unbelievable how much has changed in the past months since the "Making Love" retreat. When I think about what has happened to me, tears start running and I am infinitely grateful for these experiences and for this gift in my life. Again and again, I am confused and I keep thinking: "This can't be true. I am for sure on some sort of trip." But the trip does not seem to end. For the very first time in my life, I realize that I have treated my body badly and that I can stop this without effort from one moment to the other. The physical symptoms that come up are so strong that the beautiful sensation of having an orgasm is nothing compared to it. It is good to know the price I pay for a beautiful orgasm, and that I have the choice to pay it or not. Usually I do not feel like being totally worn out for two or three days due to having had an orgasm. So many big and small things have happened that I have for sure forgotten some of them.

Most importantly, my partner and I have come closer than ever before. Emotional moments have become more and more rare. We love to spend very, very much time with each other and have a hard time not being in each other's presence. That has been different in the past. We had moved into a bigger flat just because we could not stand living together without each of us having a room of our own. Now we have reorganized the flat and the single rooms have become a shared bedroom and office. This way we can always be in each other's presence and feel the love flowing back and forth.

My encounters with people are different. My heart is open. In the past I took a long time to develop trust in someone. This now happens much more swiftly. My connections are less language-oriented. I don't like talking as much as I did; I prefer to be simply here, feeling inside of me and perceiving what is happening. A lot of talking is strenuous for me and takes me away from myself. Whenever I used to meet a woman, an inner movie was going on: "We could have sex with each other. Do I want her? Does she want sex with me? But I have a girlfriend. Bummer!" Now when I meet a woman I feel that my heart is open, that everything is okay, that I can talk with her and feel good. I have no need for sex as my imagination used to suggest. I encounter the person in a way that has not been possible for me before. I really see her, instead of avoiding her in a way. Of course this does not always happen, but more and more often.

In the morning my lover and I both do our t'ai chi and other morning exercises together. This gives me pleasure and I'm amazed how much it helps me to stay grounded in some critical moments. My need for a career, money, fame, appreciation, exciting journeys, and meeting many friends has faded. I prefer to be with my beloved and am very content with that. If I could change my life from one day to the next, I would love to have work that allows me to stay at home every day, and not travel around all the time. Recently we were apart for ten days, and I easily lose the connection to my heart when I am alone. In the past I always wanted to be at home in order to come close to myself.

In the last month I woke up twice because I had an orgasm. I did not ejaculate. I had not experienced that since puberty. For one of these incidents I had a dream with wild sex fantasies. We have short moments with a hot kiss, but the desire for hot sex is there for only a second and vanishes before we have time to put it into practice.

I realized that my lust for sex has evolved into lust for life. Sometimes so much joy is bubbling up in both of us that we feel like exploding. My woman's menstruation is now normal, as it had not been for a very long time, and she has normal ovulation again. I can hardly believe my life has changed so much in such a short time and in such a soft and harmonious manner. Thanks a lot.

PERSONAL SHARING
Staying Connected

With tantra I often realized how my love has the effect of my going beyond myself. The union of vagina and penis is firm as a rock, which keeps reminding me of my love. As waves of hate or fear threatened to deluge me, that connection helped me to stay aware of my love. With the help of love I would then share my fear, as opposed to being trapped in it and projecting it onto my wife; as we all know, the projection of fear is the most wonderful fertilizer for fights and separations. Overall, tantra has helped me to deal with my patterns and fears. I can stay much more grounded when a pattern comes up, and name the pattern. Once it's out in the open on the table or in the bed, I can more easily deal with it constructively.

Tantric Inspiration

When you come back after a Tantric sex act, you have risen, not fallen. You feel filled with energy, more vital, more alive, radiant. And that ecstasy will last for hours, even for days. It depends how deeply you were in it. If you move into it, sooner or later you will realize that ejaculation is a waste of energy. No need of it—unless you need children. And with a Tantric sex experience you will feel a deep relaxation the whole day. One Tantric sex experience and even for days you will feel relaxed—at ease, at home, nonviolent, non-angry, non-depressed. And this type of person is never a danger for others. If he can, he will help others to be happy. If he cannot, at least he will not make anyone unhappy.

OSHO, TRANSCRIBED TEACHINGS,
VIGYAN BHAIRAV TANTRA

10
PERSONAL EXPERIENCES

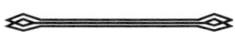

In the pages ahead you'll find a small selection of the numerous letters we have received from men and women over the past years. We can attest to the authenticity of all these letters, which are anonymous for reasons of privacy.

LETTER SHARING (MAN)
My Penis Touched Her Heart

Two weeks after the wonderful retreat, we are still deeply touched by our new experience of making love. It seems like a miracle that our relationship could change in such a fundamental way after thirty years. We could never imagine that our problems in coming together—our different ideas and expectations of having sex—would find a solution in this new, conscious, and very simple way of making love. And we are fully aware that this solution is not simply the end of an old problem, but much more the beginning of a new way of making love on a totally different level. It is a spiritual practice that leads us to our true nature, and which is able to heal us and heal the world.

Every time we feel my penis being attracted by her vagina, it is magic. We never imagined that a man's penis could immediately touch the heart of the woman. We feel the energy flowing—deep joy, peace, and love. It is a kind of coming home, of relaxing, and of pure existence. We will never forget these moments; they have already begun to change our lives. Before it was unimaginable that we would come together every day. Now we are not only enjoying our daily "quickie," but usually we also make love in the evening, in a more intense way. We both feel there is something missing when we don't come together and connect.

We both know that we are at the beginning of a long journey, and we want to continue.

LETTER SHARING (MAN)
Enjoying the Landscape

I'd like to share a picture that came into my mind: Conventional sex is like mountain climbing, straight up to the peak. Tantric sex as I learned it with other "neo-tantric" teachers is still like climbing mountains, reaching for higher peaks than in conventional sex, and then dancing for a while near the peak until you reach it.

Tantric sex, as I learned it with you, also happens in the beautiful mountain landscape. But long before you start getting exhausted by climbing to the peak, you find that there are lovely meadows, marvelous forests, small brooks with clear water you can drink . . . so you just start walking around the mountain. From time to time you can see the peak, or climb to it whenever you want, but usually there is no need to, because it is so beautiful where you are.

LETTER SHARING (MAN)
Feeling Places I Did Not Know I Could Feel

I started my career as a sexual being at age twelve. It happened during a birthday party, and although (to be honest) it was a quite short experi-

ence, it became the blueprint for almost the next thirty years of sex. All I wanted was to get back to the feelings I had when that girl touched me and let me inside her.

Needless to say, I never felt that way again. But I tried everything. And so I started traveling to some really strange places on my roadmap to fulfillment. I did things I would now like to undo, and I used some people who really loved me. I felt myself drifting away from what I was looking for, and the more I drifted, the more I fought to cling to it. In the end, I fought so hard I could not remember what it was. To cut a long story short, by the time I got to your retreat for the first time, I and my sexuality were full of disappointment, anger, and tons of aggression. By then I thought it had to be that way.

I could not imagine sex without moving, licking, and so on. No wonder I felt slightly uncomfortable when you told us about a kind of sex that included none of this. It was difficult to deal with strange things like meditation, finding a home inside myself, or massaging the perineum, but nothing was comparable to my panic when my penis was inside my wife and I had no idea what was going to happen next. The panic reached all-time highs when my penis started to shrink while inside my wife. I felt lost and powerless, as if my penis were no longer a part of me. All the anger and frustration stored inside of me turned into a huge wave, ready to drown me. There was just one solution: movement, friction, and ejaculation. Welcome, black hole.

Gradually, with the relaxation of a week of meditation, I became more and more aware of myself. I felt touches in places where I did not know I could feel anything. In fact, it was new to me to be touched without getting aggressive or horny. It was such a relief to just lie down and listen to my body. I started to feel excitement all over my body, not only inside my penis. The speed of lovemaking slowed down day by day. My body experienced that orgasm and ejaculation are not the same. Sometimes they were, but even the feeling of ejaculation changed. Good-bye, black hole.

When I came back from the week with you, I came back with the feeling that I had forgotten something really essential. All the ghosts of the past came back, and this time, hitting the floor really hurt. Once again I lost connection to myself, and no bodywork or meditation could bring me back home. We returned to your retreat to listen to you both one more time. I don't know what happened and I don't want to know what happened, but somebody or something brought us together again. There's just one word for it—grace. I'm really grateful and I hope I won't spoil it again this time.

Believe it or not, it took me four weeks to write these few sentences. If it had been a letter instead of an e-mail, there would be tear stains on it. Thank you for being not teachers, but two human beings who live what they preach. You have a place in my heart forever.

LETTER SHARING (MAN)
The Rewards of Being Present

My wife and I attended your "Making Love" course this year and completely changed our style of sex. We decided that sex has to have high priority in our lives. We make three or four appointments for making love on weekends, and two or three during the week. And in the morning we often do exercises; I like to stretch my body and get a feeling of my perinium and pelvic floor area. It is beautiful to be connected to my wife and closer through making love. We have less stress and tension around sex since we began practicing cool sex. And we laugh more while making love, for example when we change position. For me it is good that my wife always feels my penis. There is only one condition: To be present. I think my challenge is to be present and to learn to talk about my feelings.

LETTER SHARING (MAN)
Postmenopause Miracle

Since we'd been working on ourselves for more than twenty-five years and giving mental training seminars for three years, we had the feeling we knew at least the tip of the iceberg, yet you taught us much, much more.

For the past ten years, since the changes due to menopause, we had given up sexuality, but we are now living what we both call a "wonder" or a "miracle." All the doctors and the few trainer/teachers we had approached confirmed that in nature, "Women are, in fact, old models," and that we would have to live with this situation. I adjusted, but fortunately, my wife did not give up. She had the feeling that despite not being fond of sex, something was missing in our marital partnership.

Since we met you on the first night of the "Making Love" seminar, and after our very difficult and depressing experience on the following afternoon, we began making love two to three times a day with utmost pleasure and love. Although all the doctors (including a gynecologist) told us that the dry, closed, and painful vagina could only be reactivated with the help of regular hormone therapy, which my wife did not want at all, things have actually worked out to be as they were in our very young days. She is smooth and lubricated, and with love and pleasure as never before, not even at age twenty-five. For us this is a wonder. And with this completion of the circle, the love, tenderness, pleasure, care, ease, and happiness that has entered our partnership is at its very best. Nobody knows how happy we are, except us, of course.

With the easy way things are going now, we both believe your words— that this world can live in peace and happiness. We are spreading the word and hope that eventually it will reach all humans, and that all those who can see and feel the truth will live a new life with joy.

LETTER SHARING (MAN)
Making Appointments for Lovemaking

First, thank you once again for the beautiful week. It was a milestone in my personal journey toward myself. Now, after a week of practicing what we learned from you during the retreat, I notice that I feel completely different—calm, present, happy, and content—and many tensions have disappeared. Although my everyday life continues to have many obligations, I am going through it more serenely and without hurry.

The fact that I have dropped the very idea of goals in lovemaking gives me a totally different feeling in my body, mind, and emotions. Now I know that I don't need to go anywhere or do anything, but just feel and rest in the present moment. This gives me enormous trust in myself and in life, because now I know that I don't need to create anything and that I just have to wait for things to happen on their own. Also, the fact that my wife and I make appointments to make love is a totally different approach in our relationship, because knowing that we both are willing to go forward in lovemaking makes me satisfied and without anxiety. I don't need to wonder whether she wants to be with me or not; I know she wants! And this is such a relaxing feeling.

All of your "Love Keys" are so important: eye contact, slow penetration, breathing, heart opening, and so on. But one of the most important things is that lovemaking becomes like a continuous exploration, because so many things are coming to the surface. Sometimes we don't know what is going on—misunderstandings also arise—but at the end the sky becomes clear and serene and we have new insights. In any case we feel closer to each other and more loving. Of course we have just opened this door a little, and we know that we have just a little experience of what we have learned from you, but it seems like a new page in our lives.

LETTER SHARING (WIFE OF THE ABOVE MAN)
Healing Hatred toward Men

I would like to add a few things important to me. In our lovemaking many of my old fears, distrust, and anger toward men came out. It was sometimes very difficult for me to accept all my old hatred toward men, but I managed it, seeing that my husband is not that kind of man at this moment. He is full of love and compassion, and that helps me a lot. But also after those difficult moments, today we had some wonderful experiences. Feeling his penis inside, doing nothing, was such a tremendous joy, I felt that now life is beautiful, and it just goes on and on. It is some kind of miracle for me, and I thank you for that.

For me it's sometimes difficult to look at all the things that are coming up, to accept that lovemaking is like meditation, and to just watch what is coming up and not do something about it. But I like this process very much and see that I can become more aware through it, so it feels right for me.

LETTER SHARING (MAN)
Our Lovemaking Is Helping to Heal the Earth

Our lives have changed a lot in the past seven years, since we have changed a lot. We still pursue the same professions, own the same house, and so on, but within us something has changed considerably. We feel, sense, and see more, and most of all, we have learned to feel, sense, and see inside. In our daily encounters we reach physical, mental, and spiritual depths that we never considered possible.

Our love journeys have diversified. They lead us deep into our bodies, to Mother Earth, through space, to the sun, through the chakras and their colors, to temples, angels, and through previous lives. On physical, mental, and spiritual levels we are creating healing connections for our own healing and for the healing of others. We are sending healing energies to the earth, to war zones and disaster areas. We are breaking patterns from our past and from past lives.

We do all this in a deep loving connection, feeling the golden ring that streams from the penis to the breasts through the vagina, the garden of love, the kundalini line, and the organs. This golden ring stays with us throughout our everyday life. It also streams when we are not actually physically connected. It streams across continents, and we can sense our love connection physically when we are apart.

This ring, which we forged in our first tantra course, gets stronger and stronger, and we realize that the people around us can feel it, even if they know nothing about our tantric connection. We relate differently to life; we're more awake, more conscious.

Due to our healing connection we can participate in world affairs on a spiritual level, and we sense that it makes a difference. Our tantric connections are evolving. We feel this again and again with great pleasure.

LETTER SHARING (MAN)
Gratefully Relieved of a Job

I am writing to express gratitude for the beautiful and profound retreat that my woman and I attended in December 2008. For forty years I have been searching, researching, and experimenting, knowing deep down that lovemaking holds the key to the expression of love between a man and a woman. This search led me to tantra fifteen years ago, and with each workshop since, with some of the best teachers in the Western world, I ended up with just another set of techniques that focused on achieving various phenomena. Little did I realize that each of these was distracting me from what I wanted most, namely, to connect in love with my lover. What I learned in the "Making Love" retreat is that this is totally available for me in stillness in lovemaking. When my mind and body are still my heart opens and my penis becomes a vehicle of loving, healing male energy.

Also during the retreat I experienced what I can only describe as a change in consciousness around my male sexuality. Like all men that I know, since my earliest sexual experiences I felt driven by some force within me toward sexual pleasure and ejaculation. While I love sex and sexual pleasure, every so often I noticed this feeling of being out of control, as if sex had control of me. After my first tantra workshops and reading Taoist books on sex, I began to practice ejaculation control in lovemaking and conserving vital energy by not ejaculating with every experience of lovemaking. While this provided great sexual experiences and gave me the beginnings of a sense of mastery, it was still control of a strong biological urge and suppressing the habit of the intense pleasure of ejaculation.

During the "Making Love" retreat there was a shift. In our lovemaking we had the time to really experience what it was like not to move toward excitement. It was as if we created the space for something new to manifest. We had the opportunity to really appreciate one another. We experienced healing of past sexual hurts. We expressed the love that we felt. We saw and felt the beauty of male and female body joined in love. For me it was as if this deep experience of extended presence in love outweighed the fleeting pleasure of ejaculation.

There is a very practical aspect that I enjoy about this way of making love. In past lovemaking I always felt as if I had a big job to do. The first thing I had to do was to gently seduce my lover to get her interested in having sex, and then help her to awaken sexually so that she was ready for intercourse. The next part of the job was to build the level of excitement till she was approaching her orgasm. If I decided that I would ejaculate it was preferable that we try to orgasm together. Alternatively, I would have the job of withholding the energy and semen of ejaculation while she had her orgasm. That's a lot of work for a man to do. It didn't leave much time for me to experience and express love.

Now it's simple. Together we both look for the next opportunity to make love. We connect in cool pleasure and I have no job to do other than be present.

LETTER SHARING (MAN)
Opening and Closing My Heart

I will not give my power, my life-power away again. Since the workshop I feel alive, my heart is beating strongly. I am full of beans. I feel grateful for my love, my cheerfulness, my joy about a new day and about this gift. But I also feel pain for the many times when I did not, or could not, do what I actually wanted to do. A kiss with my beloved in the morning, a loving embrace, looking into each other's eyes, and sharing joy about life and about this moment cause me to laugh and cry simultaneously. It is coming from a deep place. I feel it streaming through my heart as it opens and laughs, closes down, and starts to cry.

Now I am sitting here and my heart is wide open, and in this moment I feel in touch with the silence, the joy, the love. Here, I also feel like opening and sharing it. Slowly the pain about things I did not do, about the love that was not expressed, dissolves. Yes, I am bringing light into the darkness, into the fear, and it is disappearing. Now I also understand that you can show me the way, but I have to walk it. Yes, I am walking, and sensing, and enjoying. Life is so beautiful and I am a part of it.

LETTER SHARING (MAN)
Finding a Deeper Connection

The days with you have been a refinement for us on all levels. Our lovemaking has become slower, more energetic, and less athletic. I did not have any physical discomfort with conventional sex, but often felt energetic conflict before, during, and after the sex, which had led to weird moodiness.

Now that we have become more conscious and slow, I feel more bal-

anced, ever more often finding that relaxed, flowing, powerful quality of being that I have always looked for on other paths, but never found so easily and naturally. In our hearts we are more deeply and softly connected with each other, while on the level of personality there is more space between us, which reduces the emotions.

LETTER SHARING (WOMAN)
Making Time for Breasts

Over Christmas and New Years we had a difficult time. I was not really centered and our old issues about closeness and distance resurfaced. Many emotions came up and it was not easy to get out of them. We had a shift and then we had an extra long, very relaxing time. Tantra has become a familiar form of lovemaking, and for me it is a beautiful key to come into my body, open up, and connect. If we succeed in meeting in the cool lovezone and really drop into it and connect there, I feel very nourished on a deep level and I am in bliss.

I experience our encounters as always different and sometimes very intense. I feel a lot and I've ridden the waves of energy. And then sometimes it is totally different, subtle, and relaxed. I feel very clearly how my body responds, opens, and relaxes on a cellular level, and sometimes this happens when we are simply connected, as if that is the call for relaxation. Hot love is still an issue, and if I succeed in engaging with it, staying in contact with myself, my energy, and mostly with my heart, I do enjoy this as well. The afterward time is our teacher, a beautiful experience.

I am just reading your book for women and I thank you here for it. It is really good to get background information that relates to my experiences, or to let myself be inspired by the exercises and explore them. I'm giving more attention to my breasts and I'm very happy to experiment alone with myself or during lovemaking. I have made extra time in my calendar for my breasts, and I want to deepen the connection.

LETTER SHARING (MAN)
Happy to Be Present

It was a revelation for me to finally find out how I can integrate spirituality in my relationship and my sexuality, and thereby heal myself and my partner.

I feel as if I arrive much more at home, and as if I found my true calling: to learn and live playfully and joyfully, and to share how we love and find fulfillment on Earth, thereby overcoming separation and freeing ourselves from the illusion of the ego.

It was an important part of my healing to watch how loving and respectful you two are with each other. Since I originally come from a family within which an extreme amount of fighting went on, it was very healing to see how love and respect can be practiced between a man and a woman, if we learn to understand our deeper essence. My relationship has become much deeper and more fulfilling. I am free of performance pressure and happy to see and live my part as a man—to be present.

PERSONAL SHARING (WOMAN)
You Have to Make a Lot of Love

I keep remembering your advice. When I said good-bye I was in great fear that at home everything would be different, and that all our problems would come up again. You felt my fear and said, "You have to make a lot of love." I did so, and something wonderful happened. My husband is more loving, mellower, and more tender in his whole being. The wrinkles in his face have disappeared and his skin is very soft. I believe that he let go of his difficult upbringing and conditioning during that week. I am very grateful that you guided us on this beautiful and sunny path. That's exactly what we have been looking for after our thirty-nine years of marriage.

PERSONAL SHARING (MAN)
The Bliss of Full-body Orgasm

For our love session (during the seminar) we retreated to our bungalow, which helped us to explore a totally new and healing closeness, and a new expression of our love. Since the beginning of the seminar we had been in close contact with our emotions and feelings, and we felt much more porous and sensitive than before the course. After a shower we cuddled and rested for about twenty minutes in deep relaxation. We looked long and deeply into each other's eyes. Then we put ourselves in the scissors position and connected without having an erection, and without feeling any lust.

We closed our eyes and took a deep breath in the direction of our genitals, while each of us tuned in to the inner polarity—calmly, without expecting or intending anything. After a while my woman felt very fine, short pulses of lust. My soft penis started pulsing very softly in her vagina. We both did not move. As we looked into each other's eyes, I felt as if the energy circuit between us had completed. We felt a ball of energy in our genitals. I could not tell anymore where my being, my penis, stopped, and where she started. Penis and vagina felt like one shared whole, like pure energy. Warm waves were running through my body and I thought, "This is it what it means to melt into each other."

We sensed subtle energies pulling my penis deeper inside her. She felt soft and velvety, both of us pulsing softly with each other. My penis curled deeper and deeper into her vagina, without my moving at all. We both experienced a new feeling of closeness, silence, peace, bliss, and lust at the same time. Her vagina had received my penis fully. I felt like a welcome guest in her, and realized how my penis had stiffened.

In this moment a wave of sadness rose in me. I had felt some sadness while we were making love in the days before, but this time the sadness was unbelievably strong and intense. Tears streamed steadily as I thought about what I had done with my penis up until then. It was so sad, so terrifying. All of a sudden I became painfully aware of all the unconscious sex with my woman and the women before her, how this had been caused by my goal-oriented behavior, and how the women might have felt with it. It is so painful to realize what mischief is caused by conventional sex. I had always considered myself to be a tender lover, but it is not the intention but the actual result that counts. My God, what have I done through unawareness?

It was as if I felt the pain of all women in my body. I am so sorry! I never intended that. I always intended to express my love. I simply cannot hurt the person that I love the most. While I was in tears and sharing all my insights with her, we were still united. Sobbing, I begged her to forgive each single moment in which I had been unconscious in sex with her. It was a relief when she said it had not been my fault, for it had happened without my knowing better.

Slowly I calmed down and began to feel a deep peace. I felt my heart from inside, and a connection between my base chakra and my heart chakra, which got more and more intense. My penis snaked again deep into her vagina. The intensity of the sex/heart chakra connection grew steadily, my breath got deeper, quicker, and stronger, and a powerful sensation of love rose up inside me. I stayed totally conscious with all that happened, more a watcher than an actor. I shared everything that happened with my woman. I felt how the energy in my penis started to rise inside of me. It was overwhelming. My penis and my pelvis filled with a warming energy, which finally streamed into the belly over the left side of my body up into my heart. My whole body was filled with the sensation that I usually have in my penis in moments of orgasmic ejaculation. The sensation went on and got more and more intense. It streamed into the left arm, down into the fingertips. It was overwhelming. On the left side of my body it continued streaming up to the place between my eyes. There seemed to be *no end to it; it was a permanent feeling of ecstasy. All the energy had been streaming from my penis up into my whole body. Then my penis became soft without my ejaculating.*

As previously experienced, I clearly sensed all my chakras as warming wheels turning slowly and continuously clockwise. It was a wonderful sensation. I laughed and had tears of joy, and had no idea how much time had passed. Finally, all over my body the sensation slowly faded, but in my heart I could still feel it for a long time. I was deeply satisfied. I had never experienced anything so beautiful in my whole life.

Later I asked my girlfriend what that might have been, and she said, "Darling, maybe you had a full-body orgasm."

Tantric Inspiration

The word *tantra* means the capacity of expansion, that which goes on expanding. Sex shrinks you, Tantra expands you. It is the same energy, but it takes a turn. It is no longer selfish, no longer self-centered. It starts spreading—it starts spreading to the whole existence. In sex, for a moment you can attain to the orgasm, and at a great cost. In Tantra you can live in the orgasm twenty-four hours a day, because your very energy becomes orgasmic. And your meeting is no longer with any individual person: your meeting is with the universe itself. You see a tree, you see a flower, you see a star, and there is something like orgasm happening.

OSHO, TRANSCRIBED TEACHINGS,
PHILOSOPHIA PERENNIS

APPENDIX

EXERCISES FOR IMPROVING YOUR AWARENESS AND SENSITIVITY

Practice is the best way to improve in any area, and sex is no exception. There are a number of ways to "practice" awareness by yourself and develop sensitivity skills that will enrich your lovemaking. Familiarizing yourself with some of the sequences below will help you learn how to relax and engage your attention during lovemaking, so that you can be more fully present with your partner.

⬢ Connecting with Your Own Body
Pulling Attention away from the Mind and into the Body

Becoming fully aware of your own body will make it easier to truly connect with another person's body, and this is easily done. As you sit or lie on your back you can start by closing your eyes and taking your attention to inside your body. As your awareness (attention) travels around the different parts of your body, discover a place within that feels good, restful, easy, a space that feels like home to you. This place can be anywhere below the head that helps you feel more rooted and anchored in your body, connected to it from the inside. If your whole body feels like home, this is fine, and if nowhere feels like home, this is also fine. The feeling of having a home within the body may become clearer in time, and if not, that's all right, too. This suggestion is only a tool, not a special technique.

Continue to rest and be with that part in your body, bringing awareness into the tissues. The inner realms of the body are also your flesh, guts, and marrow, and the source of your cellular aliveness. It takes practice to learn to identify and give value to finer bodily sensations, the delicious, subtle vibrations of life streaming and flowing through you. If you sincerely begin to love, honor, and pay attention to your body's inner world, it will soon become second nature. You can connect with your "inner home" at any moment of the day, while sitting, driving, eating, walking, or resting.

⬣ Becoming Aware of Habitual Tensions
Relaxing the Body from Head to Toe

It is enormously helpful to scan the body and check for tension while you are making love. Or at any other time of the day. If you've never done this in an organized way before, it might be useful to practice on your own, perhaps as you're lying in bed preparing for sleep. You can also do this sitting or standing. Begin by becoming aware of each part of your body from head to toe, and relaxing each individual part. You will notice how the body takes a deep breath as you relax, letting go of subtle tensions. Allow each part to melt down into the part below it, until it all melts out the bottom of your feet. Your crown melts down into your forehead, which softens down into your eyes, and then into your cheekbones. This continues into the mouth and jaw, and on down into the shoulders, allowing them to drop down a few inches. Continue on down through your body, taking particular care with classic tension spots such as the solar plexus (take a deep and conscious breath here), let go of the belly, relax the buttocks, and release the anus.

Breathe gently and deeply through the diaphragm and into the belly, infusing the floor of the pelvis with vitality. Maintain awareness of your breathing whenever possible and for as long as possible. Whenever you find your attention drifting, shift back to your own body and breath. Keep scanning upward and downward and notice where (and how easily) habitual tensions reassert themselves, and relax! Make scanning and consciously relaxing tense parts an ongoing process. Notice how every "let go" is usually followed by a sense of inner cellular expansion. Men report that consciously relaxing the anus and buttocks repeatedly while making love reduces the pressure to ejaculate. More "space" is created internally, and the life force is able to circulate and expand through the rest of the body.

⬢ Position for Rest and Relaxation
Aligning Your Spine for Presence, Awareness, and Sensitivity

The ideal horizontal position for relaxation is with the head, neck, and spine aligned in one straight line, not even a few millimeters out of alignment, and with the head centered and not rolled to one side. Your legs should be straight and slightly apart, and the ankles should *not* be crossed. Place a narrow, soft pillow (or rolled blanket) *directly under* the crease behind the knees to create a slight curving and softening of the knee joint. Place a flat, firm, small pillow (or folded towel) under your head. Tuck your chin to your chest and straighten your neck before placing the pillow in position. The pillow should support the lengthening stretch of your spine so there is not too much of a curve in the neck. If the chin is pointing almost directly upward and not tilted toward the chest, use a slightly deeper pillow (or give the towel another fold) to lift the head an additional few inches and create length, which reduces the curve in the neck and brings the level of the chin down. Place your open hands palm down on the groin area, on either side of your pubic bone. Allow your breathing to become deep and slow. Scan the body and relax tensions. Rest quietly with your eyes softly closed for at least twenty minutes, holding awareness in your body generally, or in the home in your body as discovered in the first exercise.

⬢ Tantric Meditation
Peace Pervading Armpits

Lie in a relaxed position, as suggested in the alignment exercise above, for twenty minutes or more. Close your eyes, taking your awareness into your body. Start just between the two armpits and with your total attention "pervade an area between the armpits into great peace." Forget your whole body; remember the heart area between the two armpits and your chest, and feel it filled with great peace. When the body is more relaxed, peace automatically happens in your heart; it becomes more silent and harmonious. Done frequently, this practice will establish peace within you and make you feel more independent, and love will be more of a giving; you'll have so much peace, you'll want to share it. You will be returning to a source in yourself that is always there.

⬢ Extending Awareness of the Physical and Energetic Bodies
Tantric Meditation for Growing in Consciousness

As you lie in the aligned position already described, you can deepen your experience by closing your eyes and imagining yourself looking backward into your body. Imagine that vision is reversed and your eyes can look inward and downward into yourself, even as far as your genitals. Breathe deeply and slowly into your belly, as if the breath is massaging your insides and touching your genitals. Continually pull your attention back into your body and use the subtle sensations in it as an anchor. Deliberately disconnect from distracting thoughts when they pop into your mind. Let them float away, and instead return home and immerse yourself in the body so that you feel a sense of resting deep within. The sensation of being submerged in yourself. Travel with your awareness to any places in the body that are tingling, pleasant, alive, or warm, or where fine vibrations are present, and be with them, dissolve into them. Notice how inner sensations expand when you take the time to feel and acknowledge them.

At a certain point, once the practice of immersing into and merging with your senses takes root, the feeling of your having physical boundaries will disappear; you will feel as if you dissolve and become as light as a feather, bathed in golden light, floating suspended in the universe. You are, but you are not. In this way you can grow in consciousness until every cell is penetrated with light. The moment consciousness touches the cells, they are different. The very quality of the cells changes. Sensuality is gradually awakened as consciousness filters through the body.

You can set a clock alarm for the amount of time you wish to devote to the experience, or you may leave it up to your inner clock to spontaneously return you to normal consciousness, with the sense of having lost all track of time. You are likely to notice that afterward you feel refreshed and rejuvenated, as though you have had a drink directly from the source of life. It is also beneficial to practice this meditation before sleeping at night and at any time during the day when you need to recharge your energy.

⬢ Awakening the Rod of Magnetism
Bringing Attention from the Head to the Perineum

This visualization will help you shift attention away from the head of the penis, where it goes automatically because it is there that intense pleasure is experienced. Envision your penis as a channel or conduit, and refocus your attention on the base of your penis, in the area of the perineum. The perineum, a small, coin-sized area of knotty muscle lying directly in front of the anus, is virtually the root of the penis and is its energetic source. It is where the muscles and tissues that form the penis initially emerge from your body. Begin to visualize your penis as a channel for potency, warmth, and love. Imagine it to be a wand or fountain of light and liquid gold that emanates from the perinium and streams along its length.

When you begin to make love and feel the heat rising, bring your attention to the perineum. Consciously relax the entire area, including the anus. When you notice your attention start to drift—there are, after all, abundant distractions—you may notice that the pelvic floor area once again contracts and tightens. Repeatedly relaxing the anus and maintaining awareness of the base, the perinium, will give you an inner feeling of your penis as a complete unit, rather than a disembodied tool for thrusting. It instead becomes a divine instrument capable of channeling subtle energies that flow or stream from the root upward to the radiant head and beyond into your receptive partner. Be aware of your breath and of the subtle sensations deep within your physical core as your inner rod of magnetism awakens. Notice how the life force rises to caress your heart into vibrant aliveness.

When you make love with your partner, take this awareness of the inner rod of magnetism with you and relax into the receptive containment of your partner's vagina, knowing that there is nothing to be done but relax and notice how energies awaken, flow, expand, simply because you put your attention there.

Personal Sharing by Man

It is like a new beginning—a tentative and vulnerable new beginning. Getting to know both in theory and in experience that by placing awareness and presence inside my body, energies begin to flow, all by themselves, and that then can mingle with those of my partner. A very important shift was seeing my penis and my role as a male as being noble and that my "task" is to be fully present in my penis and ultimately deep in the vagina. Nothing more, and this is my deepest longing.

I feel, more than ever before, that I can direct my attention into my body, my home, my perineum. Especially honoring and focusing on my perineum gave me great joy when it responded by radiating beautiful energies. Overall this attention to my body, and the fact of doing more exercise, has allowed me to relax more deeply, calming my mind, releasing chronic restlessness.

I truly see this approach to the body and sex as the deepest form of peace work for the planet. Personally and collectively I see it absolutely necessary for healing.

RECOMMENDED BOOKS AND RESOURCES

BOOKS AND RESOURCES BY OSHO

The Book of Secrets. New York: St. Martin's Press, 1998.
My Way: The Way of the White Clouds. Pune, India: Rebel Publishing House, 1995.
Sex Matters: From Sex to Superconsciousness. New York: St. Martin's Press, 2003.
The Tantra Experience. Pune, India: Rebel Publishing House, 1998.
Tantra: The Supreme Understanding. Pune, India: Rebel Publishing House, 1998.
Tantric Transformation. Pune, India: Rebel Publishing House, 1998.

For more information about Osho and to purchase books and CDs, visit www.osho.com.

BOOKS AND RESOURCES BY BARRY LONG

Love Brings All to Life. Audio CD
Making Love 1 & 2. Audio CD (Sexual Love the Divine Way)

Raising Children in Love, Justice, and Truth. London: Barry Long Books, 1998.

Stillness Is the Way. London: Barry Long Books, 1989. To purchase these products from Barry Long, visit www.barrylong.org.

BOOKS AND RESOURCES BY DIANA AND MICHAEL RICHARDSON

Richardson, Diana. *The Heart of Tantric Sex: A Unique Guide to Love and Sexual Fulfillment.* Alresford, Hant, U.K.: O Books, 2003. [Originally published by Thorsons/Element in 1999 as *The Love Keys: The Art of Ecstatic Sex.*]

———. *MaLua: Light Meditation for Women.* Guided breast meditation CD with music (English/German language). Cologne, Germany: Innenwelt Verlag, 2009.

———. *Tantric Love Letters.* Alresford, Hant, U.K.: O Books, 2011.

———. *Tantric Orgasm for Women.* Rochester, Vt.: Destiny Books, 2004.

———. *Slow Sex: Making Love a Meditation.* Rochester, Vt.: Destiny Books, 2011.

Richardson, Diana, and Michael Richardson. *Tantric Love: Feeling versus Emotion—Golden Rules to Make Love Easy.* Alresford, Hant, U.K.: O Books, 2009. [First published in German in 2006.]

To purchase books or CDs, visit www.livingloveshop.com. For further book information, visit www.love4couples.com or www.livinglove.com.

Translations of some books are available in German, Spanish, Swedish, French, Italian, and Chinese.

FURTHER RECOMMENDED READING

Robinson, Marnia. *Cupid's Poisoned Arrow: From Habit to Harmony in Sexual Relationships.* New York: Random House, 2009.

Rosenberg, Marshall. *Nonviolent Communication: A Language of Life.* Encinitas, Calif.: PuddleDancer, 2003.

Tolle, Eckhart. *A New Earth: Awakening to Your Life's Purpose.* New York: Penguin Books, 2006.

Zurhorst, Eva-Maria. *Love Yourself and It Doesn't Matter Who You Marry!* Carlsbad, Calif.: Hay House, 2007.

ABOUT THE AUTHORS

Diana Richardson was born in KwaZulu, South Africa. She holds a law degree (B.A.LL.B) from the University of Natal, Durban, South Africa, and has taught therapeutic massage since 1978. In 1979 she became a disciple of Indian mystic Osho and began a personal inquiry into tantra—the union of sex and meditation—inspired by Osho and tantric master Barry Long.

Through the integration of these different sources in her own experience, a unique body of work on "generative sex," or "cool sex," has emerged, which represents an evolutionary step for the human being. The essence of the teaching is encapsulated in the simple, practical, and highly effective "Love Keys." Since 1993 Diana has led "Making Love" seminars for couples with her partner, Michael Richardson.

Michael Richardson was born in Germany and attended the Academy of Music and Performing Arts in Stuttgart. He teaches tantra and t'ai chi—yang style as taught by Master Chu—as well as the Gurdjieff sacred dances, practices shiatsu, and is a musician. In 1985 he became a disciple of Indian mystic Osho. His thirty years experience of meditation in movement through the practice of t'ai chi planted the roots of his perception of energy within the tantric dimension.

About the Authors

Couples travel from different parts of the world to participate in Diana and Michael's informative and life-changing workshops in Switzerland. They are pioneers in the sphere of human sexuality and among today's leading authorities on the subject. They have published several books about the essence of tantra—the union of sex and meditation—and the practical ways a person can experience a more fulfilling love and life.

"MAKING LOVE"—A TANTRA MEDITATION RETREAT FOR COUPLES

The authors facilitate weeklong retreats in Switzerland and guide couples in the art of tantra. For more information on these retreats, please visit their websites listed below.

www.livinglove.com
www.love4couples.com

You may contact Diana and Michael by e-mail at the following address.

info@livinglove.com

TANTRIC ORGASM
FOR WOMEN

DIANA RICHARDSON

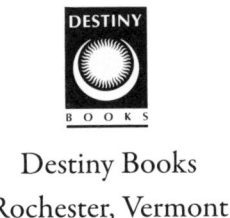

Destiny Books
Rochester, Vermont

Destiny Books
One Park Street
Rochester, Vermont 05767
www.InnerTraditions.com

Destiny Books is a division of Inner Traditions International

Text and artwork copyright © 2004 by Diana Richardson

All rights reserved. No part of this book may be reproduced or utilized in any form or by any means, electronic or mechanical, including photocopying, recording, or by any information storage and retrieval system, without permission in writing from the publisher.

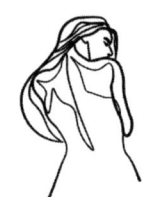

Volume I
of
Tantric Sex for Lovers
Boxed Set

Tantric Orgasm for Women

Printed and bound in India by Replika Press Pvt. Ltd.

10 9 8 7 6 5 4 3 2 1

This book was typeset in Garamond and Weiss, with Medici Script, Avant Garde, and Posterama Text as display typefaces

All Osho quotes printed with permission of Osho International

Artwork prepared by Alfredo Hernando, Madrid, Spain.

Dedicated to Love in Women

Contents

	Acknowledgments	vi
	Introduction	1
1	The Intrinsic Potential for Orgasm	7
2	Orgasm Is a Spiritual Experience	17
3	Orgasm versus Orgasmic	29
4	The Source of Orgasmic States	41
5	The Breasts: Key to Orgasm	53
6	The Vagina Is Secondary to the Breasts	69
7	The Clitoris and Excitement	85
8	Woman's Part in Man's Erection	99
9	Relaxing into Orgasm	113
10	Mastering Love and Overcoming Emotions	143
11	Woman as Lover during Menstruation, Fertility, Pregnancy, Motherhood, and Menopause	167
12	Tantric Orgasm and Same-Sex Partners	181
	Conclusion: Embracing Our True Feminine Power	201
	Appendix: The Sympto-Thermal Method of Fertility Awareness	207
	Notes	213
	Recommended Books and Resources	215

Acknowledgments

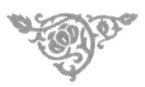

I sincerely thank the many women who have shared their experiences with me over the years, and from whom I have learned an inestimable amount. In particular I am grateful to the women who have given me permission to use their personal words of experience, which have helped enormously in conveying the true map of female sexuality, and thereby of love. In addition, I am thankful to the male partners of those same women, because their mutual experiences in love made this direct contribution possible. I have also included a few sharings by men and I am grateful to them for giving me permission to do so. I vouch for the absolute authenticity of all the personal experiences I have quoted. I have, for simplicity's sake, elected not to identify the individual contributors by name or initial.

Introduction

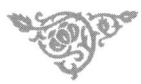

*I*n Sanskrit, the ancient religious and classical literary language of India, the word *tantra* can be likened to such concepts as "capacity for expansion" and "that which goes on expanding," and the words *continuum, web, context,* and *transformation*.¹ Tantra teaches an acceptance of who we are as a whole, from the solid density of our physical body to the refined layers of our spirit. It is concerned with the transmutation of energy, liberation of the mind, attainment of one's full potential. The balanced union of opposites is considered the way of achieving liberation of mind and body, a liberation from the supposedly endless cycle of unconscious rebirth. Tantra understood over five thousand years ago what modern science has since proven to be true through chromosome study: that woman is half man and man is half woman. The balancing of inner opposites is the way to achieve full potential. Falling fully into feminine mode in sexual union transforms woman through an inner alchemical process.

This, my second book on tantra, essentially explores tantra from the female perspective. In the pages ahead I endeavor to convey the significant role that receptive feminine energy plays in the male-female sexual exchange. It wouldn't be realistic to draw a distinct line between woman and man when talking about sex because sex is the most intimate meeting of the male

INTRODUCTION

and female elements. However, there are aspects of sexuality that apply exclusively to women, and these can be used to distinct advantage in influencing and strengthening the sexual experience—for both women and men. A woman who is without a partner can still benefit from this knowledge. It can give her a new feeling about herself and her body, and often through this new awareness she will draw the right partner to herself.

As a researcher, teacher, and writer on sex, I have been encouraged by both women and men to address sexuality from the female point of view. Women have suggested this directly; and though no men have exactly verbalized it, I have been encouraged indirectly by men's actions and what they have demonstrated, unknowingly, to me in the last twenty years.

In this time many couples have attended the "Making Love" workshops for couples that I colead with my partner, Raja. During the workshops, truly touching miracles take place every day. Many of the couples reexperience the dynamic love that brought them together in the first place, and have been able to continue into the future in loving harmony. However, not all partnerships are equally successful and sometimes couples have separated. In time, naturally, those who have separated have formed new relationships. As these new relationships begin to take hold, I've noticed something quite phenomenal and unexpected happening in the groups. The men who had attended my workshops before are returning to the workshops. It is the *men* who have been coming back to share this alternative approach to sexuality with their new female partners because they have experienced how the tantric approach can enhance love. To my greatest surprise, women (though they found the first workshops as uplifting as their partners did) have been much slower on the rebound. Only in the very recent past have women participants come back to repeat the workshop with new loved ones.

The fact that many men but few women return to the workshops with their new lovers offers two important insights. The first is that we women are afraid to talk to men about sex and are reluctant to share with men what pleases our bodies most. We hesitate to introduce our male partners to any alternative sexual approaches. The main fear for a woman is that of losing her man, of ceasing to be sexually attractive to him if she changes. Sadly, when

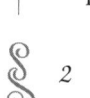

INTRODUCTION

women choose to stay with conventional sex—which is a distorted form of male sexuality—we give away our unique feminine magic and power.

The second insight is much more encouraging, and I hope it will give women the confidence to be more authoritative in the sexual sphere. The fact that men *are* bringing women back to the workshops clearly demonstrates that men develop a liking for another form of sexual expression once they have tasted it. How can a man have a taste for something he has never experienced? Often tantric sexuality has to be experienced before the longing for it can arise.

From both men and women who have no personal experience with tantra I repeatedly hear the comment, "Tantra seems to be for women, not for men." Based on my own exploration and on the encouraging response of the men who attend my workshops, I can say with all certainty, "No, tantra is not only for women. It is definitely for men too." Tantra is not simply something designed to make women happy (and men not so happy), a way of giving women the reins for a while. When a man has had one taste of the delicious depths and heights of expanded sexual energy, invariably he wants it again. But unless women make available their true femininity to men, how and where and when can men develop a taste for it?

Here and there you might find a woman who naturally has the knack of receiving and channeling masculine sexual energy upward during intercourse and can lift sex to another dimension for herself and her man. The truth is that a woman can consciously develop this art and guide her man into an expanded sexual sphere—and thereby create for herself more satisfying sexual experiences. A woman has the natural capacity to enter this realm simply by virtue of being a woman. She who is the receptive aspect in the male-female dynamic can move inward and draw or pull man along with her. This is her intrinsic power. Through receptivity, through giving way and yielding, inherent movement is possible. The opposite does not hold quite so true: generally speaking, man cannot easily initiate the experience of opening a doorway and absorbing woman into him. To do so requires great stillness and the clarity of true male authority. When the receptive (feminine) aspect gives way, actually receiving what is coming to it, its very receptivity enables the dynamic (masculine) energy to move and

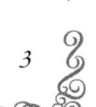

INTRODUCTION

flow. In this way man easily and naturally follows woman; he can even wordlessly flow into exalted realms with woman *if* he is fortunate enough to encounter receptive feminine energy.

Woman is the real starting point for the necessary reeducation in sex. This movement has to take root in women and spread from them out into society—through lovers, friends, one-night stands, through mothers teaching daughters and fathers teaching sons. It requires that women begin to speak up for themselves, expressing their needs and sensitivities, and that men take urgent heed of these messages. The greatest potential for true sexual fulfillment and love lies in a woman and a man joined together on a mutual journey of sexual self-discovery.

Nevertheless, a woman can do much without the conscious cooperation of a man. Sex is about as close to ourselves as we can get; it reaches, touches, and changes every cell of our bodies. Through exploring sex we will discover who we really are beneath all the social pretensions and conventions that we habitually use to cover up our deeper sexual selves.

My source of tantric inspiration and guidance is my spiritual master, Osho. Osho, or Bhagwan Shree Rajneesh, as he was known earlier in his life, teaches meditation not as a practice but as a way of life. He is a mystic who brings the timeless wisdom of the East to bear upon the urgent questions facing men and women today. He speaks of the search for harmony, wholeness, and love that lies at the core of all religious and spiritual traditions, illuminating the essence of Christianity, Hassidism, Buddhism, Sufism, Tantra, Tao, Yoga, and Zen.

There are no words to express my depth of gratitude for his profound and continuing impact on my life. Osho's interpretation of the ancient tantric scriptures creates a superior body of knowledge and insight that I have been fortunate enough to have access to since my mid-twenties.

Tantra is beyond technique; it is a profound journey of self-discovery and self-transformation, an alchemical process of transmuting base energies to higher spiritual expression. Some techniques can be used along the way, but the secret of tantra lies in bringing that which is sexually unconscious in us into full consciousness. Osho says, "Tantra is the transforma-

INTRODUCTION

tion of sex into love through awareness." This implies that *how* we do something is infinitely more important than *what* we do.

It is my privilege to include some excerpts of Osho's tantric inspiration throughout this book. It may perhaps interest the reader to know that Osho's words, appearing here in text form, were initially delivered as off-the-cuff oral discourses, completely spontaneous and without any previous preparation, at gatherings for his disciples and interested public in India. Later these were published in book form. I wish to make it clear that the handful of quotes appearing here are simply those that I chose to include. They in no way represent the full range and extraordinary diversity of Osho's spiritual insight into the human condition.

Osho Speaks on Sex

I have almost four hundred books in my name. Out of four hundred books there is only one book on sex, and that too is not really on sex; it is basically on how to transcend sex, how to bring the energy of sex to a sublimated state, because it is our basic energy. It can produce life. . . . It is only man who has the privilege to change the character and the quality of sexual energy. The name of the book is *From Sex to Superconsciousness*—but nobody talks about superconsciousness. The book is about superconsciousness; sex is only to be the beginning, where everybody is.

There are methods that can start the energy moving upwards, and in the East, for at least ten thousand years, there has developed a special science, Tantra. There is no parallel in the West of such a science. For ten thousand years people have experimented with how sexual energy can become your spirituality, how your sexuality can become your spirituality. It is proved beyond doubt—thousands of people have gone through the transformation. Tantra seems to be the science that is, sooner or later, going to be accepted in the whole world, because people are suffering from all kinds of perversions. That's why they go on talking about sex as if that is my work, as if twenty-four hours a day I am talking about sex. Their repressed sexuality is the problem. My whole effort has been how to make your sex a natural, accepted phenomenon, so there is no repression—and

then you don't need any pornography; so that there is no repression—and then you don't dream of sex. Then the energy can be transformed.

There are valid methods available through which the same energy that brings life to the world can bring a new life to you. That was the whole theme of the book. But nobody bothered about the theme, nobody bothered about why I have spoken on it. Just the word *sex* was in the title, and that was enough.

The book is not for sex; it is the only book in the whole existence against sex, but strange. . . . The book says that there is a way to go beyond sex, you can transcend sex—that's the meaning of "from sex to superconsciousness." You are at the stage of sex while you should be at the stage of superconsciousness. And the route is simple: sex just has to be part of your religious life, it has to be something sacred. Sex has to be something not obscene, not pornographic, not condemned, not repressed but immensely respected, because we are born out of it. It is our very life source. And to condemn the life source is to condemn everything. Sex has to be raised higher and higher to its ultimate peak. And that ultimate peak is samadhi, superconsciousness.

OSHO, TRANSCRIBED TEACHINGS,
SEX MATTERS: FROM SEX TO SUPERCONSCIOUSNESS
(INCLUDED AT THE REQUEST OF OSHO INTERNATIONAL)

1
The Intrinsic Potential for Orgasm

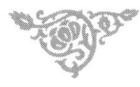

Each and every woman arrives on this earth with the intrinsic capacity to experience the uplifting joy of orgasm. Mother Nature in her unswerving wisdom has graced the female body with a special design so that this experience can arise. Women have the potential to live sex fully, as a conscious, guiding force. However, even though nature may have sincerely intended this for us, in real life very few women can say that they have genuine command over their orgasmic experiences. Instead, for most women, orgasm remains quite elusive, happening now and then, depending more on good orchestration than on an intimate understanding of our inner design. Love becomes an experience filled with ups and downs: it doesn't seem to last long enough; is as changeable as the wind; is one day here and gone the next. Women living without the ambience of love suffer tremendously, often experiencing states of acute depression and despair.

In part this unhappy situation can be attributed to a lack of insight into feminine energy and the female body. Women have no information on how to intentionally create the orgasmic state or how to embrace the gift of orgasm. In this void of wisdom, woman does not understand herself as intimately or expertly as she could. As a consequence, this naiveté about her body operates unconsciously against her better interests—in life, in love, and in sex.

Recently, at the end of a couples workshop, a man participating with his wife summed up his experience to the group: "It is quite incredible. After spending the last thirty-five years trying to become a really good lover, I discovered during this week that everything I think turns a woman on in actual fact turns her off." His observation was correct. I too have observed that the opposite of almost everything people think or say about sex has proved to be the truth. As a result of these misconceptions, women on the whole are not at all satisfied with the state of their sex lives, finding them unfulfilling for any number of reasons. Perhaps this may not be so at the beginning of a sexual relationship, but after a period of time many women report that dissatisfaction has become the norm. The body gradually closes down and a general disinterest and disappointment in sex begins to creep in. For some women this shift can occur within a few months, for others it happens over the course of a few years. The length of time involved is not relevant; what is most significant is the fact that this withdrawal from sex happens repeatedly for women.

Not knowing her body and the "how" of expanding into her feminine energy automatically places a restriction and limitation on a woman's experience of sex, and therefore of love. And if this reality is true for woman, it is equally true for man. If woman is living and loving at a sexual minimum, her male partner also exists at this same level.

For women this sexual minimum is reflected in their tremendous difficulties at achieving orgasm. So often women share with me their fear that something is seriously wrong with them because they cannot manage to experience any kind of orgasm. Or they're worried because they need an hour or more to feel a full *yes* to penetration. Or they report that sex has gradually lost its attraction, though the longing for tenderness and intimacy remains. With these negative thoughts passing through the mind, old and unexpressed feelings of unworthiness or inadequacy can ripple to

THE INTRINSIC POTENTIAL FOR ORGASM

the surface; soon insecurity begins to erode the joy of a loving heart. For a woman, unhappiness and dissatisfaction with sex can easily become the acceptable, expectable norm. Women's magazines routinely give tips on sex and female orgasm and advice about how to achieve orgasm more easily. Simply because these articles speak openly about sex (a rare occurrence in everyday conversation), they might gratify and relax a woman for a short while. But the guidance these magazines offer barely scratches the surface of the deeper sexual realm that exists for every human being. The advice found in magazines also reflects the widespread absence of concrete information on the female body. When last did we hear anything new or inspiring? When did we last hear about something that works? something that sounds right or feels right? something that resonates in the body, heart, and soul?

The truth is that your body is fully capable of experiencing deep, rich, satisfying orgasm. The key is to step inward and observe the physical sensations of your own body without judgment. How do you feel when you are having sex with your partner? How do you feel when you are having sex by yourself? Gather information about your body's responses. What do you enjoy? What irritates you? What leaves you feeling profoundly disappointed? Remember that, as long as you look at them honestly, feelings are always true. No feeling is ever "wrong."

When your partner, consumed by excitement, begins to move ever harder and faster toward his own climax (the so-called jackhammer mode), do you feel invisible, left behind, engulfed by a wave of disappointment that once again he will be all finished before you even begin to get warmed up? Or perhaps your partner dutifully feels that he should satisfy you before he allows himself to be satisfied, so he works hard to bring you to orgasm by stimulating your clitoris. He's doing the "right" thing, so you don't want to be critical. But is he rubbing too hard? too fast? Do you need more lubrication? Do you feel pressured to get on with it, to hurry up and climax so that he can move on to the "real" part of sex—that is, penetration and ejaculation? Do you worry that he's getting bored while he's stimulating you? Do you find yourself getting bored? Do you leave your body altogether and make a grocery list in your head or remember that your second child needs to take a picnic lunch for his field trip tomorrow? Or do you need to leave

THE INTRINSIC POTENTIAL FOR ORGASM

your physical body in another way and engage in a steamy sexual fantasy in order to come to climax? Do you actually feel disinterested but work hard at that fantasy, nevertheless, because your partner will be disappointed or feel diminished if he can't bring you to orgasm? Do you sometimes fake orgasm just to get the whole thing over with?

You are not alone. Unfortunately, most women in our modern-day cultures have felt some or all of these ways. And all of these scenarios miss the essential truth that your body is fully capable of a deep, sustained, fully satisfying orgasmic state. Orgasm is not a destination that we arrive at by trying—by doing the right thing or thinking the right thoughts. Rather, orgasm is a state of being that arises naturally when we are more relaxed in sex. In relaxation woman opens to her inner world, bringing herself into the focus of her attention. Doing so reveals the exquisite interplay of active male and receptive female energy, which flowers into prolonged pleasure for both the man and the woman.

You may well ask, "If this is true why don't more people know about it? Why has sexual dissatisfaction become the rule for women, rather than the exception?"

It can be said that we human beings unconsciously remain shortsighted about our true sexual selves. We are unaware of our higher potential and how to access it. As it stands, in our conventional sexual expression we are not truly physically sensitive or psychologically receptive or available enough to invite higher sexual experiences into us—or rather, to be graced by the divine, which would be a more accurate description. We are as host, and the divine is as guest, and enormous space has to be created for the divine to enter us.

These days it has become virtually impossible to shine new light on sex, to look at it and see it in a fresh, innocent, enlightened way. This is because there is an inherent limitation in our viewing situation—woman's role in the sex act is always looked at through the same spectacles, through the prevailing misconceptions about sex, the very misunderstandings that lie at the root of the orgasm issue. If you were to always look at the world through rose-tinted lenses you would begin to believe that everything was pink. If no one ever suggested that you take your spectacles off and see

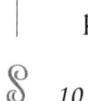

THE INTRINSIC POTENTIAL FOR ORGASM

how the world looked without them, you might continue to believe in your rose-tinted perceptions. They would become the norm for you, just as our misconceptions about female sexuality have become the norm for us in today's world.

Take, for instance, the sometimes-proffered suggestion that a woman use sexual fantasy to provoke an orgasm. In actual fact, sexual fantasy has nothing to do with what is happening in the woman's physical body in the here and now, with this particular man. It is an imagined scenario. It is a deliberate switch over from channel "body" to channel "mind," using the power granted by imagination. This can in fact trigger the response of sexual excitement in the body. But it has nothing to do with the physical penis that is present right now in the physical vagina. The issue here is that basic to lack of orgasm is a lack of connection to the body and to its internal sensitivity, its kinesthetic sense. So the advice of fantasy as a solution to orgasm—which only absents a woman further from her physical body—keeps woman circling around in the same sexual frame in which she already finds herself.

Our conventional, socially conditioned view of sex is linear and one-dimensional, lacking in balance, intelligence, and spiritual insight. Unless we are taught the full potential of sex while we are young, we inherit a sexual conditioning just by being a part of our society, by being surrounded by cultural misinformation that we absorb unconsciously. The rare person is able to access the uplifting dimension of sex intuitively; most of us are conditioned and live life in innocence of any sexual alternatives.

In response to the unconscious female conditioning of our society, the essential female qualities often become distorted: Softness can become weakness; receptivity can become passivity or resignation; the nurturing quality can become overbearing; the beauty of surrender can become submission; absorption might turn into sucking; the ability to sustain long-term waiting can shift into indolence; love can turn to jealousy and the use of female qualities for manipulation; the joy of non-doing and relaxation can express itself as the dead weight of inertia and laziness. Feminine fluidity might become a state of collapse; the free expression of individual feelings shifts toward sentimentality or moodiness; intuition and psychic abilities can slide over the line into paranoia and hysteria; the ability to allow events to unfold without trying to control them can become inappropriate indecisiveness or lack of initiative; sensitivity twists into victimhood or is used in the service of fear; appreciation for beauty becomes attachment to outer appearance; the nesting impulse can become a compulsive obsession with security; silent strength can turn to masochistic dependency; the awareness of connection to the universe beyond one's personal boundaries can go too far, resulting in an individual who is vague and spaced out and lacking enough personal definition.

The currently accepted view of "normal" sexual experience keeps women in bondage to an expression of a male type of sexuality, with no room for expression of the equally important female pole of sexual experience. The current male-oriented approach features an outward, sensation-directed expression of sexuality that effectively erases intrinsic female qualities, and in so doing firmly plants the roots of sexual dissatisfaction and dysfunction in both sexes. It is exactly the feminine, receptive qualities (undistorted by cultural misinformation) that are absolutely essential for the orgasmic state to arise in woman and also in man. Woman is required to be physically more poised and at ease so as to absorb the true male force, transform it, and channel it upward through her receptive feminine powers.

At this point in time women unconsciously, and sometimes consciously, support men in their male-oriented expression of sexuality. Many women report a high incidence of pain during and after sexual intercourse, but they endure it silently in order to satisfy their partners. Many others assume that sex will be a rough, aggressive experience with no expression of love or tenderness. I remember a woman telling me during a workshop that she had no idea that sex could be considerate and gentle. We collude with the dominant form of sexual expression simply because lovemaking has been "done" in this way for as long as we can remember. By now it seems utterly normal and we are unaware that alternatives exist.

While it appears that the conventional model of lovemaking is more satisfying for men than for women, in truth men's sexual fulfillment could also be much fuller and deeper, more sustained and more satisfy-

THE INTRINSIC POTENTIAL FOR ORGASM

ing than it is now. One reason for this is that male ejaculation is commonly understood to be the male version of orgasm. For many men ejaculation *is* the sexual experience. However, ejaculation is not the equivalent of orgasm. There is another type of male orgasm that happens without ejaculation and release of semen, an orgasm in which the energy is retained in the body, expanding upward instead of being released outward.

Women have enormous difficulties in reaching any kind of satisfying orgasm, while ironically (and yet somehow not surprisingly), men face the completely opposite problem—orgasm (or at any rate, ejaculation) is uncontrollable. It is impossible to delay or avoid. Usually it happens immediately upon penetration (or shortly before), or else within a paltry few minutes. The amount of time that passes between penetration and ejaculation is way too short for the purpose of raising a woman's sexual temperature to a sufficiently high degree that she will experience orgasm.

Once a woman discovers the art of expressing herself within the female element, with more serenity and receptivity, she will find to her surprise that she automatically reduces the likelihood of her man ejaculating prematurely. In this way, woman has the power to extend lovemaking from minutes into hours. A perceptive, sensitive internal environment can be consciously created by a woman. This environment changes the whole quality of the exchange and has the added power of strengthening the true masculine response. Distressing male sexual problems such as impotence and premature ejaculation are also symptoms of the prevailing confusion and lack of information about sex, and particularly about the female body. When woman develops the ability to shift into her feminine nature, exercising her receptive powers, many of these sexual dysfunctions and dissatisfactions can be healed.

At first most women will feel that they have little idea of how to shift into their feminine aspect or what that truly means. In reality it is easy—and it is absolutely natural. When we connect with our feminine qualities we can truly be who we are, with nothing forced and nothing acted out, we are simply open to receiving love. Relaxation, innocence, grace, and loving spontaneity are at the core of femininity. Women in my workshops frequently describe the shift toward themselves as a "coming

home" to something they have always known intuitively. Some share with me the sadness of recognizing now, so many years after their first glimpse of the truth, the insufficient trust they have had in themselves to follow through on their intuition and bring it into experience.

Feminine wisdom is nature's jewel, held deep within woman. The pages ahead are an attempt to help women uncover something they already possess, a crystal waiting to receive the light of inner intelligence.

Tantric Inspiration

Energy can have two dimensions. One is motivated, going somewhere, a goal somewhere, this moment is only a means and the goal is going to be achieved somewhere else. This is one dimension of your energy, this is the dimension of activity, goal oriented—then everything is a means, somehow it has to be done and you have to reach the goal, then you will relax. But for this type of energy the goal never comes because this type of energy goes on changing every present moment into a means for something else, into the future. The goal always remains on the horizon. You go on running, but the distance remains the same.

No, there is another dimension of energy: that dimension is unmotivated celebration. The goal is here, now; the goal is not somewhere else. In fact, you are the goal. In fact there is no other fulfillment than that of this moment—consider the lilies. When you are the goal and when the goal is not in the future, when there is nothing to be achieved, rather you are just celebrating it, then you have already achieved it, it is there. This is relaxation, unmotivated energy.

OSHO, TRANSCRIBED TEACHINGS,
TANTRA: THE SUPREME UNDERSTANDING

Awareness and Sensitivity Preparation
Position for Rest and Relaxation

Here is the ideal horizontal position to assume for relaxation: Your head, neck, and spine should be in a straight line, not even a few millimeters out of alignment and definitely not with the head rolled away to one side. Your legs should be straight and a little apart, and your ankles should *not* be crossed over each other. Place a narrow soft pillow (or a rolled blanket) directly under the knees to create a slight curving and softening of the knee joint. Place a small, flat, firm pillow (or folded towel) under your head. Pull the chin to the chest so as to straighten your neck before placing the pillow in position. The pillow should support the lengthening of your spine so there is not too much of a curve in the neck. If the chin is pointing almost directly upward and not tilted toward the chest, use a slightly thicker pillow (or give the towel another fold) to lift the head an additional few inches, so as to create length and reduce the curve in the neck. Place your open hands palm down on the groin area on each side of your pubic bone. Rest quietly with closed eyes for twenty minutes (or more), holding awareness in your body.

Tantric Meditation
Growing in Consciousness

Lying in the position described above, you can deepen your experience if you close your eyes and imagine yourself looking into your body. Imagine that your eyes can look inward and downward into your body, even as far as your genitals. Breathe deeply and slowly into your belly, as if the breath is massaging your insides and touching the genitals. Continually pull your attention back into your body and the sensations in it. Deliberately disconnect from distracting thoughts when they pop up. Let them float away, and return to your body. Immerse yourself in the body so that you feel a sense of resting deep within your body, with the sensation of being submerged in yourself.

Travel with your awareness to any places in the body where tinglings or warmth or fine vibrations are present, and dissolve into them.

At a certain point, once the practice of immersing into your senses takes root, the feeling of your physical boundaries will disappear; you may experience being as light as a feather, bathed in golden light, floating suspended in consciousness. You are, but you are not. In this way you can grow in consciousness until every cell is penetrated. The moment consciousness touches the cells, they are different. The very quality of the cells changes.

You can set a clock for the period of time you wish to devote to the experience, or you may leave it up to your inner clock, which, after a period, spontaneously returns you to normal consciousness (along with the sense of having lost all track of time). You are likely to notice that after such an experience you feel refreshed and rejuvenated, as though you have had a drink directly from the source of life. It is also beneficial to practice this meditation before sleeping at night, or at any time during the day when you need to recharge your energy.

2
Orgasm Is a Spiritual Experience

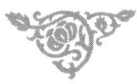

P robably most of us have given little thought to where the word *orgasm* comes from, and what it actually implies. *Orgasm* derives from the Latin word *orgia*,[1] which describes a pagan religious ceremony in which people became ecstatic—so ecstatic that their bodies were bursting with divine energy and they were able to lose themselves in time-stopping bliss. In the word *orgasm* we see our origins reflected in language, reminding us that in earlier days humans gathered together in large groups to perform rituals with the intention of deliberately moving into ecstasy. Attaining orgia was a way of praising and expressing gratitude to Mother Earth, extolling the marvel of her creation. With simple dance steps, singing to the rhythmic beating of the drum, and celebrating for days on end people became almost drunk with the divine, accessing gloriously heightened states of sensuality and sensitivity. Participants returned from the ceremonies rejuvenated, overflowing with love and zest for life.

Today few opportunities for expression of orgia exist. There has been a

shift away from emphasis on the physical body toward emphasis on the mind. Instead of sharing energy by dancing and singing together, people are more likely to meet in large or small groups to exchange ideas, discuss, argue, or gossip. We have become disconnected from our bodily sensitivity and lukewarm in our physical responses; as a result we experience a lack of fulfilling orgasm during sexual exchange. In this restricted environment sex loses its natural healing and regenerative powers. Man and woman have lost touch with the uplifting spiritual connection once regularly accessed through the physical body.

Human beings can only genuinely begin to affect or change their social environment through a dramatic and drastic reevaluation and re-evolution in sex. The repression and suppression of normal, healthy sex that has prevailed for the last few thousand years of civilization has had a severely polluting effect on the beautiful, loving, natural expression that sex is. At present it can safely be said that the source of most social disturbance and violence has its root in sex—or, more to the point, the lack of nourishing, fulfilling, uplifting sex. It is as if our society has become sexually unwell. Sex itself is not sick, but the mind—the psychology of humans surrounding sex—has become tainted, almost toxic. The sexual abuse of all kinds that occurs somewhere every minute of every day provides acutely painful evidence of the sexual distress present in society. Through widespread misinformation, sexual energy is unconsciously repressed and creativity is diminished. The prevalent lack of understanding about the nature of male and female energetic interaction means that contemporary sex rarely achieves a full expression of its spiritually regenerative potential. Although at first glance sexual perversion, sexual abuse, aggression, and war might not appear to be directly related to a lack of fulfilling and nourishing sexual experience, the rejection of an expression that is our inherent nature contributes to all of these unfortunate outcomes.

Through misunderstanding the significance of sex over and above reproduction, a woman can easily find herself forced to accept a loveless, intrusive, and abusive sex life. She may sincerely want to produce children and to love, feed, and care for a family, yet she devotes herself to all of this

heartfelt expression in the absence of any regenerative and uplifting orgasmic experiences for herself. And this lack of sexual fulfillment holds true for men, too, most of whom, even after a lifetime of sexual experiences, still believe that ejaculation equals orgasm (which, as we have already mentioned, it does not).

Biology, as the means by which life here on Earth is preserved, is without question basic to sex. Without biological sex, life as we know it would cease. Almost all forms of animal and plant life unite male and female elements to re-create life. Sometimes the two elements are in separate entities, sometimes not. Sometimes the entities join physically, sometimes not. In whatever way the miracle of fertilization occurs, sex functions to create new life, extending the collective life of all the species. Sex fully engages all levels of life in all forms in a most extraordinarily wholehearted process in order to ensure the continuation of the species.

Even though it is no novelty, human birth will forever be the most awesome of miracles. The innocence, integrity, and delicate perfection of translucent new life touches and warms the heart in the most enchanting of ways. Even so, the ability to reproduce another human being represents only our basic biological expression of sex. This is our so-called animal nature, and it depends upon a downward movement of energy. Male semen is released by ejaculation (with or without female orgasm). Fusion and fertilization of the female egg follows, and another life is initiated, a life separate from the two lives that produced it.

But there is more to human sexuality than the physical ability to reproduce. Nature did not give us the captivating mystery of sex simply for quick male ejaculation and prolonged female gestation. In humans there is a higher dimension to sex—there is more to the meeting of male and female than meets the eye.

The Upward Movement of Sexual Energy

Humans are designed to experience altered states of consciousness during sexual union—states that engender a blissful experience of union with the whole of existence. In this orgasmic ability we differ from our

friends in the animal kingdom (with the exception of dolphins, who are understood to experience higher energetic states during sexual play). Our bodies come with the innate capacity to expand energetically from the sexual center. When correctly harnessed this expansion results in altered states of consciousness: valleys of ecstatic relaxation and peaks of orgasmic expression.

The impact of upward-moving sexual energy is relatively unknown in the West and is explored by only a few. But if we turn to the East we encounter (in China) a far earlier culture whose medical practitioners urged such energy practices for good health and longevity. In India a far earlier religion also recognized and cultivated this upward-spiraling energy as the spiritual aspect of sex, as sacred sexuality.* When the energy is routed in this vertical way as an expression of the higher, generative aspect of sexuality, sex protects the body and is experienced as a rejuvenating and life-giving force in the human being.

In generative sexual expression, the intent and function are more or less opposite from the intent and function of its biological counterpart. There is no biological requirement to ejaculate semen (to coincide with ovulation). No additional life is produced; instead, the energy is retained and remains within the participants themselves, renewing lives that already exist. The lovers feel enriched, energized, loving, and joyful.

Inward and upward movement of energy during generative sexual play occurs of its own accord with the balance and alignment of male and female genitals. Energy moves according to an innate polarity, which we discuss in depth in Chapter 4. Genitals together generate energy that rises upward through internal channels eventually to reach, and return to, the "master" endocrine glands in the brain, the ultimate source of all hormonal information given to the body.

These glands, particulary the pituitary and pineal glands, themselves produce our sexual expression.[2] (At high levels of hormonal purification, the body will even release perfumed fragrances.) The pituitary gland is

---

*China (Taoism), three thousand years ago and India (Tantra), five to ten thousand years ago.

located between the eyebrows, above the nasal cavity. It is the master endocrine control gland regulating growth, gonadal function, the adrenals, and the thyroid. This gland is said to govern the forebrain, vision, and the right eye, as well as being the seat of love, compassion, knowledge, love of humanity, and devotion. It is also involved in intelligence and conceptual memory, which we use in reading, thinking, and studying. Close by is the pineal gland, located toward the crown of the head above the midbrain; its functions are related to sensitivity and to the sexual cycle. The pineal gland governs the hindbrain, hearing, body rhythms, equilibrium, and the perception of light through eyes and skin.

Given all of these functions that we take for granted, it becomes obvious that feeding and nourishing these master glands with our sexual energy—our life force—is bound to be to our distinct advantage.

When energy spirals upward it produces a vitality that radiates from the whole being. One feels cellularly drenched with contentment, love, and peace. Sex experienced in this way is empowering. Energy is not released; it is produced, strengthening the immune system and enhancing all kinds of creativity. An individual can extend her life by producing this generative energy rather than simply duplicating it, as is possible through the downward-moving expression of reproduction. Nature gives us sex so that we may have the opportunity to transcend the limits of our physical boundaries, to float as filaments of vibrating light and love. The experience of generative sex keeps a person youthful, adventurous, and responsive to whatever life brings.

It seems incredible to realize that the spiritual realm of orgasm—the most fulfilling gift human beings possess—remains unexplored during an age in which humankind has penetrated outer realms with its increasingly sophisticated technology. In spite of all of our technological know-how, we find ourselves stumbling around in the sexual arena, tethered by ignorance and by complacency. We assume that simply by virtue of being a woman or a man, we will automatically know everything about the sex act.

How then is it that woman knows so little about her body and her sexual potential? Perhaps at some time in the past this knowledge was deliberately kept secret from her, making her a more compliant slave to the

appeasement of mans' appetites. But it comes as no surprise to women that modern men are even less informed than women about women's bodies—or, for that matter, about their own bodies. Women have a longstanding affinity with intuitive knowledge—commonly referred to as "women's intuition"—which most men are less able to access as the truth residing within their bodies. By looking (and feeling) within, women need to take the lead in making a place for generative sexuality, and for the love that follows.

In the absence of a woman's cooperation in sex, the divinity of the sex act is near impossible to encounter. Generations of insensitive handling and abuse of women by men has led to situations in which sex, to a lesser or greater degree, is lovelessly imposed upon women. When a man repeatedly enters a woman's body before she is really prepared for penetration, the woman will feel turned off to sex. A certain repulsion may even begin to set in. In time, many a woman will close down physically, eventually turning away from sex if possible. When unable to avoid it, she becomes a master at submitting, enduring the minutes prior to ejaculation. Once she becomes resigned to lack of satisfaction in sex, woman can actually feel grateful for premature ejaculation in the knowledge that everything will soon be over.

Man has lost his masculine ability to "speak" meaningfully to the female body, the ability to spiral in on her in such a way that she welcomes penetration with her whole being. He has become so accustomed to woman giving in and yielding to him that he has forgotten (or has never experienced) the true taste and flair of cooperative sexual expression, the dance of male and female sexuality in perfect balance, in which woman sumptuously participates, transforming the experience into a sinuous, winding, dynamic dance between bodies. Such an experience in itself can give man the feeling of his worth as a male of the species—and for many a man it will be the first time he feels this way in his life.

Woman Is the Environment of Sex

It is impossible for man to know more about a woman's body until she comes to know a little bit more about herself. With constructive input, a woman can learn how to transform the quality of her sexual experience, even in the absence of conscious cooperation from her man. Woman's influence in the sexual realm is such that she can drastically alter the experience *if* she knows how. This gives her the capacity to make satisfying love for the rest of her life and to find the love she seeks without necessarily having to change partners.

Because a woman's body is most often judged from the outside by its shape, its proportions, and its curves, a woman has a bird's-eye view of herself. She is accustomed to seeing herself from a distance, from without; rarely does she truly feel herself from within. When a woman learns how to nourish a romance with her own body, to unite with it from the inside, alive in all her senses, she exudes a breathtakingly feminine quality that transforms the atmosphere around her.

Unfortunately, most modern women have no information whatsoever on how to accomplish such a transformation. Out of disappointment and frustration, many women today abandon sex altogether, trusting that their love for children or career will compensate for the loss. In so doing a woman commits a travesty of justice: she denies herself an essential part of being a woman. Resignation begins to settle firmly around her mouth. Often a woman feels a longing for grandchildren (for another cycle of reproduction) so that she may once again feel love flowing within her.

In an ideal world, grandmothers would inspire their grandchildren by talking freely about their most nourishing experiences with sex, guiding their grandchildren along the right track, encouraging them to give and receive love. But as it stands in our culture, our mothers and grandmothers and great-grandmothers have, like ourselves, had no access to higher forms of sexual expression. In the sexual realm, they have nothing to pass down in the way of wisdom or insight.

This does not mean that no such wisdom exists. When we look to

ancient traditional cultures of the East we find an open conduit to sexual wisdom. Central to that wisdom is the knowledge that woman is the environment, the container, the receptacle for sex. Her vagina is the space into which man physically *enters*. And, in great contrast, woman *receives* man physically into herself. These two functions—entering and receiving—are very different. Man is the guest; woman is the host.

Because of the internal design of the vagina, woman is able to exert a powerful influence during the sex act. This command that a woman has in sex, as the environment of sex, can best be illustrated by simple analogy. If you were to enter a room that was crowded with furniture and hectic with the blaring sounds of a television and the ringing demands of a telephone, this atmosphere would likely have a negative impact upon you. It would probably strike you as being frenzied, congested, chaotic, and a bit overwhelming. You might feel encapsulated by pressure and tension, and most likely your immediate impulse would be to get out into the open air again as soon as possible.

In contrast, if you were to enter a room that had a feeling of spacious emptiness enhanced by just a few essential furnishings, where the sound of a flute hung suspended in air that was fragrant with sensuality, such an environment would exude peace and tranquillity. Rather than inspiring tension, it would inspire a sensation of inner space, expansion, a feeling of coming home. The embracing atmosphere, the absence of external pressures, and the open space would give rise to an inner relaxation. As harmony and serenity descended upon you, you would probably take a deep breath and arrive fully in your body.

Now consider the event of male penetration into the female body. Just as the environment in a room has a profound effect upon the human psyche, the ambience within the female body can, and does, have a transforming effect upon man. It is extremely influential. Man is utterly affected by woman and yet he is ignorant of the extent to which this is so. Through intentionally creating a serene, receptive internal environment a woman can prolong the sex act. She can help man to delay, and even to avoid, ejaculation.

The real sadness, though, is that woman remains as unaware of her

true capacity as man does. Not knowing how to tap into it, she too fails to experience her intrinsic power, leaving her deeper realms of female sexuality unexplored. Understanding the real nature of female sexual expression can reunite woman with her god- and goddess-given power. When woman enters the sexual act within her female element, sexual fulfillment and love will be the natural consequence. Every woman possesses this natural ability to transform lovemaking into a wholly satisfying and spiritually transcendent experience. All women need is useful information on how to go about it.

Tantric Inspiration

Orgasm is a state where your body is no more felt as matter; it vibrates like energy, electricity. It vibrates so deeply, from the very foundation, that you completely forget that it is a material thing. It becomes an electric phenomenon—and it is an electric phenomenon.

Now physicists say that there is no matter, that all matter is only appearance; deep down, that which exists is electricity, not matter. In orgasm, you come to this deepest layer of your body where matter no more exists, just energy waves; you become a dancing energy, vibrating. No more any boundaries to you—pulsating, but no more substantial. And your beloved also pulsates.

And by and by, if they love each other and they surrender to each other, they surrender to this moment of pulsation, of vibration, of being energy, and they are not scared. . . . Because it is deathlike when the body loses boundaries, when the body becomes like a vaporous thing, when the body evaporates substantially and only energy is left, a very subtle rhythm, but you find yourself as if you are not. Only in deep love can one move into it. Love is like death: you die as far your material image is concerned, you die as far as you think you are a body; you die as a body and you evolve as energy, vital energy.

And when the wife and the husband, or the lovers, or the partners, start vibrating in a rhythm, the beats of their hearts and bodies come together, it becomes a harmony—then orgasm happens, then they are two no more. That is the symbol of yin and yang; yin moving into yang, yang moving into yin; the man moving into the woman, the woman moving into the man.

Now they are a circle, and they vibrate together, they pulsate together. Their hearts are no longer separate, their beats are no longer separate; they have become a melody, a harmony. It is the greatest music possible; all other musics are just faint things compared to it, shadow things compared to it.

OSHO, TRANSCRIBED TEACHINGS,
TANTRA: THE SUPREME UNDERSTANDING

Awareness and Sensitivity Preparation
Developing Soft Vision

To help your energy (which usually moves outward) to fall back in upon your own heart, it is helpful to learn *soft vision*. In soft vision you reverse the usual visual process and imagine you are receiving inwardly through the eyes rather than looking out through them.

To begin: stand, sit, or lie (in the position described at the end of chapter 1). Close your eyes and bring awareness to your body, finding a location such as the belly or heart or solar plexus that feels like "home" to you. It should be a place that easily connects you to your inner world and acts as an anchor for your awareness in the body. It is a resting place, an inner resource around which you gather yourself and from which you experience and create the present moment. If your whole body feels like home to you and there is no specific area that grabs your attention, a generalized body awareness is fine too.

When you have the sense of being rooted in your body, connected with yourself from the inside, open your eyes extremely slowly, millimeter by millimeter, allowing anything that falls into your range of vision *into* yourself *through* your eyes. It can be a flower, a candle, a plant, a painting, a view in the room, a wall, a ceiling: simply imagine that whatever appears before you—the texture, the light, the color—is *entering* you, penetrating you through your eyes. The looking becomes passive, as if vision is reversed. Your eyes are receiving energy, not dispersing energy, as seems to be the case in normal looking.

While practicing this way of seeing, the trick is to pay attention to your body and to stay rooted in the bodily home you have identified. The intention is not to lose the connection to yourself once your eyes are opened. Losing connection to the body when the eyes are open is bound to happen again and again as you make your first few attempts. As soon as you notice you are absent from your body, more involved in looking outward than directing your awareness to your inner world, close your eyes immediately and reconnect inwardly for several seconds. When settled and rooted inside again, open the eyes very slowly. Continue with this process of opening the eyes while staying connected to the body and closing when you lose connection until you get the hang of it. Practice is required in the beginning; after a while it will become easy. You can also practice soft vision in nature—with a waterfall, with a tree, with a sunset, with the moon—and you will have memorable experiences of peace and love.

Tantric Meditation
Meditating on Light

When you feel comfortable with soft vision you can make a special meditation of it using the power of light. Meditation on light is one of the most ancient meditations. Light has been emphasized because meditating on light causes something inside you that has remained asleep to start opening its petals. Through time and the collective wisdom of those seeking transcendence through the body, this process has come to be associated with the light-sensitive pituitary gland, situated in the body at the site of what yogis call the third eye.

Give yourself half an hour or more for this experience. Create a harmonious environment and sit in front of a candle. Using soft vision, allow the flame to enter you. When the eyes need a rest or you lose connection to your body, close your eyes and continue to visualize the light penetrating you through your eyes. Alternatively open and close the eyes as feels most comfortable to you.

Let light become your meditation: whenever you have time, close your eyes and visualize light. Wherever you see light, be in tune with it, be alert to it, be prayerful toward it, be grateful to it.

3
Orgasm versus Orgasmic

*T*he nature of female orgasm is not easily generalized—quite possibly there are as many kinds of orgasm as there are women having them. Even so, in order to understand the nature of feminine energy it is helpful to look at orgasm from a number of angles.

Orgasm can be loosely divided into two categories—peak orgasm and valley orgasm. Naturally there can be a whole range of experiences between a peak and a valley, but what distinguishes one from the other is the very basis of each type—the peak orgasm depends on an active buildup of excitement and the valley orgasm arises from relaxation.

Peak and Valley Orgasms

Let us consider in detail the differences in these two approaches to orgasm. From the very outset the approach and attitude is different, one from the other. First of all, we tend to intentionally seek and "go for" the peak type of orgasm, to deliberately build it up to a climax. Achieving a peak orgasm becomes a linear, goal-oriented activity requiring a mental intention to get from one place to another. We assume that we need to *do* whatever we consider necessary to reach our final destination—the peak. A valley experience is more like an invitation without an expectation or demand of orgasm. Something may or may not happen. And when it happens, it happens by itself. The final outcome is not at issue; rather, the focus is on the joy of the moment—being here and now in the body—which allows the journey to unfold without a predetermined direction. In place of pursuing an orgasm there is an openness to and acceptance of what is taking place in the body, moment by moment, which creates the sensitivity necessary for an orgasmic valley experience to emerge.

To arrive at a peak orgasm we must usually expend considerable physical effort. The aim is to intensify the stimulation and bring the deliciously exciting sensations into one glorious crescendo. This involves repeated mechanical movements of the pelvis, which get faster and faster toward the end. This activity is necessary in order to intensify energy to a peak, but at the same time it also builds up a lot of tension, which compresses the energy into the genitals. In contrast to all this customary activity, to enable a valley experience to flower we need to *be* more and *do* less, allowing everything to unfold very slowly in the most languid, easy, lazy way possible. We avoid deliberate efforts and any movements or positions that produce undue tensions. The penetration of the vagina by the penis is deliberately slow, and so are any pelvic movements. This relaxation between the genitals encourages a radiation and expansion of energy into other parts of the body.

The peak orgasm is usually quite a hot affair. In the valley things are a lot cooler. Any pleasurable moments of excitation can be enjoyed for what they are, but they will be followed by minutes of relaxation, not fed and inflamed into a climax of excitement. Through slowing down into a more non-doing approach and bringing awareness to internal movements of energy, we awaken an inner sensitivity that has little to do with excitement or stimulation. This sensitivity reveals a layer of magnetic excitation in the body that is cool, cellular, and ecstatic. A buildup of excitement is not even really required for the relaxed kind of orgasm.

Yet another way that a peak orgasm differs from a valley orgasm is in the duration of the experience. A peak orgasm is estimated to last, on a good day, around ten seconds. So we can say that a peak experience has a pretty definite start and finish. This makes it more like an event—we "have an orgasm," or not, as the case may be. In contrast, the valley orgasm is a more sustained state, a timeless experience without a specific start or finish. It can last for a few moments or a few hours—the time span is irrelevant, but the experience is the same: In a valley orgasm, an ecstatic peace descends upon us, it surrounds, embraces, and soothes us, we are suspended in it. We "become orgasmic." This is an expanded state of consciousness, not a momentary event measurable in seconds, like an orgasm.

When we merge fully with the subtleties present in the physical body, the sexual experience becomes ecstatically bodiless. This sounds contrary and upside down but in reality this is how it works. Energy turns inward and expands, streaming orgasmically upward. Rather than being discharged or released from the body, the energy gathers within the system, generating vitality and creativity. Sex experienced in this way enhances and strengthens the life force: beneficial hormones released during sex are delivered to the brain, nourishing the master pituitary and pineal glands situated there (as mentioned in the last chapter), with positive impact on good spirits, health, and longevity. Sex actually extends life.

The energy of a peak orgasm tends to work in the opposite way. In the peak experience the energy moves downward and outward, in accordance with the requirements of procreation. The intensity of excitement is followed by a pleasurable discharge of energy that is released down and out of the body. Evidence of this discharge is the fact that frequently after ejaculation a man will suffer a distinct loss of energy. He may even feel angry, restless, or disconnected from his woman. Many women observe that they too lose great amounts of energy in orgasm, just like a man but without the release of semen. Suddenly the willingness to make love evaporates; they find themselves without energy or inclination to continue. As a result of the discharge in an orgasm, a woman can often feel abandoned, lonely, sad, or depressed.

The peak orgasm is more or less experienced as a local genital experience because the sexual energy is not given the chance to expand, to touch other parts of the body. In fact it cannot expand because the very effort of achieving orgasm creates tension and thus a barrier to radiation of energy. The potentially beneficial energy is lost in release, rendering it unavailable for performing its natural healing and nourishing functions.

Special techniques do exist for deliberately extending the peak type of orgasm into multiple orgasms. By synchronizing breath and movement and relaxation, it is possible to assist energy to move beyond the automatic barriers and create expanded energetic states. Reaching these states usually requires substantial skill and focused concentration; rarely, though, do extended peak orgasms arise from an original state of relaxation.

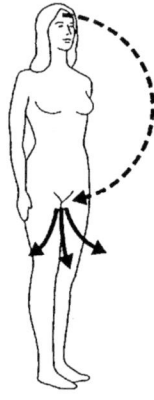

Fig. 3.1. Biological or reproductive phase of sexual energy

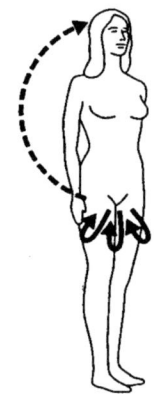

Fig. 3.2. Spiritual or generative phase of sexual energy

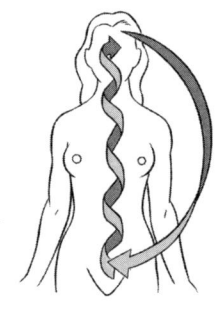

Fig. 3.3. Complete sexual energy circle with redirected sexual energy spiraling through energy centers

Opening to a New Approach

To make the sexual experience more fulfilling, in general, a woman would do well to tend toward the orgasmic approach—orgasm as a sustained state of being in the sexual exchange—rather than simply seeking out the peak type of orgasm. This approach depends a lot on the willingness to trust relaxation and intrinsic feminine receptivity. Rather than trying to make something happen, you simply receive, and *be,* and absorb energy into the core of the body through the vagina. It's natural once you get the hang of it. All the same elements of sex are present but the composition is entirely different. What makes the greatest difference is the attitude and awareness of a woman within herself, a woman's willingness to tap into her true feminine spirit. This requires a deeper understanding of her body and the courage to honor and express the feminine element residing within.

Most women associate the clitoris with orgasm; however, the vagina is more centrally associated with orgasmic states. A rising understanding of this may lead a woman to reevaluate her clitoral experiences while exploring her orgasmic potential. (Chapters 6 and 7 are devoted to the vagina and the clitoris respectively.) Please be aware that when I suggest this alternative approach to orgasm my intention is to broaden the possibilities for satisfying sexual experience. It is *not* my intention to make you think in duality, to suggest that you make a separation between peaks and valleys or doing and being. In reality one cannot exist without the other, so any separation between them is false. Included are all the delightful gradations of exploration and experience linking these two. My intention is to convey that there are choices.

I simply invite you to reflect on your experience in light of the new information I offer here, to see how it might be of benefit to you. With this new approach, the orientation is toward relaxing into being orgasmic rather than searching with effort for an orgasm. Please don't be judgmental toward yourself for your "failure" to have orgasms or for having the "wrong" kind of orgasm. There is no wrong or right way to approach sex, no one to please but yourself. Perhaps, upon reflection, you will realize that you haven't allowed yourself to turn inward during sex, to feel yourself on the inside and discover what would please you. Perhaps you'll see that you've been working awfully hard to *succeed* at sex, as though you were performing in a play or taking an examination. Perhaps you'll conclude that you're basically happy with your sex life but the idea of trying a new approach appeals to your adventurous spirit. It is my sincere hope that whatever insights you gain about yourself by looking inward can shift your perspective in a way that allows you to improve your experience.

ORGASM VERSUS ORGASMIC

Relaxation and Tension

Relaxation lies at the very base of any enhancement of experience, so relaxation and more satisfying orgasm go hand in hand. All orgasms, peak and valley, are enhanced by relaxation. Any relaxation (even briefly) of any body part invites the expansion of energy on which all orgasm and heightened experiences are based. Relaxation spontaneously leads to increased awareness, bodily sensitivity, and psychological openness. And relaxation produces qualities essential to feminine energy. Especially for woman at first, relaxation is essential because it shifts her away from the active, outward, male kind of expression required for conventional orgasm and puts her unquestionably into the receptive, feminine mode. An orgasmic state, or any orgasm achieved through relaxation, engages the genuine, deep-rooted, feminine energies of a woman, which allow orgasm to be a fully satisfying experience. This is a good point to remember when you feel unsure about branching out and exploring a new approach to sex.

Peak orgasms can certainly feel wonderful in themselves, but rarely are they deeply moving. We often feel basically untouched by them. If you find yourself reluctant to explore something other than the tried and true, remember that there is more to sex than the candles on the cake, which can be blown out at any moment. Remember, too, that countless women report problems with the conventional peak style of orgasm, with getting their candles blown out nicely. Even with every best intention, it is not always possible to build up sufficient sexual charge to produce a meaningful or prolonged climax. In our effort to "get there," our movements become faster and harder, more and more unconscious and aggressive, decreasing our sensitivity with each move we make.

The physical tensions inherent in the goal-oriented approach to peak orgasm are compounded by mental and emotional concerns about orgasm that are present even before we begin to have sex. Tensions increase with any kind of pressure and, unfortunately, most women feel pressured to have an orgasm in order to please the man. Man so enjoys the moments when a woman orgasms that he likes to make it happen if he can. Partly he likes to give his woman pleasure, but beyond that the ego issue is a very big part of the picture. When a man sees his woman orgasm, it confirms

to him that he is indeed a good lover. This is something for a woman to be aware of, and we'll attend to it more in a later chapter. It is good to know that many men are quite identified with (even addicted to) the excitement of their woman's orgasm, if she is so lucky as to have one.

I am reminded of an occasion in a workshop when, after a few days of experimenting, a woman joyfully announced that she was finished with regular orgasms. They did not really do anything for her. In fact, she even noticed she felt much better without them. (I have heard women say words to this effect more times than I can count.) Much to her surprise this woman's lover took her words very personally and reacted by withdrawing into angered silence. He unfortunately managed to receive her experiential observation as a personal insult—a message that he was no good and had been unable to satisfy her in the first place. He also felt threatened by the possibility that she would no longer be willing to have sex in the usual way, to try for peak orgasms for him or with him. Apparently he would have to sacrifice his customary approach.

Overcoming a Lover's Resistance

Be prepared for a little protesting from your man here and there, but don't let that stall you for long. Don't be too serious in exploring new sexual pathways; develop a sense of humor. Be a sincere adventurer rather than a giver of rules and regulations, a tendency that women can easily display when entering this new realm. Don't get caught up in telling a man what to do and how to do it. The tantric realm is closer to woman because of her receptive nature, so she falls into it more naturally. Man has quite some dismantling of a huge, excitement-oriented sexuality to do. He requires understanding, even compassion; instead of criticizing him a woman can become a bridge for him, a way to cross back and forth between the new and the old approaches. For a man to become tantric requires the same inward focus as it does for a woman, in order for him to contact his natural masculine responsive force and not depend on the usual male strategies. Give him space to experiment, working in cooperation with the reality (man's sexual conditioning) without getting fixated on the ideal, which will only cause tension and turn an adventure into a struggle. Of course,

many men are delighted when women take more of a commanding role in sex. Thus your man may welcome your new interest with relief, and not see it as a threat to his ego. Certainly the situation has most potential when you explore together rather than as two separate persons each intent on his or her own thing.

Nevertheless, a woman can try out many of the suggestions offered in this book without her man necessarily having to agree (although he is bound to notice there is something more enchanting about the experience of making love with her). The truth is, changing a style of making love is an individual commitment, not necessarily a couple commitment. You as an individual have to wish to be more aware, receptive, and open—not too dependent on what your partner is up to or expects of you. Otherwise you can go around in circles and never break out of the trap you find yourself in.

For example, the situation may arise that your man wants to come. What do you do? You might join him, saying to yourself, "Well then, what the heck, so will I." But this is not individual commitment; this is handing over to another person the responsibility for your own transformation. And that never works to one's greatest satisfaction. Instead you might choose to *not* come, to relax and enjoy being with him during his experience but not force yourself into coming just because he is doing so. And if you decide, in fact, that this time you do want to come, then set about it in an easier and less effortful way. Be experimental and create the opportunity to experience yourself differently. Resist falling back to the known you, the tried and tested way. Experiment for your own sake and be curious about the outcome.

It might happen that, for a period of time while making love, a man still insists on his orgasm. But in the new context this can be after *an hour of delicious lovemaking*—which greatly changes the picture. And why not? In time, he may feel that it is less important to ejaculate, that he is pretty happy with how things stand at the moment; he feels quite fulfilled and notices he is energized afterward. Through experimenting and observing the outcomes of sex, sex begins to gain significance beyond simple entertainment. This is our usual gauge of sex—did we have fun? Was it recre-

ational? In actual fact, far more telling about whether a good time was had or not is what happens *after* the experience.

Observe the Afterward

We tend to overlook how we experience ourselves after the sexual encounter. How do we feel? What is happening within me and between us? In workshops I insist to couples that "the time afterward is your teacher," not my partner and I. By keeping an eye on your postcoital states, both of you will get insights into the genuine goodness of sex and what leads you where. If after making love there is at times a feeling of distance and at other times a feeling of closeness, what does this reflect? Review your lovemaking and see how it informs you. In time a totally new vision of sex starts to emerge through understanding your experience. The inquiry becomes, "How is sex able to spread its benefit to every moment of my life, every day, in and out of bed? How do I get the best out of sex as a human being, not just a human doing?"

Recently I received an email from a couple in Australia that may serve to relax women and encourage men. After they had found a section of my first book displayed on the Internet, the male partner wrote to me saying:

> We printed the lot and took it away with us on our January break. The simple concept of letting go of goal oriented intimacy has been a revelation which has greatly enhanced the spiritual sensitivity of our lovemaking and the sheer pleasure and beauty of enjoying each moment for itself, the beauty of the feelings of each touch or caress, the moment by moment sensation of each kiss, the loveliness of each moment of body contact, instead of each action being part of the path to the goal of orgasm. Being prepared to throw away the goals and letting each moment lead to the next brings pleasure to each moment and takes away all pressure to perform. We have been married almost twenty-five years and the spiritual dimension has always been important to us, but it is easy to get caught up in our Western approach of being goal oriented in almost everything we do, and so much of the Western material we read about sex is goal oriented. Best Regards.

ORGASM VERSUS ORGASMIC

Open up to the new alternative way, so that your man too can begin to experience himself in a new way. Remember, it takes a morsel before the taste can develop. Don't just give in to going with the usual, the male-dominated sexual expression. A real woman does not stand a chance there. In giving in (or giving up), both men and women are the losers and nobody is a real winner.

Orgasm is a gift from the divine, a sip of the sweetest nectar. It is nothing to demand, expect, or chase after. If there is too much tension coming from expectations in sex, misery or frustration is bound to follow failure. Orgasms are not required every time we make love. An easygoing, innocent, unexpectant attitude creates the milieu for the orgasmic experience. So begin to change your thoughts on orgasm. As you enter sex, do something unusual: forget about orgasm. Avoid looking for sensations that could be the beginning of a climax; avoid heading for orgasm the moment your man penetrates you. Be as receptive and welcoming to the penetration as possible, paying close attention to the feelings in your vagina.

Observe within yourself the minute cellular phenomena present in the body in any given moment. As time is comprised of millions of magical moments strung together, the details are constantly changing, and these can become a constant source of delight.

Living these inner changes makes the sexual experience an organic one. Orgasm is not necessarily a huge explosion, a volcanic eruption. It can be a cool, peaceful, calm, relaxing valley where the body floats as light as a feather, dissolving into love-drenched nothingness. It can be the experience of eternity, beyond time, suspended in space by breath, one with the pulsation of life. It also happens, as if by miracle, that from this depth of relaxation a peak of energy arises, but without any effort at all. A subtle force rises slowly and steadily from the depths and moves into a sexual dance, choreographed by a divine energy passing through the bodies.

Tantric Inspiration

Relaxation is a state. You cannot force it. You simply drop all negativities, the hindrances and, it comes, it bubbles up by itself. What is relaxation? It is a state of affairs where your energy is not moving anywhere, not in the future, not to the past—it is simply there with you. In the silent pool of your own energy, in the warmth of it, you are enveloped. *This* moment is all. There is no other moment. Time stops—then there is relaxation. If time is there, there is no relaxation. Simply, the clock stops; there is no time. This moment is all. Relaxation means this moment is more than enough, more than can be asked or expected. Nothing to ask, more than enough, more than you can desire—then the energy never moves anywhere. It becomes a placid pool. In your own energy, you dissolve. This moment is relaxation. Relaxation is neither of the body nor of the mind, relaxation is of the total.

OSHO, TRANSCRIBED TEACHINGS,
TANTRA: THE SUPREME UNDERSTANDING

Awareness and Sensitivity Exercise
Partner Exercise to Harmonize the Energies

An energy-harmonizing exercise such as this one can be used to attune you and your partner to one another. Give yourselves about half an hour. It can be done as described here, as a practice in itself, or as a mode of foreplay that continues into making love. The harmonizing exercise finishes with both of you standing up, which is really one of the best ways to begin making love—kissing and embracing and gradually proceeding to the bed.

Prepare a meditative atmosphere around you and your partner. Place cushions opposite each other a little distance apart. (Use chairs if necessary.) Sit upright with crossed legs, if possible, and a comfortably straight spine. Your spine will be better supported if you sit directly on the bones of the buttocks (sitz bones), so do lean forward and pull the flesh of your buttocks slightly apart and away from you. This will create a slight arch in the lower back, which makes sitting on the floor with crossed legs easier to sustain.

Sit facing each other in the night, by candlelight or by moonlight, and hold each other's hands crosswise. Use soft vision, as described at the end of chapter 2. For about ten minutes look into one another's eyes; if your body starts swaying, allow it to. You can blink, but go on looking into one another's eyes. Whatever happens, don't let go of one another's hands. After ten minutes, close your eyes and allow the swaying to continue for a further ten minutes.

Then stand and sway together, holding hands for ten more minutes. You can have eyes open or closed, whatever feels most comfortable for you. Finish with a warm embrace. This exchange will mix your energy deeply.

4
The Source of Orgasmic States

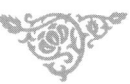

There are many reasons why the sexual exchange often does not lead to orgasm for women. One of these reasons is that the sex act is much too short, due to the chronic premature ejaculation that exists among men. A few minutes of sexual intercourse does not remotely begin to tap the orgasmic energies of a woman. The most important reason, though, is that the *real source of female orgasm is misunderstood*. We require concrete information about the delicately designed energy that exists in the female body. Orgasm should be a relatively effortless affair. Ecstasy is our natural state: we are all born ecstatic, but sadly, throughout childhood we slowly lose access to our ecstasy in becoming socially conditioned. Still, we are made for ecstasy and it can be relearned.

Equal and Opposite Forces

Too easily we assume that the energetic bodies of man and woman are in effect the same. In reality a woman's body is completely different from that of a man's and exactly to what extent our bodies differ has not been understood. Any differences between us are taken for granted, while the deeper implications are missed.

If we look at the differences that are apparent between male and female bodies—the sexual organs and associated reproductive functions—what can we see? We see the unique male ability to produce and discharge seeds containing half the blueprint for life. We see the unique female ability to receive, absorb, supply the other half of the blueprint and transform it into life within her. Reproduction demonstrates that male and female are equal forces in perfect balance: one no stronger, one no weaker; each providing a vital function. Man cannot reproduce himself on this planet without woman, and woman cannot create life in the absence of man. These two equal forces are absolutely opposite in expression while at the same time utterly complementary. There is an active force balanced by a receptive force.

Woman's body is equal to man's body while simultaneously energetically opposed to it. So, in sex, what goes for a man (apparently) is not *necessarily* energetically suitable or true for a woman. In being opposite and equal to man, woman complements man in his entirety. This equal and opposite phenomenon underpins the powerful pull of sex—we are continually drawn to the opposite sex regardless of our age and it seems that sex will not leave us in peace, or at least not for very long. Actually, sex is knocking on our door, offering a secret way to attain profound peace and love through male and female elements being rightly harnessed. By meeting, melting, and merging with the opposite force, we become complete, we become one. The sense of separation evaporates into the sense of immense union with everything that is. Most people in our societies today hold sex and spiritually far apart, and many even consider them to conflict with one another. Yet the longing for union (with the opposite sex or with existence itself) is a spiritual longing, which reveals why, in their essence, sex and spirituality are so closely associated.

Energetic Differences of Woman Compared with Man
We hear little about different energetic qualities of female and male and a lot about constitutional and emotional differences. A basic education should include a study of how our different energies manifest in our physical differences—and what significance these have in the sexual exchange. Nature intentionally instilled the female and male genitals with complementary

qualities, or polarities of energy, in order that they might interact and play with each other.

The female element is receptive and the male element is active.* Many other words can be assigned to describe these essentially opposing qualities, such as yin/yang, moon/sun, night/day, passive/dynamic. The meeting of female and male is a meeting of opposite poles, and this meeting makes a flow of energy possible between them. At the subtle energy level this complementary design produces, with relative ease, an orgasmic state. By virtue of *not being the same*, these equal but opposite forces create one vibrant unit. Only when these two halves meet is the sexual unit complete. Imagine a lock and key. A lock without a key is basically useless. A key without a lock is equally as useless. Together, through one fitting into the other, they perform an essential function. Even though each part is quite different in design, when the fit is true the unit rotates and a secret door swings open to reveal a paradise of hitherto unknown sexual experience.

In addition to the existence of this polarity, we must understand that woman is in fact half man and man is half woman. It is this inner phenomenon that forms the basis of meditation. It is helpful to use the magnet as a model to understand more fully our internal design. Although the human body is not absolutely identical to a magnet, it is similar enough to make the magnet model useful in perceiving the body energy in a different way. Poles of a magnet are traditionally assigned "positive" and "negative" to convey their essential attributes. Overall a woman is negative and receptive, but within herself she carries the equal and opposite pole of experience. In accordance with her receptive nature, the vagina, which receives man physically, is the negative pole. The opposite pole, the male pole, exists in the breasts and heart. All the male attributes and qualities—such as dynamic, active, sun, yang—then apply to the positive pole, the breasts/heart of the woman. From here she opens, radiates, expands, expresses, shares, reaches out into the world. However, through the vagina

---

*Please note the important difference between action and activity as explained by Osho in chapter 9. Action comes out of a silent mind; it is a true response to a present situation. Activity is an irrelevant pouring out of restlessness carried over from the past.

she serenely welcomes, sweetly receives, absorbs, and relaxes. Woman as passive aspect represents the negative pole, yet within herself she carries the positive.

Furthermore, between opposite poles there is a flow of energy. A channel of what can best be called electromagnetic energy, known in tantra as the *magnetic rod*, runs between the lower and upper poles of the female body. Between positive and negative is a movement of subtle electromagnetic energy that streams or spirals and becomes the source of the orgasmic experience. The ultimate source of orgasmic experience lies *within* each individual, not outside.

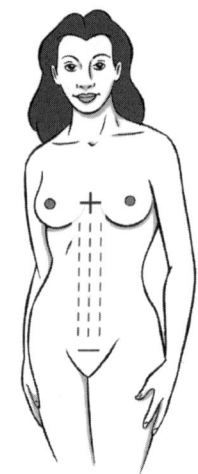

Fig. 4.1. Plus and minus poles at breasts and vagina respectively, illustrating the magnetic rod

Orgasm Is an Auto-Ecstatic Phenomenon

This means that essentially orgasm is an auto-ecstatic phenomenon that comes to pass through the interplay of equal and opposite polarities. Woman embodies the feminine passive principle externally, yet internally her male aspect balances this. In woman, the outer feminine pole triggers the activation of the inner male pole, opening a channel to the streaming of orgasmic electromagnetic energy.

Interestingly, the genital contact of the penis in the vagina is not absolutely essential for an orgasmic experience. The human being is auto-ecstatic: given the right environment, it is possible for anyone to move into states of ecstasy alone. Anyone can be blessed with an experience of ecstatic bliss *without* sexual intercourse.

In reality, then, another person is not involved in your ecstasy. It may be triggered by your partner in making love, but the inner experience, the ecstasy and joy, is yours alone. The person may or may not share a similar experience, depending on his presence and sensitivity. For instance, a woman can have an ecstatic sexual experience even while a man is fast asleep inside her without erection. In sex we are engaging with the other, having the source of orgasmic energy triggered, yet ultimately the state is experienced as our own. It is not always mutually experienced as the same thing at the same time.

Blissfulness requires only three essential elements: timelessness, egolessness, and naturalness.[1] The beauty and elegance of sex is that these three essential elements are naturally made possible by the sexual situation itself. Tracking backward and recovering our innocent, natural, egoless selves in sex, we shift into a realm where time dissolves and bliss descends.

A woman shares her experience: "I had a very strong experience of the energy field beyond the bodies, watching the bodies inside the energy space. The weird thing was that this was all happening while my partner was in total misery and couldn't feel any of it. Is this possible? It reminded me of similar experiences I've had before, lying on top of a man with him still inside me, me not moving, in bliss and joy and then the man would start snoring—he was not there with it at all (consciously at least), and then I always thought I must be imagining the bliss and energy, and I would cut it off immediately."

Two Magnets Meeting at Opposite Ends

While women are essentially auto-ecstatic, we can engage with men to galvanize our inner opposite into life—to awaken us to our inner source of ecstasy. It follows then that the male body, equal and opposite, will have the magnetic poles reversed. The positive pole is the penis, in accordance with the physical design for penetration of the vagina, and the negative pole is the heart and chest. As in woman, between these two poles there is an electromagnetic streaming, an ecstatic flow of energy. In relation to woman the male "magnet" is standing on its head in a

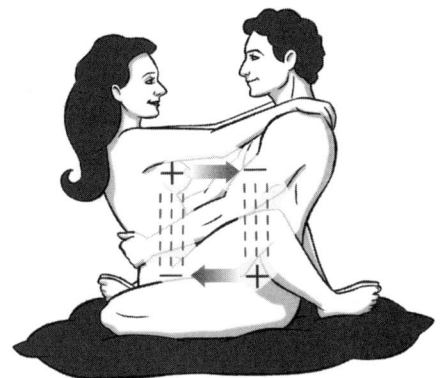

Fig. 4.2. Opposing female and male polarities, with magnetic rods and potential circular energy flow (in "yab yum" position)

reversed position. When a man stands *opposite* a woman, their inner magnets are meeting at their opposite ends—negative vagina to positive penis and positive breasts to negative chest. This is why some people avoid close hugs except with their intimate partner, and even there I see many couples keeping their pelvises withdrawn from a full-body embrace, simply out of a lifetime of habit. We avoid touch or pressure between the genitals or breasts and chest because a powerful polarity exists, and the connection is sometimes not appropriate when hugging friends or strangers.

When opposite poles are facing one another and brought into proximity, two magnets will exert a tremendously attractive force on one another. (On the other hand, magnets with similar poles facing will repel one another and push apart.) When two magnets meet at opposite poles the magnetic field is tremendously amplified. In fact, the magnetic field is then much larger and more intense than the sum of its two parts.

The attraction of magnets is due to a circulation of electromagnetic energy that is created between the two magnets, with plus flowing to minus (man to woman) and plus flowing to minus (woman to man) at both ends. Woman recirculates energy received in the vagina by channeling it upward and radiating out through her breasts to man, as the positive flows to negative. Man radiates from the penis into woman and correspondingly receives from woman through his heart. There is a reciprocal circle, a circling force of energy.

Allow Physical Contact to Be Porous

Couples will feel the power and attraction of this phenomenon when standing opposite each other, even at a distance of a yard or two apart. Some couples find it even easier to feel the energy circling from a distance than when they are in physical contact. As they get physically closer other distractions get in the way, perhaps fears of being truly open or fears of not being accepted fully, or perhaps the physical contact will be so compact as to deaden the finer sensations in the energy field between the bodies. For this reason, *porous* contact is always recommended when bodies are up against each other, as in an embrace. Bodies need to contact each other extremely delicately; otherwise, finer sensations easily get overshadowed. When a man squeezes you firmly in his arms during an embrace, you will not be able to stay in his arms for very long. After a few moments, there comes an urgent need to pull back into your own space because it is too physical, too hard, and the sensation of being hugged is not that enjoyable, not after the initial joy of the greeting and kiss. There must be a quality of porousness wherein a person respects your energy body, which extends way out beyond your physical boundaries. In the porous situation a hug can be sustained for hours as the energy bodies melt deeper and deeper into one another. Usually during physical contact we don't think about a person's energy body, but we all have one, although some of us are more aware of it and sensitive to it than others.

When we become more sensitive to ourselves and to our partner, we begin to perceive the true communion between man and woman. Man gives to woman as positive force and woman receives from man as negative force. In her very receiving she is empowered and returns that power by giving to man, and thus he receives what he himself has given. In giving, man receives and in receiving, woman gives. When he knows how to speak to the body of a woman through polarity, the love a man gives returns to him through his woman. It is recorded that an actual circle of light can start to move between a couple, and they will begin to emanate light. This is an interesting image to have as inspiration; however, reaching such heights requires much preparation and loving patience.

The Circling of Love Energy

The energy circle as an image can help you. With practice and in good time, this circle may be an outcome, but it can never be a goal. When a man is able to experience his woman as his equal and opposite, love is created in her and returned to him through breasts and heart. The second part of the magnetic circle is complete. The inner magnets and outer magnets are in accord. This unfolds by itself when a man and a woman put the basic elements in correct alignment. With magnetic rods meeting at their opposite ends, the circular energy can flow.

This circle is more likely to happen spontaneously when a man and a woman are in love. If they are not in love, it will be a meeting of sex centers—one positive pole with one negative pole. There will be an exchange of energy, but it will be linear energy, not circular. This is the reason why sex without love is never very satisfying.

Femininity, arising through inner awareness, is magically magnetic. The inner focus, the joy of resting within herself, compels the male, who is equal and opposite in every way. A man will feel himself overwhelmingly and irresistibly drawn across a room to a certain woman. Suddenly there is a space, a vacuum, a receptacle into which his energy can flow effortlessly. In man a deep restfulness and satisfaction arises when his energy is received and absorbed and returned to him. Woman, in being loved, becomes love as the heart center grows more and more vibrant. Orgasmic states begin to arise when you relax into electromagnetic cooperation within and between female and male bodies.

The Seven Chakras

The positive and negative poles also fit into the esoteric system of the seven energy centers (chakras) that are present in the body. These are connected to five further energy centers that bridge us with universal consciousness, the energy of creation. The first energy center is located in the perineal/genital area of the body. The second, sometimes called the *hara,* is a few centimeters below the navel. The third is the solar plexus. The fourth is the heart. The fifth is in the throat. Sixth is the "third eye" between the two eyebrows. The seventh is at the top of the head and is called the crown chakra.

In the female body the first chakra is negative (vagina), the second positive, the third negative, the fourth positive (breasts), the fifth negative, the sixth positive, the seventh negative. The male body is opposite, starting with the first chakra as positive (penis), alternating upward with the fourth chakra as negative (heart).

The Healing Power of Magnetism

Magnets basically create order around them by aligning objects in their presence. You no doubt remember the earliest school science experiments

demonstrating this. When iron filings are scattered on a sheet of a paper with a magnet lying underneath, the magnet demonstrates the field around it as the particles align themselves with the flow of magnetic energy between the positive and negative poles. When two magnets are placed apart under the paper with opposite poles facing each other, you can see the magnetic field in the circle of iron filings between the magnets themselves. In addition, the overall magnetic field surrounding the two magnets is infinitely greater than the field formed around a single magnet.

Plants and animals respond to a magnetic flow of energy through them that is induced by magnets. Today the use of magnets for their healing properties is becoming more and more respected.[2] They can be worn, for instance, as insoles, wrist bands, or kidney belts. Healing occurs because magnets provoke the magnetic flow of energy through the body. For example, photographs of unhealthy blood will initially show the individual cells in a random and chaotic arrangement. A second photo taken after a week of magnet therapy will show a semblance of alignment emerging between the cells of the body tissue. A week later again, the tissue will show an increasing order and formation developing in the cellular arrangement. The subject usually feels a relief in symptoms and an increase in well-being.

With all of this understanding of magnetic energies, the inner human magnet remains underdeveloped and unexplored. This is a sad state of affairs because the source of the orgasmic experience is precisely the same magnetic streaming between the female and male aspects within us. As these poles are gradually brought back into action and reestablished, energy organically flows between the positive and negative, bringing the body into a rare state of vibration. Realigning these magnetic poles in our bodies is a healing process in itself, and it starts with beginning to respect the feminine polarity within. Instead of playing out a male idea of how a woman is, our healing comes from being an actual woman: allowing ourselves to fall into the female element of receptivity and absorption—in other words, more being and less doing. With this *being* we discover what happens in the body when we focus on the vagina and the breasts. In conventional sex the vagina and breasts are sorely misused and this is affecting woman's orgasmic capacity. Right attention to the breasts and the vagina will be our focus in the next two chapters.

Tantric Inspiration

How to manage it [ecstasy]? Out of this question the whole science of Tantra was born. How to do it? It can be done. It cannot be done *with* the beloved outside—it cannot be done *without* the beloved outside, remember that too, because the first glimpse comes from the beloved outside. It is only a glimpse, but with it comes new vision that, deep down inside yourself, there are both the energies present—male and female.

Man is bisexual—every man, every woman. Half of you is male and half of you is female. If you are a woman, then the female part is on top and the male part is hidden behind, and vice versa. Once you have become aware of this, then a new work starts: your inner woman and inner man can have meeting and that meeting can remain absolute. There is no need to come back from the peak. But the first vision comes from the outer.

Hence Tantra uses the outer woman, the outer man, as part of inner work. Once you have become aware that you have a woman inside you or a man inside you, then the work takes on a totally new quality, it starts moving in a new dimension. Now the meeting has to happen inside; you have to allow your inner woman and man to meet.

OSHO, TRANSCRIBED TEACHINGS,
THE BOOK OF WISDOM

Awareness and Sensitivity Exercises
Partner Exercise to Awaken Polarity

This exercise can be done complete in itself or as a preparation for making love. Give yourselves at least thirty minutes.

Sit opposite one another on cushions situated a little distance apart so that you are without physical contact. (If sitting cross-legged on the floor is too uncomfortable, sit upright on straight-backed chairs facing one another.) Close your eyes. Inwardly tune in to your positive poles: woman tune to the breasts and man tune to the penis.

After a while imagine your breasts are radiating energy and light and warmth toward your man's chest and heart. Your partner should imagine himself receiving the love into his heart and at the same time channeling energy out through his penis, radiating warmth, light, and love. Imagine you receive all this energy and absorb it into your vagina. The imagination can be supported by radiating outward on the out breath (woman–breasts, man–penis) and absorbing on the in breath (woman–vagina, man–heart). You can breathe out together and in together.

After a while, begin to have eye contact with receptive, soft vision and continue circling the energy as before. After five to ten minutes, you (woman) can move across the space and sit with your legs wrapped around your man's waist while sitting in his lap. (This is called the yab yum position; cushions can be used to support the woman.) This brings genitals into closer proximity and the breasts and chest into correspondence. Again, keep working with your imagination, and this time you can experiment with synchronizing your breathing—as man breathes in through the heart, woman breathes out through the heart; as woman breathes in through the vagina, man breathes out through the penis. This practice will intensify the sensation of a circulating force between the bodies. If you do not feel this right away, after a time you will probably begin to feel it happening because energy follows imagination.

If yab yum is not comfortable to sustain for a period of time, you can move into standing position, or if yab yum is not at all possible the whole exercise can be done standing, to great effect. Standing allows for greater dance and fluidity of movement between bodies.

Spontaneously the wish to be penetrated may arise, and if your man is willing, continue with making love. Otherwise, when there is a sense of completion in the exchange, very, very slowly disconnect and move away from each other while maintaining eye contact. You can complete with a bow of the head with hands folded in a prayer gesture, or rest your foreheads together and then lie down on the bed or floor, side by side without contact (holding hands at most), and each rest within yourself for several minutes, keeping awareness on the inner streamings of the body (the magnetic rod).

Tantric Meditation
Peace Pervading the Armpits

Lie in a relaxed position as suggested at the end of chapter 1 for twenty minutes or more. Close your eyes, taking your awareness into your body. Start just between the two armpits, and with your total attention "pervade an area between the armpits into great peace."[3] Forget your whole body; remember the heart area between the two armpits and your chest and feel it filling with great peace. When the body is more relaxed, peace automatically happens in your heart; it becomes more silent and harmonious. Done frequently, this practice will establish peace within you and make you feel more independent, and love will be more about giving—you have so much peace you want to share it. You will be returning to a source in yourself that is always there.

5
The Breasts: Key to Orgasm

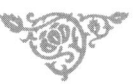

The breasts have the power to bring woman to the deepest of orgasmic experiences. The breasts are central to a woman's experience of sexual ecstasy, not merely an appendage for breast-feeding and without implication for the female energy system.

It is true that, for most of us, breasts are not directly associated with female orgasm, although certainly many women are aware of an internal hook-up to the vagina that is quite sensational. This connection between breasts and vagina happens via the magnetic rod (as explained in the previous chapter), the ultimate source of orgasmic states.

Orgasmic moments transpire when essential elements align themselves. Tantra is based on the science of the body and its energy centers, with their electromagnetic polarities. On the psychological level an individual requires a certain innocence. Heightened states are not accidental, although people may accidentally slip into a heightened state naturally perhaps once in a lifetime, without actually knowing how it happened. With information about the role of the breasts in orgasm, a woman has more command over her orgasmic experiences. She can consciously begin to create those experiences, rather than leaving it all to man's actions or to chance.

Energy Raised from a Positive Pole

The significance of the breasts in female orgasm is enormous in that, generally speaking, *energy can only be raised from a positive pole,* not a negative pole.[1] This means that energy is awakened or activated from the positive pole *before* it flows toward the negative. In the female body, sexual energy flows *from* the breasts *to* the vagina. When breasts are pulsating with aliveness, the spontaneous overflowing of energy results in a vibrational resonance in the vagina, the opposite pole. Only when the vagina is vibrating in this magnetic response is it truly available for the beautiful event of penetration; is it truly sensitive and perceptive. A woman will experience a genuine *yes,* a deep willingness to make love, a willingness not only to yield and give in but to participate fully as an equal and opposite—which changes everything, as if lifting sex to a higher octave.

The sexual route conventionally taken is very different because in it the vagina is regarded as the doorway and is approached directly (this will be discussed further in chapter 6). Indeed, while the vagina is the physical entry point, to energetically enter a woman the breasts must be given priority and consciously incorporated into the sexual exchange. Breasts are quite often ignored by women and men; certainly they are misunderstood in terms of their true role in accessing female sexual energy. If a man is into breasts, more often than not he uses them for *his* stimulation, to turn *himself* on, to fulfill some fantasy of his own, often treating the breasts very roughly in the process. The effect can even be to turn a woman off, causing her whole body energy to shrink into an unwillingness for sex. The naked truth is that regardless of the appearance of a woman's breasts or a man's personal interest in them, breasts represent the key to women's sexual fulfillment through orgasm.

Sadly, many women carry complexes about their breasts for any of a hundred and one reasons—the size, the shape, the hang, the fullness, the balance, the texture, plus all the variations possible in nipples. This lack of self-acceptance creates a tension and distances a woman from the delicate inner sensations present in her breasts. Emotional injuries, heartbreaks, and childhood wounds also can create energetic shields across the positive

THE BREASTS: KEY TO ORGASM

pole. At first these tensions and repressed feelings can make it more difficult for a woman to feel into her breasts, until she learns to access the power lying within them.

When a woman allows this magnetic phenomenon to come into play, she begins to truly enjoy sex—sometimes for the first time. Not with the feeling of having to fulfill a duty, submitting and enduring it, but with a joyfulness that enables her to flower into a dancing sexual being. As the breasts are brought more into the sexual forefront, orgasms will happen more easily. Many different kinds of delightful orgasms will follow from the breasts being lavishly included in lovemaking. Naturally, this involves man—how he caresses and touches the breasts—but only to a certain extent. At the deepest level it involves a woman's interest in herself as an expression of the feminine.

You are encouraged to start feeling and sensing your breasts from within. Do not be distracted by how they look from the outside, but instead focus your attention on the breasts themselves. *It is best to keep attention on both breasts at the same time.* Avoid long periods of focus on one breast only. Spread your awareness over both of them: feel them, love them, accept them as they are. Negative thoughts separate you from their feminine qualities. Place your attention on the breasts, not with fierce concentration, but more with ease and relaxation, with the sense of melting *into* the breasts, merging with them, becoming one with them. Massage them, hold them, feel them from within at any time during the day—as you set about working on the computer, cooking, gardening, or whatever you happen to be doing. Whenever you remember, make an effort to sense the breasts *from within*. And especially enter the breasts with your awareness while making love. You will have to remind yourself of this again and again, as our attention tends to stray easily to other things. The breasts are the gateway for woman and need to be showered with all the attention they can get—in and out of bed.

Even though most women do realize that the breasts are connected with sexual pleasure, few really grasp how central and how intimately linked their breasts are to full involvement in the sexual act and orgasm. As mentioned earlier, fresh insight into the breasts puts a woman in a

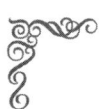

better position to orchestrate events to her advantage, so as to let things flow in accordance with her feminine nature. A surprising number of women tell me that they always knew, intuitively, the truth about not forcing orgasm and about the role of the breasts in orgasm. Because of the pressures of conventional sex they had overridden their inner voices, not trusting themselves or their bodies. Some women have stood before me, eyes brimming with tears in the awesome realization that for twenty or thirty years they had been acting in direct opposition to their very essence. They feel so much time lost, opportunities missed, misunderstanding, and unhappiness as a consequence.

Fortunately, as far as the body is concerned, it is *never too late* to start changing our approach. The body welcomes all respect given to it, and in acknowledgment responds in beautiful and unexpected ways. The body is innately sensitive (our own insensitive and callous ways with it notwithstanding) and extremely responsive to *awareness*. Awareness means the sensing of the body from within; it means getting in there and feeling oneself on a cellular level.

Some women say they find it quite easy to sense the energies and sensations present in the heart area but not in the breasts, and they wonder if it is favorable to go directly to the heart. Even if the heart center is easily available, I nonetheless suggest that they tune in to and slowly awaken the life energy of the breasts. Ignoring the breasts and going directly to the heart may seem the easiest strategy, but it is a rejection of the essential feminine nature. Breasts access exquisitely delicate energies and surround a woman with the fragrance of femininity. Through the breasts the heart center is activated. In a sense a woman does not have to concern herself directly with the heart center. The heart opens as a by-product of the breasts becoming alive, and through this expansion of energy woman becomes increasingly loving, feminine, graceful, and elegant.

When you first begin to experience the breasts in a different way it is possible that some sadness or tears will surface. This is not at all unusual and is actually a good sign—a sign of your positive pole beginning to cleanse and free itself of earlier unexpressed feelings from hurts and heart-

breaks that have accumulated energetically around the heart center. These tensions are released and the body purified automatically, through its intrinsic healing capacity, when a woman begins to amplify the positive energy present in her breasts. In this framework of cleansing, any tears and crying are to be welcomed, not shunned. Allowing them can bring profound healing of earlier unresolved issues. With each layer of tension that leaves the breasts and heart there will be a noticeable increase in the sensitivity and receptivity of the breasts. Some women carry a sensation that they describe as feeling like a metal plate of some kind across the heart. Energetically such a shield exists, but it is quick to melt when the environment is favorable. Past tensions can show up for release at any time—before, during, or after making love—so maintain an openness to yourself as much as possible.

The two nipples are the highlights of the positive pole, super alive and sensitive. Nipples have the ability to emit and radiate energy, making them similar to the head of the male penis. *Always bring both nipples into the focus of your attention* when feeling into the breasts as a whole. The nipple should be in the foreground of your awareness. Nipples are extraordinarily, deliciously sensitive and should be treated with love and respect.

Often nipples are twisted and turned roughly, like a couple of buttons. This can be very stimulating in effect, especially when a woman is younger. As women get older (and numerous women have reported this to me), they frequently find themselves rejecting almost all touching of the breasts, particularly of the nipples. Breasts and nipples that once were gloriously receptive and alive, that loved to be touched and played with, slowly become hypersensitive and overcharged, or deadened. A form of repulsion sets in because the rightful place of breasts (in the role of awakening female sexual energy) is not granted to them. In time a woman's instinctive reaction is to turn away from man's hands as they approach the vicinity of the breasts.

Touching the Breasts

Creating new experiences naturally involves the cooperation of the man to a certain extent, so encourage your man to touch your breasts in a way that feels good to you. Help him learn how to treat the breasts with love and awe. Some men are hesitant to touch the breasts because of earlier reactions and rejections, either by you or by a previous woman. This makes it really necessary to show him *exactly how* to touch your breasts in the way *you best* like your breasts to be touched, as suggested in the partner exercise at the end of the chapter. This is an intimate and beautiful step in taking responsibility for your own sexual expression. Show your man how to touch (or suck) your nipples and how to touch your breasts, separately and together. A man's two hands are not always available while making love. If only one of your man's hands is at your breast, touch the other breast yourself to give a feeling of balance.

Seek always that your man touch you in a way that *makes your body energy expand*. This sensation becomes the guideline for how to evaluate touch—look for an expansion of energy rather than excitement or stimulation. Avoid types of touch that create a contraction, withdrawal, or closing of your energy body. Light (and extremely featherlight), caressing touches have the effect of expanding and bringing sparkling sensations, while a heavy touch can reduce and deaden the pleasant sensations already present.

Touch your own breasts as often as possible while making love, any time it feels right or when you wish to deepen the connection to your inner experience. Touch your breasts simply and in the way that *you* most enjoy. This is the beauty of self-touch—you can do it however *you* like it, which brings a certain relaxation.

Cupping each breast lightly with your whole hand is a simple, loving way to touch the breasts. You can also cross your arms and cup each breast with the opposite hand (the right breast in the left hand and the left breast in the right hand). Keep your hands and fingers relaxed and open, shaping to the form of the breast. Give the breasts space; avoid squashing them too much. The palm of your hand automatically touches the nipples, which is a good thing because it will intensify the experience of the nipples. Soft

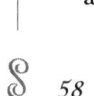

caressing and stroking of the breasts is very nice, and especially erotic are the sides of the breasts as you lightly stroke upward from the armpit or side of the ribcage toward your nipples. Cupping and vibrating your breasts very gently from time to time also works wonders! Whenever you like, lightly stroke or squeeze the nipples just enough to produce fine sensations. A little saliva enhances the nipples' sensitivity. As you keep touching yourself in different suitable ways, you will feel the breast and heart awakening, filling up with energy and creating a pleasing response in the vagina.

There is another advantage to touching oneself that is completely unrelated to sensation. It can easily happen when another person touches us that we unconsciously and reflexively go on guard in fear of a touch that is uncaring or painful. Memories of these kinds of touch can come up. This fear, this tension, this contraction blocks the ability to deeply receive from the touching hand, to absorb the warmth and energy and love. With touching oneself there is no likelihood of this withdrawal happening.

Perhaps you feel a bit shy or self-conscious about touching your own breasts in front of your lover. But breasts have been the domain of the man until now, and it's time for a change. The effects are surely worth the risks. Gather courage and begin to express yourself in a different way. *Take risks each time you make love and you will be rewarded with love.* Every occasion you make love is an opportunity to experiment and explore, to check things out to see where your curiosity brings you. It really is best *not* to wait for *next time* to be adventurous. This postponement will continue as days all too quickly accumulate into years. If you wish to get out of the male-oriented sexual routine of today—and it is possible—you absolutely must take risks. Don't be overawed by man, by what he thinks or what he likes. Woman has been pleasing man in sex and moving away from her female expression for far too long. It is time for woman to take her place as the true counterpart in lovemaking that she is, and begin to please her body and cooperate with its inner mechanisms. Lucky is the man whose life will be enriched through her adventurous spirit.

THE BREASTS: KEY TO ORGASM

Breasts and Excitement

A certain kind of touch or stimulation of the breasts by a man can produce a sudden surge of excitement or a desire to have a peak kind of orgasm. You might experience it as a real compulsion, an overwhelming urge that you simply *must* go with the desire and follow it through to the end. Touch or stimulation provoking this effect should be avoided or modified a little, perhaps offered more softly or with less intention. A relaxed, easy, caring touch will enable the deeper magnetic response to gather in woman and not flip her over into a state filled with desire for excitement and conventional orgasm.

Any hard squeezing, sucking, and stimulation of the nipples will often have this instant turn-on effect. But it can also have the entirely opposite effect—of turning a woman *off*, suddenly leaving her with no wish to go further. Which way she will react depends on the individual woman, her age, and how she has been handled by men in the past. Each unpleasant experience leaves a cellular imprint, a memory in the cells of the body, that creates a subtle barrier and layer of protection. (We will consider this again in chapter 6, in relation to the vagina.) Conscious melting of a man's hands into the breasts without squashing or squeezing them—not doing anything special other than sensing the breasts, feeling the energy of the breasts, loving them—works wonders. Avoid overstimulating the nipples, especially in the early stages of lovemaking or foreplay. *It is appropriate to touch and squeeze the nipples with more firmness when sexual arousal is complete and lovemaking well underway.* When the energy is flowing freely, the pressure to the nipples can cause delightful things to happen.

Direct and invincible evidence of how crucial the breasts are is that loving stimulation of the breasts encourages and increases lubrication in the vagina. Almost all women experience this. Through the magnetic link and overflow of energy, the lubrication glands in the vagina respond abundantly. In fact, there is a great deal more lubrication when the breasts are lovingly touched compared to when the vagina or clitoris is touched directly in foreplay prior to penetration.

Women who have had a breast removed for medical reasons report that the positive pole continues to be active *even in the absence of the physical breast.* The same filling up and spilling over into the vagina happens, as does the lubrication of the vagina. This remarkable feedback bears witness to the integrity of the body. The breast is more than just juicy flesh; it deeply embodies an energy dimension that remains active even in its physical absence.

A woman with one breast removed shares her experience: "When I touch my right breast in a delicate, quick, patting way, my vagina responds—it twitches and quivers and a wonderful wavelike, joyful current of sexual energy flows through my vagina, from the womb outward right to the vulva and clitoris. I can even feel the spot of my nipple and its connection to the vagina, although on the right side there is no physical breast anymore; there is only a thirty-centimeter scar.

"I am happy! It is so beautiful. With conscious loving touch and holding of the right breast 'in the air' as it were, it is fantastic. Sometimes I even feel the sensations more strongly and more vaginally than with the left breast. Interesting enough is that this most often occurs when sex is happening with heartfulness. With 'horny sex' I experience the touching of my scar as stimulating, often in the clitoris, but definitely much less than with the left breast. My partner is very sensitive; he can even feel the vibration of the nipple on the outside of the absent breast. I experience the energetic touch as a deep vaginal opening, and it creates a longing of the heart for deep touch.

"Since we discovered more about sexuality our sexual life has clearly moved in the direction of the heart and is creating a supportive, loving, divine atmosphere. One time after a deep union of hearts my lover shared, 'In the beginning it mattered to me. I was having thoughts about your having only one breast, particularly because I am attracted to big breasts. But now I feel everything is totally fine, as long as the heart is present and can be felt between us.' Sometimes my mind becomes doubtful, thinking: 'This isn't possible; this is just a scar! You're crazy, you're just imagining things!' And then I observe that in tandem with the negative thinking, the

pleasing sensations are instantly gone. Then I feel into my body, into my vagina, and the moment I am able to accept my situation, and my lover touches *both* breasts a little more quickly, I again feel a strong twitching in my vagina. And there they are again: my two breasts! One time, lying naked in the sun after a deep penetration by my lover, I could distinctly feel my right breast when I touched it energetically, "in the air" so to speak. Because I am a skeptic, I immediately tried to just imagine being touched. I could feel something then too, but the sensation was much less than compared to the energetic touching by a conscious, loving hand.

"I received my diagnosis of breast cancer in 1993. My life had been ruled by fear, abuse, many years of drug use, a heavy and closed heart, and a certain longing to die. By means of awareness, with the help of countless workshops, meditations, and therapeutic groups, my life has transformed into conscious enjoyment, into a deep love of the universe, of life, with often a childlike joy and ease. My longing for real love, letting go, trust, flowing, inner peace, and connectedness has come true."

Deliberate Interference with the Breasts

It is extremely fashionable for women to have their natural breasts altered; in some countries it is considered normal to have artificial breasts, and a woman who has not had a breast enlargement is something of a rarity. As body piercing gains popularity around the world, some women choose to pierce their nipples, others their lips, and others their labia. And it seems that as the sexual confusion increases generation by generation, these types of enhancement and ornamentation are done at an increasingly young age.

In light of the crucial role of the breasts in female sexual energy circulation, cosmetic surgery to breasts raises certain issues. Fortunately, it is clear from the personal experience reported here that interventions do not ultimately destroy the energy intrinsic to breasts. It is also true that a woman's incentive and wish to be proud of her breasts is quite possibly a reflection of her intuition that her breasts play a dynamic and creative role in the sexual exchange, and therefore in her life. The urge to display her breasts to man naturally follows, and so the media and fashion world use

exposed breasts in any way possible. One might say it's a good thing that men have greater opportunity to appreciate breasts through such displays. A woman's intention to display the positive, radiant pole is laudable—but sadly, her focus is misdirected. She is focused outward toward man, not inward toward herself. Breast enhancement surgery fixates a woman on the *outside* of her body, on her external appearance, not on how she feels internally. It then is not so easy to turn around, look within, and access the inner sensations of living breast tissue.

Some women have breast reductions because their breasts are so uncomfortably large that they become a physical and psychological burden to live with. In these circumstances, reducing the size can be considered a medical intervention and of psychological benefit. It can also be argued that increasing the size of the breasts puts a woman more at ease, gives her more confidence and trust in herself and her powers of attraction; in other words, that it benefits the woman herself. The added fullness of the breasts may result in attracting the male attention that a woman wants, but at a subtle level she might unconsciously begin to protect her breasts because they feel delicate. As a result she may be perhaps not so willing to let a man touch them. Men have shared with me that they can sense this, and that they will stay away from touching a woman's breasts in these situations. The breasts can feel uncomfortable; scars are sensitive, some never really healing properly. Artificial breasts have been known to explode during air flight! All these disturbances can easily affect the expansion of energy from the positive pole.

A woman might question whether encouraging a man to lust after her perfect breasts really serves her orgasmic potential in the long run. When a woman loves her own breasts and allows a man to love her breasts, they respond to the positive attention. Many women report an increase in breast size after they begin to make love according to female and male polarity—through bringing the breasts into their rightful magnetic alignment. Uncalled-for intervention of the breasts is a disturbance that interferes with the delicate magnetic system given to woman by nature.

A young and quite beautiful woman I met in a workshop told me she had enhanced her breasts two years earlier, saying, "You know, it was one

of those things I just had to do, and after I did it I realized that I need not have done it." She had been thinking of reversing the operation, but after receiving the information on the importance of the positive pole, she decided that for the present she would finally accept her breasts as they are now and not interfere a second time. She was pleased, and relieved, to observe an overflow from her breasts to her vagina when she began making love using tantric principles.

Tantric Inspiration

This concentration at the breasts, melting into them, will give a new feeling to the female meditator—a new feeling about her own body, because from the center now she can feel the whole body vibrating. Just by loving the breasts of a woman she can be brought to a deep orgasm because the negative pole automatically will go on responding.

If you start from the breasts, meditating on the nipples, don't follow the route that you have read in books because that is meant for men. You simply don't follow any chart; allow the energy itself to move. It will happen this way; just a vague suggestion that first your breasts will become filled with energy, they will radiate energy, they will become hot, and then immediately your vagina will respond. And only after your vagina responds and vibrates, kundalini for you, for women, will start working. And the route will be different and the way the kundalini will arise will be different. In man it arises very actively, forcibly. That's why they have called it the serpent rising. Very forcibly, suddenly, with a jerk, the serpent unfolding. And it is felt on many points. Those points are called chakras. Wherever there is resistance the snake forces itself. It is just like the penis entering the vagina: the passage is similar for man. When the energy arises it is as if the penis inside is moving.

This will not be the feeling for a woman. The feeling will be quite the opposite. When woman feels that the penis has entered in the vagina—the melting sensation, the welcoming, the vagina giving way, vibrating very, very delicately, in a very receptive mood, loving, welcoming—the same will be the phenomenon inside. When the energy rises, it will be a receptive, passive rise, as if a passage is opening—not a serpent rising, but a door opening, and a passage opening, and something giving way. It will be passive and negative. With men something is entering, with women something is opening, not entering. Everything will be just the opposite. It must be so. It cannot be similar. The ultimate thing will be the same.

OSHO, TRANSCRIBED TEACHINGS,
THE BOOK OF SECRETS

Awareness and Sensitivity Preparation
Self-Massage of the Breasts

Massaging the breasts on a regular basis helps to reinforce the feelings of life force (also called *chi, energy,* or *prana*) present in the breasts. You will notice them becoming more sensitive and receptive. You will find it easier to get a feeling of them from the inside any time you put your awareness in them. Self-massage also helps you get to know your own breasts, to accept them, and to love them. Use body lotion or massage oil if you like. Breasts are ideally always massaged upward or in a circular motion, the left breast counterclockwise and the right breast clockwise. Lift the breast tissue upward as much as possible and include your chest and throat.

This practice is also a natural way of monitoring any changes in the breast tissue. If anything feels abnormal, is painful or itchy, is not associated with the onset of menstruation, and does not disappear after a short time, report it to a doctor immediately. It is not necessarily a cause for alarm, but have it checked as soon as you've detected it.

It is also beneficial to include with the breasts a deeper massage on the rib cage. Using your thumb or first two fingers braced together, make little circling movements that reach through your skin to the bone. Start with the breastbone (sternum), traveling up and down two or three times. In the center of the breastbone, on a line with the nipples of upright breasts, is the "love-spot"—an important energy point that lies over the thymus gland. Massaging here stimulates the immune system and is also a doorway to the heart. On each side of the breastbone is a series of little hollow spaces between the ribs, where the ribs join the sternum. These are called the intercostal spaces. Massage of these points encourages the growth of the breasts and also relaxes physical and emotional tensions. Massage the intercostal spaces using the fingertips in the circular way described above. It is also good to extend the massage to the ribs themselves, using a circling motion on the bone and between the bones; you can track the ribs with your fingers as they run behind the breasts and into the armpit area. You can also reach certain parts of the ribs by getting your four fingers under and behind the pectoralis muscle (the muscle that forms the front of the armpit and runs across the chest). You can use this massage sequence as complete in itself, as foreplay before making love, or followed by the tantric breast meditation below.

Partner-Exchange Exercise
Partner Exchange Massage for Breasts and Penis

It helps to show and teach each other how you like to be touched, communicating what opens and resonates in your body. Focus on touching with warmth and love; avoid the kind of touch that is intentionally stimulating and therefore has different effects. The aim is for the body energy to expand and flow first, not to arouse the body into excitement by touch. Put aside forty minutes or more for this exchange, depending on whether you wish to make love afterward, which is quite likely to happen.

Take several drops of unscented massage oil (such as almond or olive oil) in your hands and begin to touch and massage your own breasts with oil, showing your partner what pressure your breasts enjoy and what they do not respond well to. Show him how you prefer the nipples to be touched—or maybe not touched, perhaps just held by the palm of the hand. Share in this way for a few minutes, explaining as you go along, and then pour a few drops onto his hands so that he is able to continue massaging you in the way you most appreciate.

Lie back or sit up and absorb his caresses into your breasts for fifteen or twenty minutes. In general, the lighter the touch the greater the sensuality; featherlight works wonders. After completing this part, your man should do the same by showing you how to touch his penis and testicles, and then allowing you to take over the massage.

The orientation in this exchange is toward increasing feelings of aliveness, of awakening, but not directly toward any stages of full-blown excitement, where we get overwhelmed with desire. After a further fifteen to twenty minutes of the woman loving the penis with her hands, if it feels appropriate continue with a very slow penetration. All subsequent movements should happen in an unhurried, lazy manner.

Tantric Meditation
Meditating on the Breasts

Lie down alone in the ideal position for relaxation suggested in chapter 1, with about twenty minutes for yourself. Breast meditation can be done daily and will greatly support your breasts in coming to life and encourage the opening of your positive pole. If you have a lover, you can also use it as a part of foreplay or preparation for love, either on your own or with your partner lying in bed beside you.

If you wish, place a slightly cupped hand on each breast. Touching will enhance the feeling within the breasts, making it easier to bring awareness into them. If your elbows become uncomfortable at any time, change the position of your hands, placing them on the groin or lying with your arms straight at your sides. Close your eyes and take your awareness into your body, sensing your breasts and in particular your nipples. "Feel the fine qualities of creativity permeating your breasts and assuming delicate configurations."[2] Move into your breasts; let your breasts become your whole being. Melt into them, merge into them. The whole body can become secondary to the breasts; the body can fade into the background as you bring the breasts into the foreground. Your inner emphasis is on the breasts, totally relaxing in them, moving in them. Do this for twenty minutes and then simply rest for a few more minutes. True feminine creativity arises when the breasts become active.

6
The Vagina Is Secondary to the Breasts

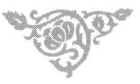

The vagina plays a secondary role in a woman's orgasm—secondary to the breasts but not secondary to the clitoris (which is the subject of the next chapter). Breasts are the positive pole in the female body and the vagina is the negative pole. Energy from the breasts overflows and internally ignites the vagina, which creates the full *yes* for penetration by man. The breasts are a little detour away from the vagina for man, a trip through the female energy system before he approaches the physical port of entry. Instead of forced or quick penetration without enough knocking on the door, there is a waiting at the threshold for the deeper invitation to man, which awakens in woman through the breasts. When a woman's vagina vibrates in magnetic response to her breasts being loved, she instantly recognizes her moment of sexual readiness—she knows without any doubt that she is ready. There is an involuntary movement toward the man, a seemingly magnetic attraction to his body, a yearning for intimacy, for penetration, a deep longing to unite. This moment is not a mind decision or a submission to someone else's desires or wishes. It is instead a completely spontaneous, energetic happening: from the depths arises an utter *yes* to man. To man the difference is electrifying and immediately perceptible. This welcome, this wholehearted and full-bodied response, shifts sex into a higher dimension, a dimension in which it becomes an electromagnetic celebration that leaves you satiated and radiant with love.

Energy Flows from Male into Female

The intrinsic properties of the vagina are passive and receptive, welcoming, silky, serene, sensitive. The vagina is not an external organ like the penis; it is an inversion, a canal providing flow into the body, a delicate muscular recess. It is not designed to take direct action but to exert an influence on the penis through the quality of energy present in its tissues.

The physical correspondence of the penis fitting into the vagina is not accidental. The design is like this *because energy flows from male into female,* not the opposite way.* This is the direction of flow—from penis into vagina, from plus to minus. Through a balance in polarity a doorway opens; energy streams upward through our internal energy channels.

The penis is therefore to be appreciated as a conduit for vital energy as well as for semen. Likewise, the vagina is the receptacle for this force as well as for the semen necessary for reproduction. Woman as the feminine, receptive force has the capacity to draw the male energy upward through her vagina, as if raising it to a higher frequency. The vagina melts around the penis and drinks the energy radiating from it. When the penis and the vagina are united in penetration they form one complete unit, one dynamic force and one passive force, a live electromagnetic circuit.

However, women report that the vagina is rarely involved in their experiences of real sexual pleasure. The presence of the penis alone is seldom sufficient to create any kind of heightened experience. Very few

---

*In advanced stages of tantic lovemaking, in which a heightened balance has been achieved between male and female poles, energy can flow back and forth between the two poles in such a way that woman will alternate between active and passive phases of sexual expression, and man will be correspondingly passive and active.

women report a type of vaginal orgasm in which the vagina reaches an extraordinarily heightened state of sensitivity, in which the penis produces an experience of pleasure that is infinitely prolonged, utterly ecstatic. The vagina needs to be reincorporated in lovemaking, to take its rightful place in accessing pleasure and the flowering of orgasmic states. In a manner of speaking, until the moment of penetration man walks around as half a unit, half a circuit, and woman exists as the other half of the very same circuit. We must begin to ask ourselves in what way these two half circuits can meet so as to maximize the built-in energy circuit.

It is here, at the level of the genital interaction, where perhaps the greatest confusion in sex lies. How should the vagina best relate to the penis? How should they conduct themselves when they get together? What would *they* want for themselves if we did not force our personal expectations on them? These are questions we don't normally even think of asking because our sexual past has proved to us that the backward and forward movements of the penis in the vagina is what sex is all about. Without this rubbing interaction between them we think sex is not feasible, and so it is a stretch to imagine that other pleasures really do exist.

The truth is that the vagina, as passive pole, ought to be maintained wide and easy, available to receive the maximum impact of the male energy. When the vagina is physically and energetically open, man is finally able to flow *into and through* woman, following the direction of energy flow from positive to negative.

The Vaginal Consequences of Conventional Sex

With no choices available to us in sexual expression we stick to one style of sex, a style that has many unfortunate consequences. The greatest disadvantage for a woman is that the vaginal tissues are adversely affected, their receptive qualities gradually deadened. In the first place, a man usually penetrates a woman well before her sexual temperature is sufficiently high for her to invite him in. Man basically wants to enter as soon as he has an erection, and this forced entry makes the vagina reluctant and defensive rather than welcoming and willing.

Second, once man has entered, the repeated friction of the penis against the sensitive, silky vaginal walls has another negative effect: the vagina changes from a highly perceptive and receptive canal into a toughened, protected one. With time an increasing lack of sensitivity develops within the vaginal cavity itself. When the vagina toughens up this way, its magnetic perception of the entering male half circuit is drastically reduced. The receptive, absorbent tissues are instead literally covered over with thickened skin. The tensions held in the vagina, which can show up sometimes as sexual excitement, form an artificial screen of positive charge, almost male in character, that hinders a woman from absorbing male energy.

Third, the physical movements of the pelvis that go with the usual sex routine add to the increasing insensitivity within the vagina. Extremes of pelvic movement amount to a woman using her vagina in an active way rather than a passive way. Movement converts the vagina into an active, doing, outgoing organ. And the vaginal canal gets physically restricted and narrower, which disturbs the subtle, receptive energies of the vaginal environment. We use the penis and the vagina to have a nice rub together because we do not have the sense of how they communicate and exchange energy through their magnetic polarities. When the vagina becomes shy because of forced visits, hardened through friction, and tightened through movement, all the necessary passive complementariness to the male dynamic is obscured.

It's important to realize that simultaneous to this desensitizing of the vagina, the penis is *also* becoming less and less perceptive. With accumulating years the male organ becomes highly congested, tense and overcharged, excessively positive. In the same way that the vagina cannot absorb, the penis fails to function as a transmitter of pure positive male energy. This distortion of our given polarities is the root cause of our lack of deep, moving sexual experiences. The good news is that the polarity is not destroyed—it is hiding beneath this screen of tension. Overcoming the sexual habits and patterns responsible for this step away from polarity is the most direct route to reclaiming femininity (and masculinity) and regaining our inborn sensitivity.

Preserve the Vagina as a Sacred Place for the Penis

The first disconcerting observation a woman may have is that when there is no movement in sex, she cannot feel very much at all going on with the penis in the vagina. This is clear evidence that her vaginal walls have toughened up through excessive stimulation; through aggressive, hard thrusting of sex; and also through fingers and synthetic objects being inserted into the vagina. A woman is encouraged to respect and preserve her vaginal sensitivity and to take special care about what enters the vagina and how. It is best to consider the vagina as a sacred place for the penis. Too many uncaring visits and invasions lead to loss of vaginal sensitivity, and from there, to reduced capacity to perceive vaginal pleasure and delight.

In the short term, most forms of direct stimulation inside the vagina may increase pleasure; but in the long term, more and more stimulation will be required to produce the same effect. Increasing numbness sets in as the body gradually forms a protective layer and becomes less and less sensitive to the stimulation. With objects and fingers there exists no real energetic correspondence, as there is with the penis during penetration. Objects can produce an effect through stimulation and resulting excitement, but they cannot possibly substitute for the profound effect of the living penis. A woman can resensitize her vagina through changing her style of lovemaking and learning to trust the power of receptivity.

Accessing Deeper Reaches of the Vagina, the Female Epicenter

It will interest women to know that the most meaningful part of the vagina is not the tighter entrance area, with its rings of muscle (which men like to focus on for stimulation), but the higher parts of the vagina, especially around the mouth of the uterus. It is here that the feminine pole is most negative and most receptive. This is where a woman is more likely to experience quite heavenly sensations and access altered states of consciousness. A woman will experience this phenomenon even if she has

had her physical uterus and cervix removed. But this upper part of the vagina is usually not touched by the penis because the vagina is restricted and tense, in part to protect and guard against fast deep penetration. Most women, whether they are conscious of it or not, hold the upper part of the vagina tightly closed because it is *extremely* painful when the penis aggressively hits up against the cervix.

To allow a man to reach this most sacred focal point in woman—a place that can be thought of as the garden of love—she must keep the vagina relaxed. Essential for this is the prerequisite of a loving penis and, initially, an exaggeratedly slow penetration of the vaginal canal, millimeter by millimeter. One penetration to the very depths of the vagina can easily take several prolonged minutes, and even then perhaps the lovers will remain still for some minutes more before the need for further movement arises.

This style of deep penetration will bring the epicenter of the female pole, the area around the cervix, to correspond directly with the head of the penis, which is like a highly sensitive magnet. If the penis is unable to reach as high as the cervical area, women have reported that the cervix itself draws closer to the head of the penis. Between the negative cervix and the radiant positive penis head, a powerful interaction on an electromagnetic level occurs, with a catalytic discharge of the accumulated tensions that are lodged in the tissues causing insensitivity. The penis will have this effect in the vagina as a whole, and particularly in this upper region.

Healing Sexual Traumas with Deep Penetration

Many women carry forward into their lives the devastating emotional pains and tensions resulting from sexual abuse they suffered as young girls. Courageously they piece themselves together again to enter the sexual domain, sometimes as deeply wounded beings. Some fortunate women are able to get therapy to process the past, to work the feelings out of their energy system. While this is certainly helpful, there still remains a residue of the memory stored on a cellular level in the body, particularly in the vagina, the lower belly, and the ovaries. These disturbing memories may on occasion unconsciously get triggered, resulting in recurring emotional out-

breaks and unhappiness as the woman reexperiences the negative vibrations of her past, still active inside her. (See chapter 10 for a more detailed discussion of emotions.)

All the old memories and feelings, stored as tensions, can be discharged by the penis—the very organ that did damage in the first place. Unconsciousness caused the damage; consciousness can heal it. Lack of love was the cause; love can heal it. The penis is able to gradually break up and discharge tensions and return vaginal tissues back to sensitivity and aliveness. In fact, most women will notice that the vagina has many painful places that only become discernible and evident when the vagina is more relaxed, having given up its guard, and when the penis is slow and loving. Pain almost always reflects tension, or it reflects a memory or an inner holding of some kind. The releasing of old tensions enacts a profound healing for the female psyche. (And the penis experiences the same kind of healing through this process.) The partner exercise at the end of this chapter provides practical details on deep penetration.

A woman shares her experience: "When we did the deep penetration I had a big energy release at my womb. It was very painful but at the same time it felt very good; it was almost unbearable. I understand now about how energy is stuck inside. I felt lighter afterward and I can feel my womb pulsing. But today I was even more aware of the tension. It is as if I'm noticing this tension for the first time, and the more I feel the release, the more aware I am of the tension."

A woman shares her experience: "About the deep penetration around the cervix—at first I felt beautiful sensations and joy and I had the image of having a very small gold treasure box in there. But that was very short-lived. After, it became an unbearable physical sensation right at the cervix. We had to stop many times because I could not take it, and all the time I was having an electrical discharge all over the body. It became more unbearable when we made love later that night. I had great discomfort, I was tense everywhere. Then I started to have the feeling of being at the doctor and I connected with the actual fear of physical pain right at the cervix. I remembered gynecological visits, where they touch there to take samples for tests, and the painful insertion of an IUD. As I talked to my lover about it the pain calmed down. In the morning I experienced total relaxation, silence, presence, and stillness as we made love."

A man (partner of the previous woman) shares his experience: "The lovemaking was very powerful in that a lot came up for my partner. It would be so intense for her that I had to come out several times. Finally something released and it was beautiful to feel her vagina relax and suddenly I started crying."

A woman shares her experience: "Today there was much pain released during the penetration, in my vagina and my heart. All the rapes came back. I had a big emotional outburst and found it difficult to accept that nevertheless it happened—and my vagina is feeling more alive and still very painful—so is my heart. For me right now it is an emotional phase. Cramps and pains, release in the vagina, vivid memories of different abuse stories, abortions, sterilization. Often tears come up and a deep mistrust and for the first time I see how the sexual abuse has wounded me, made me vulnerable, and much is opening up in my heart. I see the tendency in myself to trash that vulnerability with jokes and power games."

A woman shares her experience: "When I open, there is a flower in my vagina, deep inside, like at the cervix or thereabouts. I can speak from there. It is a welcoming. It is like another heart in my body. I have experienced this before but I never valued it."

A woman shares her experience: "Whenever the movements get too much for me, I say 'stop,' and my partner waits for a while and later begins moving again. We have found a form that is feeding our basic hunger, caring for our tissues' needs for exchange instead of friction, and we have become much more sensitive. When we go for friction sex every once in a while just to see what it's like, we both get so sore and itchy we have to wait a week before we are back to normal. All we need for our physical healing is simply putting the penis in the vagina! Speaking of which: the medicine

I had bought before our first workshop to heal my heavy fungus has been sitting in the refrigerator unused ever since. My vagina has never had fungus again!"

Healing is usually a process that happens in layers, sometimes gradually and sometimes more quickly. Do not expect immediate results or even instant ecstasy. Healing depends a great deal on how willing a woman is to relax into her nature and to release the past that she is carrying. When old feelings arise it is not essential to understand the source of trauma; if you do, great, but you need not search around for the reason why your tears are falling—simply dive into the feeling and express it. Otherwise you can get lost in thought and lose contact with the feelings welling inside. Women also carry pain on a collective level, for all of womankind and the tragedies of humanity.

Following a period of cleansing of old memories and pains, the polarity will be fully restored. Women will feel an ecstasy generated by the luminous, beaming penis head corresponding in its rightful way with the epicenter of the passive, absorbent vagina. In these moments a woman can also feel a vibration in the opposite end of the magnetic rod: in the heart and breasts. And many women report the experience that as the energy moves upward to reinforce the opening in the breasts, it is as if the penis actually penetrates the heart, the female positive pole. It becomes a full-bodied experience, radiating through arms, legs, and head—at times the sensation extends beyond the body, giving rise to a bodiless, floating sensation. The experience of penetration is not limited to sensations localized in the vagina. The vagina is the physical entry point of the female energy system, and as such the vagina is only part of the total experience.

The Breasts Impulse the Vagina and Expand Energy

When first "in" love, women report that they more easily have experiences of orgasm. This is true because the heart is naturally open, chest and breasts alive and vibrating in love energy. The vagina, at the other end of the magnetic rod, automatically begins resonating and answering.

As years pass lovers can lose their initial sensitivity and aliveness to themselves and to each other. Slowly, sex becomes more routine; each starts to take the other for granted and forgets to appreciate his or her partner's good qualities. This process is often accompanied by a diminishment of energy vibrating in the heart center. Sometimes this corresponds with the common experience of the "honeymoon being over," where suddenly something radiant but invisible evaporates. The sensation of being *in love* with a man becomes one of loving *him*. This in itself is fine, but life can become full of habits that distance us from the heart center and from our partner. For a woman, this distance can also affect her orgasmic capacity.

Fortunately, the converse is also true. When a woman approaches the sexual act with her breasts, in their organic sequence, the female positive pole vibrates, generating orgasmic states. *Being* in love becomes a daily reality.

To summarize, there is a circular movement in the female energy system that flows down first and then upward. Following polarity, the sexual energy awakens initially in the breasts and then overflows to the vagina before turning upward again to return to the heart. Any intensification of touch or awareness at the breasts at any time will create further overflow and intensification of experience, and will even enhance male erection. (See chapter 8 for woman's part in erection.) Sex that does not harness these body polarities becomes a linear experience leading to frustration and unhappiness, because the innate ecstatic potential of the meeting is completely forgone.

Tantric Inspiration

So just relax into each other and forget about the mind. Enjoy the very presence of the other, the meeting, and get lost in it. Don't try to make anything out of it; there is nothing to make. Then one day there will be a valley orgasm, there will be no peak. There will be only relaxation, but that has its own peak because it has depth. Some day the body will trigger itself into a peak orgasm but that will also be coming; you will just be there.

Sometimes there will be a valley, sometimes there will be a peak . . . and that is a rhythm. You cannot have a peak every day. If you have only peaks, then the peak will not be very big. You have to earn the peak by going into the valley. So it is half and half. Sometimes it will be a valley orgasm. Then get lost in the darkness of the valley, the coolness and the peace. That is how you earn a peak. One day the energies are ready: they themselves are going towards the peak. Not that you are taking them. How can you? Who are you and how can you manage to? By being in the valley the energy accumulates; the peak is born out of the valley. Then there is great orgasm; your whole being is suffused with a joy.

OSHO, TRANSCRIBED TEACHINGS,
THE OPEN SECRET

Awareness and Sensitivity Exercise
Building Consciousness in the Vagina

While standing equally balanced on two feet, relax and contract the pelvic floor to build awareness in the vaginal cavity. The pelvic floor refers to all the muscles surrounding the vagina and anus. These stretch in one direction between the coccyx to the pubic bone and crosswise between the two sitz bones. They form a web of muscles with the perineum in the center, situated between the anus and the vagina, as the focal point.

Slowly pull up and slowly relax, with your attention at this focal point of the perineum. You can also highlight the vaginal muscles at the front or the anal muscles at the rear. While doing so it is important to also relax the belly muscles, as many women unconsciously tighten the abdominals to give an impression of a flatter belly. A relaxed belly, one that protrudes, is of great advantage in that it maintains the balancing integrity of the arch in the lumbar spine. Allow the stretch in the lumbar area to come through the relaxation of the abdominal muscles and not through simply sticking out the buttocks, which is a form of tension. Search for this balance within yourself, and then consciously contract the muscles of the vagina for about 60 seconds of slow, rhythmic contractions.

Slow means *slow,* and you are likely to feel this as quite an effort. In time you can increase the number of contractions. When finished, immediately lie down with eyes closed and rest for five to fifteen minutes. While resting you can also get in tune with the magnetic rod running between your vagina and breasts, and relish any spreading of energy and warmth that may follow.

At any time during the day, make it a practice to bring awareness to the area around the vagina (and the belly) and relax it, wherever you are and in whatever you are doing. Tighten, relax, tighten, relax—no one can see, and it feels really good. With your awareness begin to focus inside the vagina to awaken the life already present in the tissues. You will notice again and again that the vagina is tightened (through unconscious fears and tensions), so simply keep relaxing whenever you remember to. When the channel upward is clear and open, any contractions are likely to result in ecstatic sensations pulsating upward to the top of the spine.

Partner Exchange Exercise
Deep Penetration and Healing the Vagina (and Penis)

You and your lover should develop deep penetration as a style of lovemaking, with your man focusing deep in the vagina whenever possible. The way to set about this is to ask your man, when he has an erection, to enter your vagina extremely slowly and to go as far in as he is able. Then hold still for a while, as described earlier in this chapter. Before your man penetrates you, open your labia (the vaginal lips) and hold your vagina open while he penetrates. Doing this will make the penetration smoother and more powerful.

In addition, it is an excellent idea to reach between your legs from time to time during lovemaking and open your outer labia. It really enhances the feeling of the penetration because of the increased correspondence—it is like a deepening kiss between penis and vagina. Simply reach your arms between your legs (your man may have to pull his body away a tiny bit, but without losing penetration), lay each hand alongside the vulval area, and with the fingers pull the labia apart, clearing the way as it were, pulling open the folds of tissue at the entrance of the vagina (inner labia) as well as extricating any pubic hairs that may have strayed there. You can keep your hands in this opening position for a while before withdrawing them from your pelvic area. When you have withdrawn your hands, your man can deepen his penetration by a few centimeters (which is worth more than it may sound). This procedure may seem like a bit of a disturbance, as your man has to back off for a few moments, but the increased sensations of pleasure in depth are clearly worthwhile.

With extremely slow penetration any painful places are likely to become apparent as the penis moves, or even lies still, in the vagina. Remember, pain anywhere is usually an indicator of some inner holding, and pain can be present at any point of the vagina, even right at the entrance. We must seek out these painful points with intention, with the penis, and bring the area into correspondence with the magnetic penis head. As mentioned already, the penis will still have an impact even if penetration is not to the full depth of the vagina.

Ask your partner to hold still when the head of his penis is touching any place that feels painful. Travel internally with your awareness to the area and feel into it from the inside. It is essential for the penis to have "porous" contact with your vagina, which means the head must not push with force into any tender area. Rather, once you have identified the discomfort—the point where you tell your partner to hold still—he should draw his penis back about a millimeter or two, a hairbreadth. This minuscule amount of space allows for an interchange of energies; otherwise the pressure of the penis will further compact tensions instead of loosening them.

You can contact your partner's eyes with soft vision or you can close your eyes, whatever feels appropriate at any given moment. As you rest in yourself, just see what you feel and allow whatever wants to happen, be it feelings of sadness that come up, any shivering or shaking—a gale of laughter may even suddenly erupt out of you. The deep penetration may only last a few minutes; sometimes the penis will relax down after it has done this work, and if you both remain relaxed and easy and allow it to lie in the vagina, resting, it might surprise you by rising up again into erection.

Possible Positions for Deep Penetration

A variety of positions are suitable for deep penetration. You can try them all. Each position allows the penis to engage with the vagina from a variety of different angles, giving the opportunity to explore every corner of the vagina. It is most useful for a woman to place a folded pillow or a small square cushion under her pelvis (as shown in figures 6.1 and 6.2) so as to raise the pelvis and increase the depth and angle of penetration.

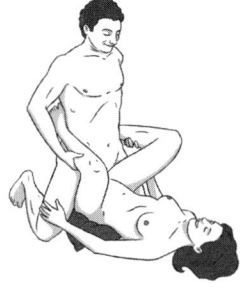

Fig. 6.1. Middle position, man kneeling (with pillow to raise woman's pelvis)

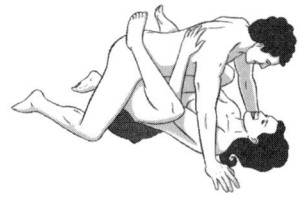

Fig. 6.2. Middle position, man on hands and knees (with pillow to raise woman's pelvis)

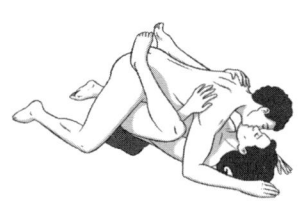

Fig. 6.3. Middle position, man lying forward, half kneeling (with pillow to raise woman's pelvis)

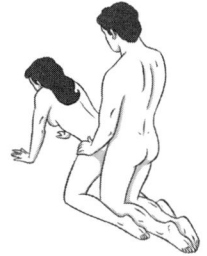

Fig. 6.4. Rear position

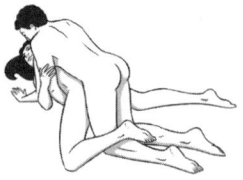

Fig. 6.5. Rear position with man lying on top of woman

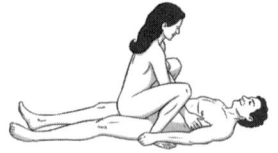

Fig. 6.6. Woman sitting on top

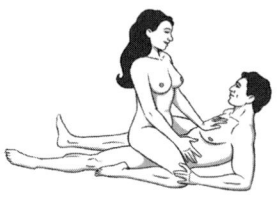

Fig. 6.7. Woman kneeling on top

7
The Clitoris and Excitement

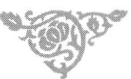

The clitoris has a beautiful place in the sexual exchange, but even with an incredible fifteen thousand nerve fibers that penetrate the pelvis and connect with the clitoris, it is not the center of female sexuality (as believed by most women today). The clitoris does not even rank a good second place; the breasts and the vagina are the true source of the orgasmic state. For many years now, we have placed undue emphasis upon the clitoris for female orgasm because we lacked wisdom and insight into the receptive aspect of the vagina.

Today more than 70 percent of women report that the vagina has little to do with their experience of orgasm and pleasure; instead, they rely on the sensations of the clitoris. This reality reveals the fact that male penetration is not very significant to most women, as far as their sexual satisfaction is concerned. It also implies that man has lost his ability to communicate meaningfully to woman through his penis. Instead of bringing her to heightened states, penetration usually leaves a woman high and dry, with no orgasmic experience at all. In the face of this situation, both men and women have resorted to directly stimulating the clitoris with the intention

of producing a peak type of orgasm for the woman. The goal-oriented pressure and tension needed to "achieve" an orgasm (especially when the woman feels pressured to climax to please the man) can make it hard to climax at all or to do so in a satisfying manner. When we understand more about female sexuality, we can see that the clitoris acts as a great diversion for a woman. In seeking orgasm via the clitoris she is distanced from the feminine, receptive qualities of her vagina in relation to the penis. As a consequence, fulfilling sexual experiences become more and more elusive. The clitoris can certainly contribute intensely pleasurable experiences, but it is the vagina, which actually embraces the penis, that leads most directly to orgasmic states. To access these finer levels of sensitivity a woman needs to be willing to steer away from the clitoris and develop an interest in the vagina, the deep receptacle of her femininity.

Excitation Versus Excitement

It is essential to understand that direct stimulation of the clitoris produces sexual excitement, which is a form of tension. Tension causes contraction and inhibits energy from spreading, so it is not basic to the expansive orgasmic design. Perhaps differentiating between *excitation* and *excitement* will be helpful here. Excitation is a state of aliveness, of refined vibration, tingling, and inner delight. If such pleasing sensations are played upon or intensified through continued touch or stimulation, excitation can quite easily change character and shift into excitement coupled by an overwhelming urge for orgasm. Excitation is beautiful, wide, of the here and now, without direction—the pleasure is enough unto itself. Excitement is narrower; it has a direction and it rouses a compulsion to take the sensations to some overwhelming conclusion.

A woman is advised to stay with excitation as much as possible and to avoid excitement, especially during penetration. Woman's excitement has a peculiar effect on a man, with dire consequences—intensity of sexual excitement in a woman encourages early ejaculation in a man. Premature ejaculation is fostered when women get too excited either before or during the sexual act. If a woman always wants or needs a great deal of stimulation

during sex, her partner is more likely to have a premature ejaculation problem. When a man attempts to arouse his woman through a lot of stimulation, he is ensuring that he will ejaculate soon. Some men ejaculate immediately before the much-dreamed-of penetration, totally overcome with excitement and anticipation. Others ejaculate within a few minutes. As we well know, loss of erection usually follows ejaculation, and man is disabled from staying inside woman for long enough to make any impact on her. (As to his experience, with this quick ejaculation man does not deeply sense that he has made love and so he begins longing for sex again, fantasizing about it, dreaming of the moment when he will penetrate again. As mentioned earlier, the mere discharge of semen does not grant a man the satisfaction that comes with deeper orgasmic states.)

Thus, a man is seldom inside of a woman long enough for either of them to experience the pure channeling of energy into the woman, and the glory of this. When the sexual energy is able to move in a circular way according to polarity, the penis is functioning finally as a conduit for male energy. However, because of his premature ejaculation, the man is unable to remain present in the vagina; this has made his woman dependent on her clitoris, and thereby on excitement, for sexual satisfaction.

If both parties to the sexual act remain relatively "unexcited," they can delay ejaculation for a long time and prolong the lovemaking. Ejaculation becomes a choice, not a necessity. To reduce the incidence of ejaculation *prior* to penetration, a woman should cool down during foreplay to ensure that her man stays relatively unexcited—that is, if she wants him to enter her. By reducing excitement she naturally makes her man more potent, putting him in more of a position to satisfy her.

The same principle of keeping it cool applies during penetration: keep the excitement level down so that man can continue to avoid ejaculation. When the excitement level and tension in the vagina get too high, a man will ejaculate, especially when the woman moves her pelvis in an active way in order to engage and stimulate the clitoris. The excitement of this is instantly communicated to the penis. Any sudden, urgent rushes of excitement should be avoided because these will virtually "pull" an ejaculation out of a man. Unless a man has authority, unless he is relaxed and

THE CLITORIS AND EXCITEMENT

in control of himself, he almost has no choice but to ejaculate. Men report in particular an uncontrollable discharge when a woman shifts gears and tries to intensify excitement so she can pull off an orgasm. One man described how he experienced this pulling sensation as a kind of dark substance entering and overwhelming him. Men themselves are amazed at how quickly an ejaculation can happen in the face of a woman's increasing excitement. Of course, if a man loses his erection, it hardly matters to the 70 percent of women who in any event rely on the clitoris; but this conventional approach limits female experience because it is removed from the penis and vagina—the organs of love themselves.

The Inclusive, Polarized Vagina

The vagina is an electromagnetic cavity, and *included* in it, not separate from it, is the clitoris. One pole ("positive") is found at the clitoris and the other pole ("negative") is found in the deepest part of the vagina, around the mouth of the uterus (cervix) and upper regions, as explained in chapter 6. An electromagnetic connection exists between these two poles, which runs through the so-called G-spot. (The G-spot is named after the gynecologist Ernst Grafenberg, 1881–1957, who was the first to offer a theory concerning this area.)

The G-spot is a highly erogenous cushion of tissue located just a few inches inside the vagina on the front wall, almost up behind the pubic bone. This is where the vagina wraps around the urethra (the tube that carries urine from the bladder). The area is connected to the sphincter muscles of the bladder, which may be one reason for its sensitivity. Added sensitivity can be attributed to the fact that the area forms the back end of the clitoris, which has nerve roots that run very deep.[1]

Recent research has established that the tissues of the G-spot contain an enzyme also found in the male prostate gland, suggesting that the urethral sponge may be the female version of this gland, which is also rather sensitive to pressure and touch in men. The existence of these tissues in this place may also explain the fluid secretions many women experience during or after G-spot stimulation. Sometimes called female ejaculation,

copious sexual juices can be released from the G-spot. For some women, ejaculation happens in heightened sexual states; for other women, ejaculation is not accompanied by any special sensations.

There can be no question that every woman possesses a G-spot; what differs is whether or not she feels it. Each woman carries her personal sexual history, made up of individual physical and psychological factors that can interfere with her sensitivity. However, by now we know that the penis has the capacity to heal the vagina of past aggressions. This means in reality that, in time, any woman ultimately has the capacity to experience the joy of the G-spot. While this is true, it is rather hidden away inside the vagina—though most women can feel it if they probe gently into the vagina with a forefinger and explore behind the pubic bone/bladder area. During lovemaking the area can sometimes get engorged, making it easier to feel. In any case, the G-spot should not be made a separate focus of attention and thus interrupt the awareness of a woman from the *whole of the vagina.* All these mysterious parts *together* make up the incredible wonders of the female genitalia.[2]

And so it follows that the G-spot, like the clitoris and like the vagina itself, should be approached in a passive, easy manner, not sought after or hunted. Perhaps in certain angles of penetration the G-spot or the clitoris may come into play. A little further on we will consider how women can make use of clitoral possibilities. However, neither the clitoris nor the G-spot is the real source of orgasmic ecstasy for women.

Integrating the Clitoris without Disturbing the Vagina

We need to reevaluate the clitoris and find its place in deep, moving orgasm. We also need to appreciate the vagina and give value to the event of penetration—the conjoining of male and female poles—which will lead to higher experiences. The real art for women lies in integrating the clitoris without distracting from the vagina. To do this it is usually best to avoid stimulating the clitoris before penetration. As mentioned, excitement builds tension in the vagina. The vaginal environment physically contracts—

some women report a slight, dull ache—while turning slightly positive and unreceptive, which inhibits the potential electromagnetic streaming from the penis into the vagina.

I frequently ask women in my workshops if they notice whether the vagina is less sensitive or more sensitive to the penetrating penis after a bit of clitoral stimulation during foreplay. The overwhelming majority of women raise their hands to say that in fact they notice the vagina is *less* sensitive after the clitoris has been played with. They perceive the sensation and pleasure of penetration as tremendously heightened when the vagina is in a more innocent and passive state, undisturbed by any previous genital touching. (Remember, with tantric sex the vagina is already streaming with receptive energy from loving focus on the breasts.) This clearly demonstrates that stimulation of the clitoris creates tensions that make the penetration much less sensational. The stimulated clitoris seems to disturb the composure of the vagina, creating a restlessness, a wanting, a kind of hunger for orgasm that dramatically reduces the significance and intensity experienced in penetration itself. And once the penis is inside, the excited woman's tendency is to want to go for the orgasm (again by way of the clitoris) rather than to stay with the actual reality of the penis in the vagina.

If you choose to engage the clitoris during sex, it is much better to do so much further down the road—certainly well after penetration, perhaps even after an hour or two of making love. This time gives your body a chance to open fully via the energy channel between breasts and the vagina. Then, if the clitoris is approached in a relaxed, easy, passive way—as an extension of the vagina itself—it can deepen vaginal awareness, greatly intensifying sensitivity, and adding to orgasmic states.

The clitoris can therefore be used in two opposing ways: The first is as a direct doing, an active stimulation—with the outcome of making woman a bit pushy and easily orgasm-oriented, which reduces her awareness in the vagina. Or the clitoris can be used in a non-doing, more passive, softer way, which makes a woman more receptive and open and increases awareness in the vagina. One way leads to discharge, the other way leads further into her ecstasy and femininity.

So in general it is advisable to leave the clitoris unstimulated to a certain extent. The temptations of the clitoris are enormous because it does feel delicious, but in truth the clitoris should serve as a bit of fun now and then, not as the basis of your orgasm or sexual experience. On occasion the clitoris will unexpectedly, happily chime in with everything else and further heighten your experience. But without an orgasmic base—the vibration of the magnetic rod between the breasts and vagina—the clitoral orgasm is not usually deeply moving, and can leave women in an emotional state.

The Clitoris as Bridge to the Vagina

Certainly peak orgasms do feel good in themselves; but they beckon us away from the orgasmic state—the relaxed expansion (of the same energy) that lies at the other end of the spectrum. However, some women report that through stimulating the clitoris and having a quick peak orgasm, they can relax more into their orgasmic nature. The quick release skims off tensions present in the system, and this can have a relaxing effect on a woman. And relaxation is basic to orgasm. When relaxed, a woman will suddenly feel more sensual, feminine, and receptive, with the vagina more available. So a woman *can* use the clitoris as a bridge to the vagina, but if she peaks in this way during penetration she gets there at some risk to herself. As we know, man easily ejaculates with the final onrushes of female excitement, thus ending the approach to her deeper orgasmic state.

Some women also say that a bit of clitoral stimulation can raise their temperature to a full *yes* to penetration. Some women, in experimenting, say it is a relief to turn away from the imperative to go all the way for a peak orgasm with the clitoris; instead, at some point it feels right to say, "That's enough, I want you *in* me now," and then to relax into penetration without effort.

Many women prefer oral stimulation of the clitoris to other types of clitoral stimulation because it's wet, it can be sensuous and silky, and there's no irritation from rough, calloused fingers. Even oral stimulation is not appreciated so much when it gets hard and fast and rhythmic—it builds too much tension, too much pressure to climax.

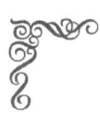

THE CLITORIS AND EXCITEMENT

Oral (or any) stimulation of the clitoris requires a new attitude: it should be like a short visit just to say a loving hello and then to move on. Oral sex can be used in support of awakening the energy but not to produce a full-blown orgasm; it can be used in support of remaining in excitation states without getting overexcited.

As we know, many women don't even expect to reach orgasm during actual intercourse, with the penis in the vagina. Their peak results from some form of direct oral and/or manual stimulation of the clitoris, which is in fact most easily achieved without penetration. Or it comes from pelvic rocking to stimulate the clitoris during intercourse. (A woman might think, "Of course he's going to come before I do once he gets in there. That doesn't mean I need to give up peak orgasms. It just means I need to have a quick orgasm before he goes in, or manage one after he's come.") On top of this, clitoral stimulation is generally assumed to be essential to female orgasm.

But here is new information: One of the biggest differences between conventional sex and tantric sex is that, in the latter, women *can* experience orgasmic states with the penis in the vagina. In fact, penetration is a necessary part of how the polarities work together to bring us into the orgasmic state. Leaking the sexual energy through momentary experiences, pleasing though they may be, is ultimately not enriching or uplifting and neither is it empowering for a woman.

If a woman is curious about her clitoris and about exploring it from a completely different angle, it will be interesting to know that tantra recognizes the existence of a subtle nerve that connects the clitoris to the little hollow above the upper lip.[3] Gaining control over this secret nerve route can enhance the pleasures of lovemaking for woman and man. (See the awareness exercise at the end of the chapter.) During lovemaking this subtle channel can be activated through visualization. Then, a man can greatly enhance this activation by kissing the upper lip of his woman, gently sucking and tugging on it, thereby stimulating one end of the channel. At the same time the woman can, if she wishes, take the lower lip of her man into her mouth and do the same.

THE CLITORIS AND EXCITEMENT

Identifying Desire and Separating from Urges

As you make love and monitor your excitement in an attempt to keep the climate cool, it is important to identify the precise point where the tide changes for you—where you suddenly feel an urgency for orgasm. This point is significant because here something creative can be done, if you are interested in transforming conventional sexual patterns. If a desire arises within you, tantra does not tell you to fight it. It is futile to fight with desire, but that doesn't mean that you become its victim or that you indulge in it. Instead tantra gives you a very subtle technique.

"When a desire arises, just at the beginning, just at the first glimpse, the first flicker of desire arising, be alert. Bring your total awareness, the entirety of your being to look at the arising desire."[4] Don't do anything, just face the desire squarely, in full consciousness, and relax back into yourself. Nothing else is needed. The energy falls back inside you, wells up, and expands powerfully through the body, lifting you to another level of experience and sensitivity. When desire disappears without a fight, it leaves you powerful, filled with immense energy and tremendous awareness.

The problem with desire is that when it has arisen—and even five seconds of entertaining desire is too much—you cannot do anything about it. Then desire will have to take its full course; it will complete its circle, and you will be carried away in its grip. Only in the beginning can you do something about it: burn the seeds of desire right then and there. When you identify the point of rising desire, then you can begin to separate from the urge and choose to go through relaxation instead. The response to go with our desires is a conditioned response, as if we flick into automatic-drive mode, so naturally it takes some practice and experimentation to steer away from the excitement track. After a while of separating from desire, the heightened feelings you experience will cease to translate into desire but will transform themselves into expansion and deepening of sensitivity. A little excitement in the beginning is always good to bring the body into excitation, but then there is a corresponding need to relax and allow the expansion of that very same energy through the system. In reality, desire and horniness are *not* prerequisites for sexual

congress; in fact, more can happen when two bodies meet as relatively unexcited beings.

A woman shares her experience: "My husband and I decided to do an experiment with the clitoris without penetration. When he first touched me on my clitoris, it felt as if a button was pushed. As he touched me and moved his finger around my clitoris, I started to feel horny. I got hot; the previously slow and fine sensations and energy movements in my body suddenly changed. I started to move up against my husband's body with urgency. My breasts went out of my awareness. They seemed not to be at all important anymore. My focus was now totally on my clitoris. My vagina changed from relaxed and open to contracted and narrow. I got into a certain stress, started sweating. I moved faster and faster. I had the impression that I *had* to go toward an orgasm. My body felt tense and my vagina got more contracted. The contraction went even more up toward my stomach. I started using exciting words. It was a stress. I could not really feel my body as a female body anymore. The deep connection I could feel with myself was gone. The deep love I could feel toward my husband was almost gone. The connection seemed to be cut. Joy was gone. It seemed more like stressful work, like a satisfaction I needed to have, a clear goal. It had nothing to do with love or my heart.

"There was a point when I could not and did not want to go on. I asked my husband to take his hand away from my clitoris. I tried to relax my body, my vagina, to get back with my awareness to my breasts. I closed my eyes to return to the connection with myself and by that to my husband as well. I realized how difficult it was to relax my vagina. My husband and I then touched my breasts in a nice and soft way. By doing this I could relax more. But I could not really relax my vagina for a long time. It felt like cramps. This feeling stayed for hours. When we got together again with a soft penetration, it felt like a healing process starting from my breasts to my vagina and expanding to the rest of the body. I felt so good and connected again. My female part could start living again.

"We also did this clitoris experiment another time with penetration. My man did not have a real erection yet but he was inside me and it felt very

nice. After stimulation of the clitoris it turned out that my contraction of the vagina got so strong (I would even call it horrible) that the penis did not have any chance to stay inside. It seemed it was kicked out. I am happy that we did these 'experiments,' as we have learned a lot. . . . I am not so ready to go for this experience of intense focusing on the clitoris again, as I know now that it hurts me on a very deep level; besides, my body does not like it anymore. I had not noticed this before. There is lots of very loving joy when we are together."

Tantric Inspiration

Excitement seems to be equivalent to ecstasy; it is not. Excitement is a state of tension; it feels good because the old is disappearing and the new is coming in. A new breeze, a new experience—it is good to welcome it with an excited heart. . . .

Excitement is only a welcome, but the welcome is not the whole story. Then the coolness has to come, and coolness is far deeper, far more valuable than any excitement can be. So jumping up and down has to stop. Sit silently, be calm and cool. Ecstasy is coolness, it is not excitement.

If you accept coolness, then only will the deeper experience of coolness give you the experience of ecstasy. It will be full of life, but not childish. It will be full of joy, but with deep contentment. The joy will not be against sadness, the joy will be beyond sadness.

OSHO, TRANSCRIBED TEACHINGS,
THE OSHO UPANISHAD

But excitement is not joy, it is just an escape from misery. Try to understand it very clearly: excitement is just an escape from misery. It gives only a pseudo experience of joy. Because you are no more miserable you think that you are joyous—not to be miserable is equivalent to being joyous. Joy is a positive phenomenon. Not to be miserable is just a forgetfulness. The misery is waiting back home for you: whenever you come back it will be there. When excitement disappears, one starts thinking "Now what is the point of this love?" In the West love dies with excitement, and that is a calamity. In fact love had never been born. It was just love of excitement, it was not real love. It was just an effort to move away from oneself. It was a search for sensation. You rightly use the word "fun"; it was fun but it was not intimacy. When excitement disappears and you just start feeling loving, love can grow; now the feverish days are over. This is the true beginning.

OSHO, TRANSCRIBED TEACHINGS,
LET GO! DARSHAN DIARY

Awareness and Sensitivity Exercise
Awakening the Secret Tantric Nerve

Give yourself twenty to thirty minutes on your own. At first it is suggested to do this meditation alone so that you can get the energy moving through the channel. Later you can use it as a kind of foreplay, as well as tuning into it while you are actually making love. You can also experiment with your partner sucking your upper lip, as suggested earlier in the chapter.

Lie down on your back, or sit upright with a straight spine. Visualize a subtle nerve running from your clitoris to your upper lip. You will be able to awaken it and consciously channel sexual energy upward through this nerve channel. From the clitoris, it runs upward through the center of the belly and chest to the base of the throat, and then through the neck to the occiput (the hollow at the base of the skull). Looping up to the crown of the head, then down through the center of the eyebrows, ending at the palate and the little hollow above the upper lip. It is like a serpent with mouths at both ends.

Visualize this nerve as an empty but vibrant tube, with a conchlike shape at the vagina/clitoris and a mouth at the upper lip/palatal region. Link some deep, slow breathing to a very gentle tightening of the vagina; this will awaken the nerve. Remember that strong contractions of the vagina during lovemaking can encourage male ejaculation, so be aware if you choose to do this, and do it very delicately so as to be almost imperceptible. Once you have connected with this path energetically, it awakens without any vaginal constrictions.

Partner Exchange Exercise
Exploring Excitation, Excitement, and the Full *Yes*

Give yourselves about forty-five minutes to do this exercise. Lie on your back side by side with your partner, with a space of about three feet between you and with no physical contact. Each of you take your awareness into your body and find a place of rest within yourself.

When you feel connected with yourself, slowly turn onto your side and face the other, allowing your eyes to meet in soft vision. After a few minutes, gradually move across the space that separates you. Place your hands on each other's genital area (one or both hands, depending on your comfort) as consciously and gently as possible, and fill it with your awareness and love. You'll find it extremely helpful in your exploration if you can report to each other in a few succinct words what you are experiencing in your body through the different kinds of touch. (See chapter 9 for more information about sharing the "now" during lovemaking.) If a certain touch arouses horniness, observe this, share it with your partner, and look to see how the touch can be modified so as not to create excess excitement.

You, the woman, want to avoid stimulating your man's penis, so don't do the usual masturbatory movements, with your hand copying the way a man would masturbate. Instead, hold his penis softly by wrapping your whole hand around it at first, and then a bit more firmly; then squeeze your hand and release it gently, slowly and lovingly moving up and down the penis squeeze by squeeze. From time to time simply hold still and embrace the penis with the warmth in your hands. With one hand you can also hold the testicles, firmly yet loosely, and delicately roll them around in your fingertips without squashing them in any way. Then hold the testicles with one hand and the penis with the other hand and melt into your hands, filling the penis with energy. Your man can very lightly rest his cupped hand over your pubic mound and follow this with a little tapping on the pubic bone and then resting still for a while. Then he can very gently pull one or two pubic hairs so as to cause a sensual little tug in the root of the hair. Again, he can rest his hands in a cup shape over your pubic mound. Continue for as long as feels right. The art is to create aliveness and excitation while bypassing overwhelming excitement that leads to desire.

8
Woman's Part in Man's Erection

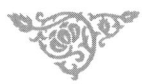

We generally consider an erection to be necessary for sex, and we place the responsibility for erection exclusively on the man. With erection sex happens, without it sex is impossible—or so we think. At the same time, for a woman a man's erection is a delicate issue, and it can be an excruciating experience when a man does not respond with an erection, in spite of every loving affection. Easily a woman will take this personally, intuitively sensing that in some mysterious way she too is part of the erection phenomenon. But exactly how erection functions is not so clear.

Because sex is thought to be out of the question in the absence of erection, whenever erection *is* present every attempt is made to keep it up. The woman overcomes her insecurities by keeping the situation juicy and interesting for the man. She adds to the level of excitement by deliberately stimulating him or by getting excited herself, indirectly exciting her man. As we know, excitement in high doses will encourage—in fact, it will virtually guarantee—a man's early ejaculation. So when a woman actively assists with maintaining a man's erection through stimulation, she steps onto a tightrope. It is definitely in woman's best interests to prolong the sexual act and

either prevent or delay her man from ejaculating. Lengthy lovemaking suits women because the more passive female body requires time for the sexual temperature to rise. By relying on excitement and stimulation, woman opens the door to premature ejaculation and suffers frustration instead. However, when a woman learns to be *more tranquil and serene* she can extend the lovemaking and also have a profound influence on male erection.

Woman Is Equally Responsible for Erection

We know that woman is the receptive element within the male-female dynamic, and this extends to the level of the vagina. Because of the equal but opposite polarities of the vagina and penis, exactly 50 percent of the erection response is an outcome of the environment surrounding the penis—the vagina itself. And really, when you think about it, this is as it should be: erection happens due to an interaction between the male pole, which is half of a circuit, and the female pole, which is the equal and opposite half of the very same circuit. When the magnetic poles are joined or lying within their spheres of influence, the poles exert a force on each other and erection is the outcome. The electromagnetic qualities of the male and female bodies build an erection through dynamic interplay. The positive male energy extends outward as it is simultaneously drawn inward by the negative female. This electromagnetic phenomenon makes the degree of femininity present, especially in the vagina, vital in determining true erection. The significance of this is enormous—a woman's influence on a man's erection is more profound than she ever imagined.

Thus, erection is not simply a matter of getting excited and staying excited. The presence of the opposite pole is required to trigger the mechanism in man. Excitement can be enjoyed for what it is—it is a choice we can make at any time—but it is important to understand that it is not the *source* of the male erection. The subtle electromagnetic properties of the penis and the vagina exist *beneath* the level of excitement, as an energy reality in the physical body. It is actually easier to perceive the interplay of opposite polarities in the absence of excitement, because with excitement

the delicate deeper polarities are easily overridden and obscured. An erection that arises through polarity can be maintained for an hour or more without the usual efforts. An erection of this kind is a totally different sexual experience for woman and for man. It is like an inner earthquake that awakens every cell in the body. It is the most extraordinarily organic happening, full of the delicious sensations of the penis lifting and twisting its way into the vagina, writhing upward snakelike, touching woman to her very core.

Penetration without Erection

Because erection is possible at this delicate, organic level, we can begin to think about penetration (which usually requires erection) in a completely different way. "Soft" penetration offers us an interesting alternative style of lovemaking. It is very relaxing to begin penetration while the penis is soft. A woman can easily insert an unerect penis into her vagina, once she learns how. A man can also do it, but it is more fun all around when the woman actually puts the penis in the vagina—perhaps with a little help from the man, if necessary, who can join in holding the penis at its base. Often by this stage the penis has already started to respond to all the loving attention with the beginnings of an erection, and this makes the penis even easier to slip in. Soft penetration is a useful skill that, with a little practice, can be quite artfully done, thereby opening up a whole range of what hitherto were impossibilities.

With this new skill of putting the penis inside the vagina without erection, the lovers bypass the usual need for excitement or stimulation. This is an excellent way to begin intercourse, because it means the poles meet in a relatively undisturbed state, from zero so to speak. In the optimum scenario, of course, the woman has experienced an overflow, a showering of energy, onto her vagina from her breasts prior to the soft penetration; however, this is not absolutely essential. Quite okay, too, is to place the penis in the vagina after a short kiss and cuddle. Without excitement there may be a lack of lubrication in the vagina, and this is easily rectified with lubricants. (See more about condoms and lubricants in the partner exercise for soft

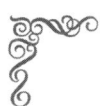

penetration at the end of the chapter.) Once penetration is achieved, the woman can begin to bring her breasts into the foreground as elaborated in chapter 5, touching them, sensing them from within, or having her man touch them with love. And then it is a simple matter of waiting to see what wants to happen. In any event, the unerect penis can feel very delicious, and it is good to relax into whatever radiating sensations are present, *remembering that awareness at this level is what creates an environment conducive to erection.* A man is also able to sense his unerect penis, if not at first then certainly after a few attempts at diving into awareness in his penis. Most men in my workshops report that the penis is a great deal more sensitive by the end of a week, after being more conscious in sex.

In an unpretentious meeting of the vagina and penis, a natural kinetic of positive and negative follows from which erection can potentially unfold. I say it *can* because it does not always happen like this; it takes a bit of time for the penis and vagina to become accustomed to communicating at this level. On the other hand, it may happen on the first try! It really depends on the sensitivity of the individuals—and this will change at each moment and day by day. It is most likely to occur when a man and a woman are loving, intensely present, and relaxed in their general approach. Certainly when lovers achieve an erection in this way it is not by physical effort or fantasy. It is more likely a by-product of love, respect for the body, intimacy, and physical tenderness and is not something that should be expected *every* time. In this atmosphere the penis will naturally expand and wind upward and perhaps after a while relax and unwind. This is not cause for anxiety: if you wait without interfering, often the penis will rise once again.

In fact, starting out with soft penetration can be a tremendous relief to a man because it takes the immense pressure off him about *having* to achieve an erection before he can make love. This relaxation in itself helps his erection potential.

Healing Impotence and Lost Sensitivity

As explained in chapter 6, conventional sex causes the vaginal walls to toughen up and thereby lose sensitivity and receptivity. So on the first few

occasions a woman may not feel as much of the delicate and divine vaginal sensations she is in reality capable of. Usually, though, she *will* feel herself and she *will* feel the penis in her vagina *before* the man can actually feel his penis himself. The penis, too, has become insensitive and overcharged, the tissues hard, tense, and dense. In this state of congestion it is very difficult for man to really perceive his penis without movement, let alone be a channel for his masculine force to flow into woman. So this lack of sensitivity is quite normal. But the good news is that relaxing together with the genitals in electromagnetic connection is a powerful healing force. The body responds very quickly and, depending on sincerity and the frequency of lovemaking, the penis and vagina soon begin to feel increasingly sensitive and alive to each other, whether erection is present or not. The unerect penis in the vagina is also a delight, and increasingly so as sensitivity is reawakened. Orgasmic states can happen as easily with an unerect penis as with an erect penis.

Impotence, the inability of a man to get an erection, is a mammoth problem facing men and women these days. Generally speaking, impotence can largely be attributed to the tensions, aggressions, pressures, heat, and excitement brought on by conventional sex. Man's dependence on stimulation and sensation means that with the passage of time he may eventually lose all capacity to respond as he slowly loses his sensitivity to himself and to his surroundings (woman and the environment). In addition, men frequently are disconnected from their true inner feelings, which include feelings of inadequacy and hopelessness, and repress them instead. Repressing feelings only makes matters worse. On top of the physical congestion is emotional turmoil and sexual confusion, and so a man can lose all potency.

Through soft penetration and the gradually returning sensitivity of the genitals, impotence really can be overcome. The healing of the penis and likewise of the vagina is something that can only be done together. Each needs the other half for healing energy to arise. In a relaxed atmosphere the penis (and the man behind it) is more able to perceive and sense the surrounding environment, which is the source of his erection. Healing impotence takes time and patience, communication and expressing inner feelings, and it can be done.

The key for a woman is to continually develop awareness within her vagina. Each time of making love is a new chance to dive deep within and feel the vagina from the inside; to start to perceive it differently and treat it differently; to imagine it as a receptive canal and will yourself to absorb and be receptive. It may take a few attempts to trust yourself, but the outcome will be sufficient encouragement to spur you on your way. This can be an ecstatic journey that lasts a lifetime.

Receptivity and Fear of Not Feeling

Women generally carry a great fear of feeling nothing—no interesting sensations in the vagina *at all*—if they relinquish the movements of conventional sex. This fear is something to be squarely faced, because behind the barrier of fear of inadequacy lies a world of feminine experience. All kinds of fears are instilled in us through an accumulation of insensitive sexual experiences; but now, in this loving, tantric context, a woman can let go and allow herself to receive man, allow herself to be healed by him and with him.

The more present and conscious a woman is in her vagina, the stronger the man's erection response is likely to be. Remember also that the breasts are the route to the vagina, so these must not be abandoned and overlooked in favor of the vagina. It's best to be aware of both places at once. If that is a bit of a stretch (which it will be at first), then choose the breasts as the focus of your awareness and trust that the vagina will respond. If the sensation in a woman's breasts are suddenly intensified, for instance when she or her partner touches them, there is often an accompanying surge of energy experienced through the penis as it rises and burrows deeper into the vagina. The same effect results through breast awareness itself, without even the need for physical touching. When a woman increases her intensity of awareness or begins to melt with the breasts and really enters them from the inside, it serves to encourage erection or even retrieve an erection.

Man, as he is now, is easily overwhelmed by woman (who is a bit "male," herself), and especially easily loses his fragile erection response

when woman's sexual overtures seem more like hungry demands than gracious invitations. Man needs space to fall back into himself in order to truly realize his masculine qualities. And woman needs time to relax into her element in order to have the required alchemic effect on man. With our habit of taking action in sex, right now it may seem far from natural to relax and absorb; with practice and commitment it will soon begin to make all the difference to the sexual exchange.

Some emphasis is given to woman strengthening the muscles of the vagina, or using contractions or pumping the vaginal muscles during sex to squeeze the penis. Usually she does this with the intention of encouraging and maintaining erection. It will be most interesting for women who use this strategy to hear that in exactly the moment a woman contracts her vaginal muscles intentionally, men report that they immediately begin to sense that they are losing their erection. The moment a woman makes a demonstrative, positive, male-like expression, it has the opposite of the desired effect. The flow of energy between negative and positive poles is disturbed; suddenly the complementary component is absent, and erection begins to fail. The penis will begin to shrink back and both man and woman will feel it instantly.

A natural flow occurs when there is an ambience of vaginal relaxation creating space for the delicate, organic phenomenon of erection. And essentially, woman is the space in which everything takes place. When man feels this magnetic flow emanating from his penis, as if drawn out of him and absorbed by woman, it gets easier to change conventional ideas that sex equals getting excited and coming. When a woman is more feminine—poised and centered in herself, relaxed and receptive in her body, with awareness in breasts and vagina—it happens spontaneously, without thought, that male energy extends outward in the form of an erection, without great effort or great excitement. A spark jumps across the space and the bodies follow in unison. At a certain level of sensitivity it is possible to lie and be enthralled by the magnetic goings on of the penis snaking up and down the vagina for many hours with no movement at all. Remember: making love frequently enables the sensitivity to return and the electromagnetic finesse to develop between the penis and the vagina.

A man shares his experience: "Making love has become a part of my daily life and the fulfillment of my deepest longings. More and more I reach that incredible space of no-mind, of endless love, of inner expansion without boundaries, of great bliss. To me it still is a miracle, every day again. The wonderful thing is to be able to reach that space as a couple, but also alone. I can feel how the stillness and depth of that state of being infiltrates my ordinary life in a very subtle way. And I realize that I have become much more conscious about the moments when I lose contact with myself. And I can quite easily return back in and down. How can life be so easy? For me it has become a deep meditation to be together with my partner in this way. It nurtures my whole being in a wonderful way. The way I go back to my daily habits has changed. I feel much more connected with that still-point in me."

A man shares his experience: "I am learning to trust myself. Many of the things we have spoken about I have felt or done before sometimes, but I didn't understand or trust it. Simply to be there, naturally, waiting—this is very relaxing. I can watch what happens between me and the other. All the little fine movements of energy I don't normally recognize while I am excited—the excitement is what stops me from relaxing more and trusting in my energy. I have noticed that I don't have trust in excitement. There is always this fear of losing the erection. This does not happen when an erection comes out of a natural energy flow, by itself."

A man shares his experience: "Today I experienced the interactions of male and female energy. I always felt responsible for everything that happens in lovemaking, but at the same time I always had this feeling that it is not true—there is something else that creates the situation as well. Each day now my trust, acceptance, and relaxation grows. I begin to feel what happens on the other side for my partner, that something in me activates something in her, and this activates something in me, and so on and on. It is the feeling of creating something together, and the ability to receive love grows."

A man shares his experience: "In the beginning a lot of conditioning came up. It was going so far that I couldn't get an erection. But as soon as I found the door out of my mind, an erection was there. The process brought me back to myself. The more I can relax in lovemaking the more I feel my sex energy. When I notice I am outside of myself with my energy and I bring it back inside of me, the energy increases and spreads out in my body. The energy that wants to flow out of my penis, the pressure that wants to ejaculate—if this energy comes back to my body, it spreads out in my body and relaxes me very much. The fear of ejaculating early, all the tensions there—the pressure falls away if I can own back this energy. It's softening to my body; I feel myself fluid, like waves in the ocean. The more I relax, the more the energy takes over. Suddenly a wave of feeling, of energy, comes and moves my body, then it slows down and I feel a soft energy flowing out of my sex center toward my lover. This is combined with beautiful feelings in my belly. Then another wave comes and carries me away. There is no fear of ejaculating, no pressure—the awareness is not only concentrated in my penis."

A man shares his experience: "This approach strengthens me immensely, gives me trust in myself, gives me self-acceptance, freedom to express myself. It makes me feel more worthy."

A man shares his experience: "I see that most of the time I am outside of myself with my energy in making love. I'm a doer. I want to give pleasure, to satisfy. The first days I missed an orgasm—the feeling that lovemaking was incomplete, the urge to masturbate was there. While making love I have to be very aware—I come so quickly to the point where I ejaculate because the pressure is so strong. This is changing now. The more I bring my energy back to myself, having no ejaculation, the more I am myself. It makes me more and more sexual. The longing for my lover increases—to be loving, soft, gentle, more sensitive. Going into my mind I destroy all this. If I can stay in my energy all feelings increase."

A woman shares her experience: "We plugged in again last night just to charge our batteries, and just as I was falling asleep B. went 'boom' and

kept on going while I slept. He said he felt high almost the entire night, in and out of sleep, and that it was a totally new experience for him. Naturally we plugged in again this morning and amazingly he kept right on going. It was beautiful to see and hear him talk about it . . . but I am just a tiny little bit envious. For some reason I have problems holding my presence within my body these last days. I was more relaxed these last two times—I am juicy all the time, even when we are not plugged in, and I enjoyed just being with my man in this relaxed atmosphere."

Tantric Inspiration

And while making love, forget about orgasm. Rather, be in a relaxed state with the man, relax into each other. The Western mind is continuously thinking about when it is coming and how to make it fast and great and this and that. That thinking does not allow the body energies to function. It does not allow the body to have its own way; the mind goes on interfering. . . .

Relax with the man. If nothing happens there is no need for anything to happen. If nothing happens then that is what is happening . . . and that too is beautiful! Orgasm is not such a thing that it has to happen every day. Sex should be just being together, just dissolving into each other. Then one can keep making love for half an hour, for one hour, just relaxing into the other. Then you will be of utter mindlessness, because there is no need for the mind. Love is the only thing where the mind is not needed; and that is where the West is wrong: it brings in the mind even there!

OSHO, TRANSCRIBED TEACHINGS,
THE OPEN SECRET

Partner Exchange Exercise
Soft Penetration

See Figures 8.1, 8.2, 8.3, and 8.4 for suggested positions for soft penetration. The easiest starting position is 8.1, in which the man lies on his side, facing the woman. The woman lies on her back, bringing her pelvis close to his. Both open their legs, and the genitals will be naturally lying opposite each other. Bring the genitals together and wrap the legs around each other. If the man is lying on his right side, the woman places her right leg between the man's legs keeping her knee bent and her foot resting on the floor. and brings her bent left leg to rest on his pelvis. This is called the scissors position because of how the legs interlock in scissorslike fashion. The

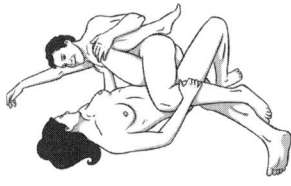

Fig. 8.1. Scissors side position for soft penetration

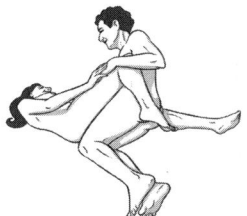

Fig. 8.2. Couple rolled to one side

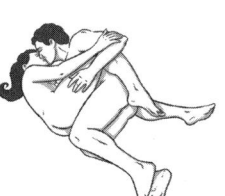

Fig. 8.3. Couple rolled to one side and kissing

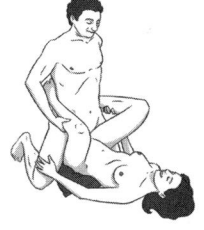

Fig. 8.4. Man in middle position for soft penetration

woman may have to move her upper body away from her lover's (to more of a 90-degree angle) in order to make the pelvises fit more snugly, or she can angle her own pelvis upward to the same effect. Experiment and find what is most comfortable (positions 8.2 and 8.3 make nice changes once penetration is achieved).

Once you are positioned correctly, pelvises close together and the vagina opposite the penis, the woman can now proceed. First take the penis in your hands. If you want lubricant, now would be a good moment to apply it. If you need a condom, now is the right time to put it on, while the penis is still soft. After the condom is on you can apply lubricant* and proceed directly with penetration as described next. Condoms do not interfere with electromagnetic sensitivity.

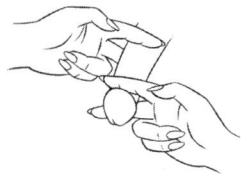

Fig. 8.5. Finger position holding penis for soft penetration

First take a moment to open your labia to make the vaginal entrance accessible. Then gently pull away the folds of foreskin wrapped around the head of the penis, exposing it even more while pulling the skin away and down toward the root. Next, make a two-pronged fork with the first two fingers of each hand (short fingernails to protect the vagina as well as the penis). Place one finger fork (try the left hand) firmly around the base of the penis and hold it there. With the other hand (the right hand) place the fingers directly on either side

---

*Use condoms only with a pharmaceutical lubricant, such as KY Jelly, absolutely not with a vegetable oil. Suitable oils for lubrication when no condom is necessary are almond oil, sesame oil, and olive oil. All oils and lubricants should be without perfume or scent.

and behind the rim, encircling the head of the penis (see fig. 8.5). Squeeze the fingers together so that you have a gentle grip on the penis and then pull the penis toward your vagina. When it arrives at the entrance, begin to insert it. You will be able to push the penis in and up into your vagina a little way. Release the fingers of your right hand and do the same thing again a little further down: grip the penis between your two fingers and direct it into your vagina, pushing it inward. By repeating the finger movement again and again, it is as if you're feeding or walking the penis into the vagina, gently pushing him inside a little more each time. Once you have pushed the penis inside you (or as much as you can manage to insert—even to get the head in is a good start), remove your hands, bring the genitals together as closely as possible by wrapping your legs around each other, and lie back. Use pillows for support anywhere you need them, and make yourselves as comfortable as you can. If the man tends to lean backward, wedge a pillow behind his pelvis and lower back.

You *absolutely must* keep your vagina relaxed during the soft penetration, or it will be like trying to force the penis through a closed door. It doesn't work. As you insert the penis, you most likely will want to look between your legs at what you are doing. Doing this will contract the belly musculature. When the belly contracts, so does the vagina. To avoid this tightening you will have to send your awareness downward into the vagina in order to intentionally hold it relaxed and open. The easier alternative, once you have the penis between your fingers, is to lie back for a moment and to stop looking at your hands. Then consciously relax the vagina and widen the vaginal muscles prior to attempting insertion. When open, slip the soft penis in, as described. Soft penetration can be a way of approaching lovemaking every time, or use it when you need it.

The scissors position may not work for every couple. In the middle position (figure 8.4) it is quite easy for a man to insert his penis himself—a good alternative. The man should position himself almost kneeling between the legs of the woman, who has her pelvis raised by a pillow. After pushing the penis into the vagina bit by bit (perhaps with the help of the woman), he can lie forward on her, and together they can roll onto the left or right side from time to time.

Tantric Meditation
Meditating on the Spine

You can experience this meditation lying on your back or sitting upright with a straight spine. Usually during sex, imagination is used to take the energy downward, but this pattern can be broken. The same imagination can be used to turn the energy upward. It can help to give the spine divisions according to the energy centers present in the body: at the genitals, below the navel, at the solar plexus, heart, throat, third eye, and the top of the head. These divisions can be used by the mind to help the energy move upward in fragments. If, however, you can connect with the spine as a whole, no divisions are needed.

Close your eyes, reverse your vision, and look back into your body, down into the pelvic area. Sense the bones of the pelvis and slowly bring your awareness to the sacrum and coccyx, which form the base of your spine. Visualize rays of light rising up your spine. Imagine yourself as particles of light, electricity. "Imagine your essence as light rays rising up your spine, from center to center, through the vertebrae, and feel 'livingness' arising in you."[1] Concentrate at first on your sex center and imagine that golden light rays are moving in an upsurge toward your navel center. Let the energy gather there and extend toward the solar plexus like a river of light. Feel warmth rising in you as rays begin to move up toward the heart center, filling you with warmth.

Travel gradually upward through your spine until you reach the top of your head. Feel your spine streaming from the sex center to the crown center. If you wish you can extend the connection beyond your body, imagining the light reaching about one meter above your head—and if you wish to travel further, reach out to the moon.

9
Relaxing into Orgasm

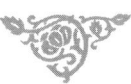

Relaxation, the foundation for new experiences, has many applications and implications for a woman on the quest of regaining her femininity. Relaxation creates an immediate aura of femininity around a woman. She becomes porous, delicate; her whole being extends an invitation to man in her presence.

The deep power in being a woman lies in her quality of being—in her capacity to influence a man by responding to him from *within the female element*. From a place of receptivity, from poise, from rest and ease within herself she exerts a force on the space around her and on anyone who enters it. She has the ability to transform her environment through receiving the male force, be it by an embrace, a touch, a kiss, or penetration; to receive, drink, absorb man as he penetrates her, with his touch, his body, his lips, his penis. The more a woman can melt into her body and experience herself from within, the more she will feel ecstatic. Relaxation and melting into the moment become natural because there is no investment in a specific goal, so an unhurried, easygoing interaction is possible. There is plenty of time to perceive what is happening in the body as it is happening—to register it in the depths of your being.

Pulling Awareness In and Down into the Body

The initial step for a woman in exploring the role of relaxation in lovemaking is to place the attention on herself. Her intention is to be more aware of herself and to be open to herself, to be curious about what is happening within. Without meeting herself in this way and passing through herself first, she cannot meet man in any profound way.

To relax means to pull your awareness away from the outside (and from doing), to pull it in and down into your body, to be awake in the senses, to feel your body's internal sensations and sensitivities. This requires a quiet atmosphere and a certain alertness—an atmosphere in which you have a chance to feel yourself rather than focusing attention on your man. To a large extent you are even ignoring your man. Not that you are oblivious to him; certainly you are not. You are vitally aware of his presence while holding the prime focus of your attention on *your* internal reality. When a woman begins to experience herself from within, she naturally becomes more still and receptive and immediately creates a feminine milieu around her. In other words, woman is required to turn her energy inward, not to project it. The true male (not the conditioned male, caught in hyperactivity) projects energy; he extends outward while woman moves inward, so as to be in a position to absorb male energy.

As receptive principle, woman is able to create a serene environment. Through relaxation she easily steps into her element and becomes an irresistible invitation. Her very presence invites the positive force and her desire is no longer a frustrated demand. When she learns to become an opening space, a fully present emptiness, she will experience that male energy is equally fully available to being received and absorbed, and transformed into something dimensional and completely fresh. In this alchemy between male and female elements an electromagnetic, attractive force arises. As a woman falls into the feminine principle the true meaning of sex dawns on her, and the real joy of being with a man begins.

Once the art is learned, she can exert her influence on any man she chooses. It is irresistible, magnetic, magical. A simple, sustained, lingering meeting of the lips can shake a man to his very foundation. Or a hug

involving every cell in the body can last and last and last forever. Relaxation creates a kind of slipstream effect where man can effortlessly slide into place and connect with his equal and opposite. In my experience, man simply cannot maintain an aggressive, macho, goal-oriented stance when he meets a force that simply invites him to melt and merge through his body and penis. The presence and allure of the female body is tremendously amplified when relaxation is embraced in place of the physically strenuous activity normally occurring in intimacy.

Scanning and Sweeping the Body

There are many different levels to relaxation; it is a very subtle and multi-dimensional experience. On the basic level is actual physical relaxation. Habitually we hold many parts of the body tight without realizing it. Learn to scan your body continuously for unnecessary tensions. While embracing, while kissing, while making love, while moving or assuming any position, scan from head to toe and again and again relax any superficial layers of tension—consciously let them go. For instance, release the clench in the jaw, the tightness around the genitals; soften and let go of the belly and solar plexus; drop the shoulders a few inches; relax any curling at your toes and feet. Undoubtedly, a certain amount of tension is required to maintain any position in space; tension is a prerequisite for physical and bodily integrity. It holds us together. But we can drop all the extra tensions around that central tensegrity.

Sometimes relaxation is mistakenly interpreted as a sort of collapsed, absent, floppy doll state. This is a misunderstanding. Relaxation increases inner aliveness and vitality, it brings grace to the body and a radiance to the being. Relaxation is an attempt to make less effort; to start being, instead, more inner, more present to what is happening rather than chasing the idea of orgasm.

At a more subtle level, beneath this kind of immediate physical relaxation exists a deeper layer of relaxation that happens through employing awareness. Use awareness to filter through the body and to "sweep" through it, or to linger in certain areas, diving deep into the cells, becoming

sensitive to the warm, tingling, streaming, glowing, vibrating sensations present in many places.

Delightful waves of inner expansion as well as a deeper level of relaxation follow this kind of lingering with the awareness, marked by a spreading of inner warmth and expanding sensations. Sensitivity becomes heightened. Body tissues get more porous as they are penetrated with life force. In particular, the vagina and breasts respond to such awareness, and a woman can greatly sensitize these two poles and thereby increase the magnetic flow between them. Inner awareness awakens the auto-ecstatic potential of the body through the magnetic rod—the source of orgasm (as explained in chapter 4). Essentially, relaxation implies presenting and opening oneself, not absenting and switching off to oneself. Woman can create an exotic ambience simply through expanding her awareness and being present throughout the slightest of any and all of her body movements and positions. Relaxation is a beautiful experience in that it finally allows a woman to be herself, present as she is, in all her glory, here and now. By adopting an easy, graceful attitude, not doing anything special, not going anywhere special, the enormous energy normally devoted to chasing the known pleasures of sex suddenly becomes free and available to expand into other areas. Instead of moving in an outward direction, the same energy is turned inward, rechanneled as it were, creating an intense awareness of the subtle, ecstatic cellular happenings within the body.

Relaxing the Vagina

Basically a woman should hold her awareness in the breasts as much as possible before and during sex, remembering that energy overflows from the breasts to ignite the vagina. At the same time it is good to ensure that the vagina is wide and relaxed. Linger with the awareness in the vaginal canal and sense into the tissues, entering them on a cellular level. Relaxation and sweeping with the awareness enhances the quality of "emptiness" of a receptive, welcoming vagina. This in turn reinforces the positive, active "fullness" of the penis present in the vagina. Once penetration has taken place the porous, absorbent, welcoming emptiness of the

passive pole should be maintained for the duration of lovemaking. When these positive and negative poles are in balance (within your own body and between the penis and vagina), the passage opens, energy flows. The delight of this electromagnetic streaming within the core of the body is quite removed from the sensations we conventionally associate with sex.

Awareness naturally creates slowness, and so being unhurried becomes easy. Especially recommended are slow movements within the vagina to prevent an unconscious defensive reaction of the vagina as it attempts to protect the cervix. As mentioned in some detail in chapter 6, a tight, constricted vagina is a hindrance to orgasmic experiences. Instead of tight and narrow the vagina ought to be soft and supple, which immediately gives it the sensitivity to feel the energy radiating out of the penis. Encourage relaxation by keeping the vagina wide and open; there is no need to constrict or tighten it around the penis. The feeling of space and porousness is necessary for the electromagnetic qualities to be activated. When both poles are physically restricted, the plus and minus cannot meet, mingle, and interact.

Many women carry a fear of having a loose vagina with a widened channel after giving birth, but this is a misconception, a result of the conventional picture of sex. I was horrified recently to hear from a gynecologist that it is not uncommon these days for a woman to choose cesarean section instead of natural vaginal birth even when a cesarean is not medically required. Women are trying to bypass vaginal birth in a misguided attempt to preserve their supposed vaginal integrity.

Having mentioned the no-no's of intentionally flexing the vagina during sex, exercise of the muscles of the pelvic floor and vagina outside of sex is *highly* recommended as a means of maintaining the tone and health of the genitals and even of encouraging deep relaxation, as related in the exercise at the end of chapter 6. Exercising consists of consciously contracting and relaxing the pelvic floor, as if you were trying to stop the urine flow. Consciously done, these exercises will encourage an awakening in the muscular walls of the vagina, which increases the general tone and chi. They should not be done mechanically or absently, as this just creates hardening and insensitivity.

Combining Movement and Relaxation

To incorporate relaxation into the enjoyment of physical movements is an art—and a great deal of fun. In chapter 6 we considered the fact that when a woman moves her pelvis backward and forward, the very efforts of doing so contract the vaginal environment, usually making it less sensitive and receptive. With each forward thrust the vagina contracts and effectively squeezes the man out in the very instant he is trying to get in. This gives little chance for the plus and minus poles to meet, correspond, and exchange energies. As your man is thrusting I advise that you not thrust back. Instead, angle and hold the pelvis still, in a receptive position, and focus intensely on receiving the penis into the vagina. Also, encourage your man to make the penetration very slow, because this enables the vagina to be more available to the incoming penis. The slowness definitely highlights the delicious sensations in the vagina. If you wish, penetration can be sustained without an immediate reverse movement. As suggested in chapter 6, the optimum is to have prolonged minutes in the depths of the vagina before your man withdraws his penis and penetrates afresh. In this way your man reaches to your most receptive part, your garden of love, where divine, orgasmic sensations are contacted.

Not to contradict any of the above suggestions, movements back and forth are by no means excluded from the range of choices for a woman. Movement with awareness raises a whole different quality of perception in the body. It is not what you do but how you do it that counts—almost anything you do with awareness is going to be great. It is the lack of awareness that causes the obstruction. The main guideline is to avoid mechanical movements, as these tend to compress the body's energy and are usually done without inner feeling. This is how the connection to the inner world can easily be lost.

As mentioned, when a woman deliberately squeezes the vagina to stimulate the penis into erection, her action is slightly misguided. Erection is easily lost or ejaculation encouraged. Some techniques are a bit more advanced, for example when the woman attempts a pumping action with the pelvic floor muscles to push energy upward in the body. The amazing thing is that

this kind of pumping action will in fact on occasion happen by itself. The body, given a chance to operate without our interference, does this from time to time. The body knows perfectly well how to respond with its own intelligence. (Perhaps the practice of conscious flexing of the pelvic-floor muscles originated as a mimicking of the body's response in the first place.)

While making love, sometimes just lifting the neck and head to meet the lips of the beloved is enough tension to introduce into the vagina, and this will increase sensitivity. Placing a pillow under the pelvis, as shown in the figures in chapter 6, is also excellent for creating an interesting tension in the vaginal cavity while keeping it receptive. Add these subtle tensions to kissing, and the interchange between the penis and vagina is wonderful.

Isolating and Relaxing the Vaginal Muscles while Moving

We can begin to think about movement in a few alternative ways. One way of moving is to change positions frequently without losing the contact between the penis and vagina. The penis-vagina unit is the central point around which all movements happen. (See figures 9.1 and 9.2 on the following pages for two sequences of positions that rotate around the penis and vagina.) When you want to move the pelvis, attempt to isolate the vaginal muscles and keep them relaxed and open while moving the pelvis itself. The pelvis is actually moved by a muscle in front of the spine (the iliopsoas), so when moving the pelvis, try to connect with that area behind the belly and in front of the spine. This is not so easy; it demands awareness. Check to see what other muscles are *not* needed for the movement (there are many, such as the buttocks, belly, and thighs), and be sure to use the muscles that *are* needed in a relaxed, slow, easy, conscious way. Slow movements guarantee awareness and increase sensuality. At times the two bodies will unexpectedly take off and move of their own accord in a rolling fashion as an outcome of the magnetic attraction and a circular movement of energy. Also, a whole range of reduced or smaller movements of the penis within the vagina are possible that do not result in much rubbing of the penis against the vaginal walls, and these are delightful to do any time or all the time.

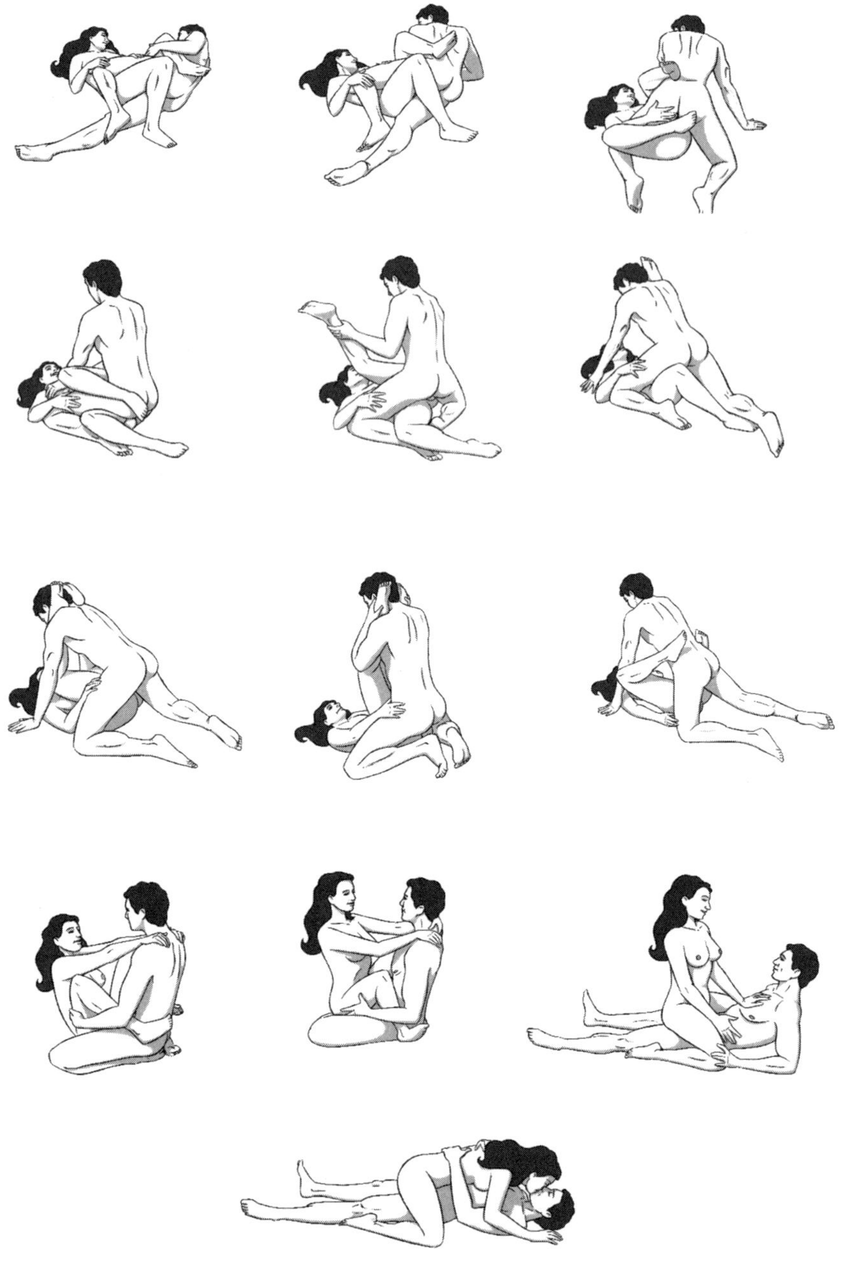

Fig. 9.1. Sequence of rotating positions through front

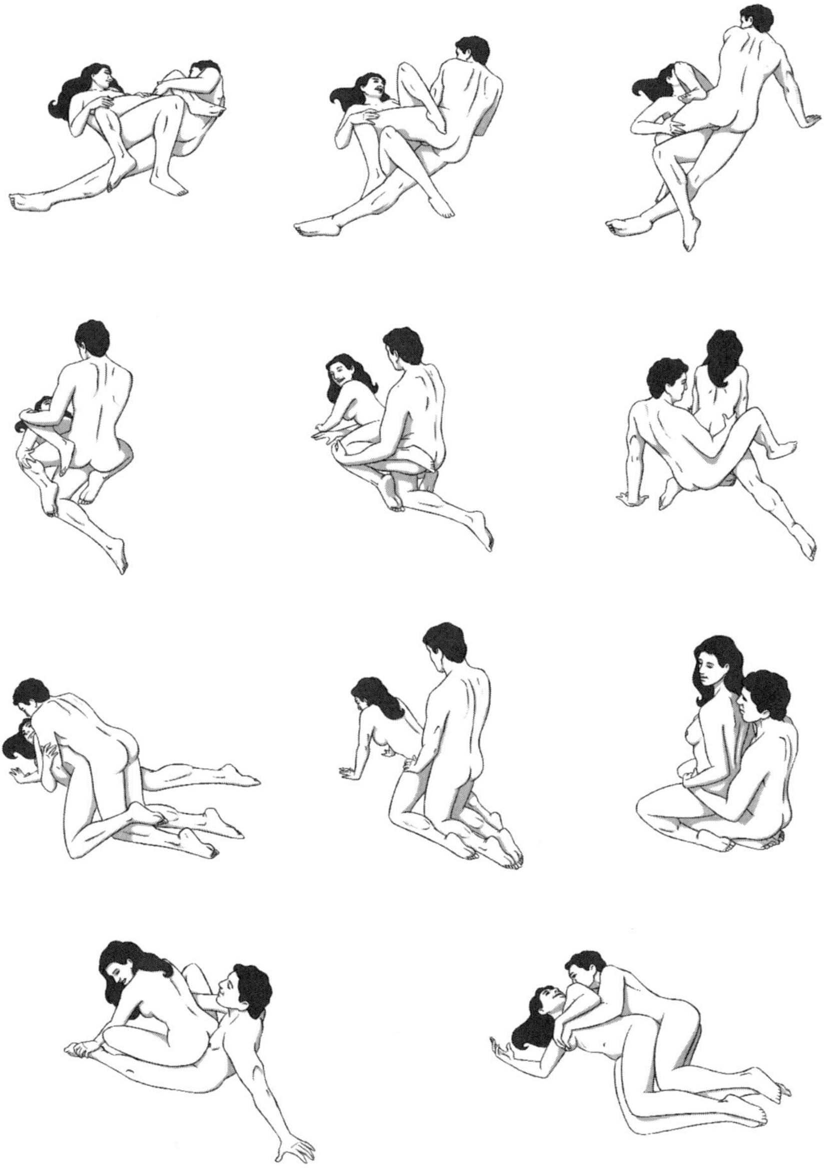

Figure 9.2 Sequence of rotating positions through rear

The essential thing to know is that tensions in general do not invite the deeper experience of orgasm, and can even work against it. In conventional sex there is a fair amount of activity and movement because we believe this is a prerequisite to sexual pleasure. But relaxation, not tension, is at the source of female orgasm as a prolonged, sustained state.

Using Breath, Words, Eyes, Lips

Relaxation hails the present moment, with nothing to do and nowhere to go. Lovers can greatly intensify the here and now in a few significant ways. They can use breath, words, eyes, kissing, and embracing all of the senses—each of these has an impact on the sexual exchange. Breath in itself is enough to lead to the orgasmic state. Breath keeps you in the present in your body, which is a good thing because you won't easily have an orgasm while you are in your mind thinking about something else. Breath helps you to merge with the body and become one with the source of life.

Ideally, breathing should be rhythmic, deep, and slow. Attempt to take the breath down into the belly; avoid taking it into the chest. Breathing through the nose is a more refined breath; however, breathing through the mouth is at times more comfortable or appropriate. Take the breath in the direction of the genitals to expand your sensitivity there.

You have probably noticed that, in practice, it can be extremely difficult to keep attention on the breath—especially while you are so involved with awareness on other levels. However, do return with awareness to your breath whenever it strikes you that you are not present to it. Consider your breath as a best friend that can help you out whenever you feel a bit less than alive and present. Breath always has a positive impact. If you are interested in pursuing the breath more deeply, it is helpful to create a balance between the length of the in breath and the length of the out breath. Count along with the exhale and the inhale for five or seven counts each way, or for whatever count suits you. With practice you will establish deep and regular breathing. Balancing the breath will also bring awareness to the moment between breaths, the *no breath*—a moment in which, floating ecstatically in the gap between the out breath and the next in breath, we glimpse eternal life. You can intensify the effects of the breath by using imagination too, which works wonders for some people. Imagine golden light streaming from the breasts on the out breath and golden light being drawn in through the vagina on the in breath.

Kissing brings a tremendous feeling of unity, in your own body and with your partner. When lovers' lips come together it is as if a circle has been completed, so the body sensations will intensify. Kissing helps a woman merge with her body. Kissing with the tongue penetrating the mouth easily leads to excitement, especially for a man, so it is a treat to be saved for rare occasions. But far more interesting than the tongue are the lips themselves. Keep your mouth closed and bring the lips together in a relaxed way. Infuse them with your awareness and then bring them into juicy contact with the lips of your partner, who with luck is doing the same thing with his lips. Make good, succulent contact, not a light and airy touch. Be as present as possible in your lips; imagine you are drinking from one another. I was touched in one workshop I led when a woman told me she and her husband had learned to kiss after twenty years of marriage. She was ecstatic about it—a new level of sensuality had opened up through the effects of truly kissing to her heart's content.

At times when you are not kissing, keep scanning with your awareness at the lips and mouth, because habitual tensions gather here very quickly. The habit is to pull the corners of the lips down. Experiment with this setting of the lips and pay attention to your mood; you will notice that you start to feel a bit miserable. Numerous people display this unconscious tension, especially women, because it is here that disappointment in life begins to reflect itself. To offset the drooping lip corners you can consciously raise your lip corners a few millimeters, into the tiniest hint of a smile. If you are observant you will notice an immediate sense of well-being: a contentment and a lightness rises up, lifting the face, and you may even experience the energy circling into the third eye area between the eyebrows.

Finally, speaking out loud what you are experiencing in your body is a way to amplify inner experiences immensely. Simply say what you feel and where you feel it. Start with the words "I feel . . ." and only talk about yourself, not your partner. The moment the words are spoken, your body will instantly respond with a spreading of the sensations already present. It is as if they answer to the acknowledgment with a kind of applause. We probably have all had the experience of putting a name to something and having a sense of ease follow. The same thing happens in making love. First, in communicating this way you are acknowledging your own body with your awareness. Second, sharing and speaking up has the benefit of informing your partner about what is going on for you. This in turn relaxes him because he doesn't have to guess. Through sharing in the sexual exchange, a man is able to learn from his woman what suits her and how it suits her.

"Sharing your now" means giving a short, concise report, a few words describing your inner experience. It does *not* mean having a long conversation about what is going on—on the contrary, the shorter the better. And you do not need a reply, although hearing your partner share *his* now in that moment, or any other, is wonderful. But if you turn a "sharing of now" into a conversation, you divert attention away from the intensity of the present moment, which leads to thinking and then, all too easily, to talking about old experiences that are not really relevant to the moment. The brief body reports help us keep track of what is happening moment by moment, without fantasy or imagination, past or future. Expressing tears or any feelings (again, simply) are also ways of sharing that increase body sensitivity.

A woman shares her experience: "Sharing so far has been the major key for me. From the beginning we shared anything that disturbed *the new*. As the sharing was mutual it helped me to drop all judgments and really share *everything*, which feels like a revolution. It makes me aware of the collective, and the depth of my conditioning—how much my ego, my self-worth is related to sex, to my pussy."

Communication is also greatly enhanced by the use of direct language; indeed, getting closer to one's own experience in sex, and that of your lover, requires the use of direct terms. For this reason I continually use the biological words *vagina* and *penis*. Often people will use more romantic or euphemistic words for the male and female genitals, like *yoni* and *lingam*, but this still keeps us in slight mystification and distance from ourselves. Experience has shown that it is helpful to communication to use the culturally accepted biological terms.

An event in a recent workshop in Europe may serve to illustrate this point. During the translation of my words from English into German, the translator (a man) twice used a crude but commonly accepted German slang word for the penis. On the third occasion of my using the word *penis*, I leaned over and whispered quietly to him, asking him please to use the actual German word for penis. It was difficult for him to do so the first time, and later a few times he made the same slip, quickly correcting himself.

On the final day of the group a man came up to me and said how important it had been for him that I had insisted that the translator used the word *penis*. He said that for him this marked the start of real communication with his wife. For the first time they were really able to talk about sex. Over the course of the workshop they became comfortable using a common and shared language, and so suddenly they could describe and share many small details, which before was impossible. When I shared this feedback with my partner, Raja, he said, "It's true, you know. You can say *penis* and *vagina* happily a hundred times over and over and it sounds fine, but for sure you can't keep saying *pussy* and *prick*. It just sounds wrong. Even *yoni* and *lingam* again and again is too hard." Unfortunately, many of the slang words associated with sex are degrading to women (and some are degrading to men as well). We would do well to slowly ease those kinds of words out of our daily expression.

The moment is also tremendously intensified if you allow a meeting of your eyes while making love. The eyes should be used in the way of soft vision as explained in the exercise at the end of chapter 2—no hard and fast staring, but a passive, receptive, inward vision. This inverting of the energy that is usually dispersed in actively looking allows that energy to fall back and flow onto the heart, opening it. Closing your eyes is also fine—it enables you to sense more deeply into yourself in certain moments—but keep them open as much as you can. The eye contact helps enormously in releasing old patterns of self-consciousness, being embarrassed by sex and the like. At first it

can be challenging to be confronted by our limitations, but usually some tears or laughter, even a shiver or a shake, will do the trick and burn up our sexual confusions.

Women Sharing Experiences

"It is beautiful to keep eye connection. It makes it easier for my body and vagina to receive my partner. I experience energy moving from my eyes to my heart and from my vagina to my heart. I feel very good, very happy."

"I was a bit apprehensive about the eye contact as I have been used to keeping my eyes closed a lot of the time—but actually I liked the space it brought me to. It definitely added another loving flavor to the flow with my partner."

"I realize the importance of being *inside* first, centered in oneself before connecting, and then *staying inside* while connecting—the more the better. It's also important for me that I do not feel my partner 'coming out,' becoming disconnected to his own center. Then his desire can feel like a demand, a wanting. Feeling connected this way is a delicate space to get to. It requires practice when we are not so used to it."

"Something exquisite is happening for me. I often feel, as I look in my partner's eyes while we make love, that I am looking in the eyes of a Buddha. I thought such an unconditional love could only exist between me and my Master. Now it is right here."

"I find more peace in me. I discover my female side more and more. I feel this quiet happiness. I feel there is a healing process occurring on many levels. Old patterns come up once in a while, but as long as we stay open about them I can deal with them. The awareness of the eyes receiving images instead of looking outward helps so much to relax us. The energy is so different. We have not experimented so much with different positions yet, but we did experiment with small changes in one or two positions. It

is amazing how a small change in a position or a small change in the movement can change the energy so much. How or where my lover is touching me is changing my own energy flow."

"We are very well, feeling happy and fulfilled, our love warm, tender, and wonderful. We're having fun experiencing more and more about lovemaking. For me it's mainly experiencing the expanding orgasmic waves up to my solar plexus/heart area, which feels so ecstatic when it happens. It's also great to feel that it doesn't matter if it doesn't happen because I can experiment again next time and again and again. It's a wonderful release to experience that lovemaking has become an important part of our lives and has gained so much priority. This helps me a lot to relax and just be with whatever happens. My man is still ejaculating often, but we stay together for a long time before he does. I am really improving being in the here and now and enjoying what is instead of looking for something else to happen. Sometimes, in lovemaking, it's like unseen doors are opening up, giving me deepest insight into questions I might have about life or death. It's like getting flashes of stunning clarity—comparable to experiences I've had in deep meditation. So it is wonderful, and I am very happy."

"I must tell you my wonderful progress. I have had my first truly wonderful orgasm with my man's penis in my vagina . . . with no pain! This has so far been unachievable in our twenty-three-year relationship! I still cannot believe how much has changed for us. We will keep going this way because it works—it is a healing process. It can change everything in the way we perceive ourselves and it makes us conscious in making love."

Letting Go of Tensions, Masks, Protections, Efforts, and Projections

As you can see, when moving into relaxation and opening up to the moment, the outcome is a great deal *less* tension and the dropping of

masks, protections, efforts, and projections. What you gain is vitality, a physical porousness, and a psychological openness that expands the energy body. Orgasm always requires openness, so the tiniest bit of relaxation on any level, however achieved, is a good thing. As we know by now, relaxation is basic to orgasm, even a conventional orgasm. The orgasmic state tends to follow upon being more natural, dropping parts of our artificial, social selves. A woman often thinks that she is required to be open to a man before she even shows herself or can relax in sex or explore sex. But this is a misunderstanding. When people are open they are open *to themselves* first of all. By virtue of *their being* open, they open up to another person. So opening to ourselves comes first and foremost, and as we open up we become aware of the many unconscious tensions in the body: where and how we hold ourselves so tight. Many women's bodies are extremely hard to the touch, with contours that are not at all feminine. Tensions act as a subtle form of protection and defense against vulnerability. We fear an unloving reaction, based on previous experience. Even though these reactions may be absolutely valid in their own way, reimagining yourself, perceiving yourself from another angle, and opening into your femininity all require a vulnerability and healing of past wounds that is liberating and revitalizing.

A woman shares her experience: "I begin to love being present more and more, just as a means unto itself. I notice over and over again that I actually feel more satisfied after two hours of soft penetration than after a so-called fuck. Today I felt very horny twice and then realized I did not feel anything in my vagina; the source was absolutely in the mind. When the wanting comes, a key for me is to bring the energy back to the source of the wanting, and I am again flooded with energy."

To explore unknown territory always requires courage, but the rewards are huge. We step away from our inherited ideas to discover that simple relaxation is quite thrilling. It takes us far beyond the enjoyment of sexual pleasure by providing the possibility of sexual ecstasy.

The Difference between Lust and Passion

In doing research on sexuality I have found precious gems of insight along the way. One comes from Barry Long, the Australian spiritual and tantric master who has made an immeasurable contribution to returning men and women to their true, loving, sexual selves.* While he does not incorporate some of the polarity insights that are basic to the ancient tantric teachings (for example, he ignores the breasts), Long does give women a tremendous amount of support and inspiration. His specific guidance in sex is that a woman should remain very still and very present. And he uses the beautiful phrase "passionately undemonstrative" to describe the state to which women should aspire. At first glance these two words appear to be opposing, and an inevitable question pops up—how on earth can passion be undemonstrative? To us it may seem that passion is demonstration itself—the ultimate demonstration.

To understand fully what Barry Long is suggesting, we need to clear up our confusion about lust and passion and what these two states represent. Interestingly, Long says that "passion is pure presence." In conventional sex, when we are not present because of our interest in orgasm, most of us experience lust and mistakenly think it is passion. In reality, lust is linked to stimulation and excitement and somehow being out of control. Lust almost always has a direction and an end point. In contrast, passion is the experiencing of the intensity of the moment with inner stillness—not necessarily without movement! A highly passionate state can be stepped out of at any time in case of emergency (to take an important call, for example) without any "ruffling of feathers." But lust that is not completely satisfied will leave you frustrated and upset, more like a bird that just got all its feathers wet. Passion is not necessarily active or outgoing; it is a state of being in which every cell in the body is vibrant, flowering with life. When a woman becomes passionate she falls into alignment with her

---

*More than twenty years ago, Barry Long produced two audiotapes entitled *Making Love*. The revolutionary content on man and woman and sexual love has made a lasting impression on me and substantially furthered my personal journey toward demystifying sex.

inner body polarity, becoming utterly present in every cell, exuding an invitation but taking no direct action. This is the state of being passionately undemonstrative. In this state, a man is able to truly respond as man. When a woman is able to get herself into some semblance of inner "order," then a man can stop running around in sexual circles like a dog chasing its own tail. When a man experiences his energy being received by a woman, moving through his woman and thus through himself, his life is changed, something deep falls into place. He has been waiting for that moment all of his life.

While heeding and exploring Barry Long's insight, Osho says, "be wild, but do not become unconscious."[1] Notice that Osho's words warn against unconsciousness but certainly not against wildness. Wildness in this sense means a state of passionate wildness, not lustful wildness as we commonly experience it. He says that in that state, wildness is beautiful and there is nothing wrong in it; because the more wild, the more alive. "Then you are just like a wild tiger or a wild deer running in the forest . . . and the beauty of it!"

The Solar Plexus and the Third Eye

True passion arises in a woman through the solar plexus being open and free of hindering tensions. The solar plexus is a tremendous source of the love force and of genuine spontaneity. For this reason it is a highly significant area to become attuned to, connect with internally, and hold in your awareness while making love. For many people the power of this third energy center is blocked, through tensions from controlling, struggling with others, and suppressing feelings. (The negative effects of these will be covered in more depth in chapter 10.)

In much the same way, the third eye—the sixth energy center, situated between the eyebrows—has power in influencing the sexual energy to rise, although for women it should not be a point of extreme focus, especially in the initial phase of exploration. Far more important for woman is the connection to the breasts, the expansion at the heart center. From here the third eye (so called because its tissues resemble the retina of the real eyes) will open as a by-product. With the third eye activated, a woman becomes a visionary and a source of true wisdom. In the awareness and sensitivity exercise at the end of the chapter are tips on how to connect internally with the solar plexus and third eye. These techniques can also be used while making love, amplifying a woman's internal experience.

Ecstasy Is Cool, Not Hot

For a woman with an inner openness to herself, sex becomes a cool experience, even if it can get wild at times. Our ideas inherited from conventional sex leave us with the imprint that ecstasy is a hot, steamy, and overwhelming affair. But in reality, bliss and ecstasy engender the ultimate experience of coolness.

It is important to grasp that the word *cool* does not mean cold, with its negative connotations. *Coolness* is the experience of being rooted in yourself first and foremost. Eternal bliss is sometimes described by the enlightened ones as being cool as the eternal snow on the Himalayas. Certainly every blissful person I ever met was never hot and excited and jumping up and down all the time, but instead was wonderfully serene, inwardly composed, and simultaneously passionate and alive. To reach such a state of blissful passion might seem light years away; but any journey can start with a few tentative steps. The key is to relax into oneself first. This naturally places woman in a more passive role, where she *responds* according to the polarity and does not *react* according to the personality. Being passionately undemonstrative produces a dynamic, attractive force that draws man toward you as you repose in body and being.

As we have come to realize, for orgasm to unfold and flower into a meaningful experience, a woman needs *time*—for preparation, for opening up—before the actual sexual exchange begins to appeal to her. The female body requires loving foreplay, with prolonged kissing of the lips, sensitive and featherlight caressing, and touching advances to awaken her yearning to make love. Real clock time is required, though when an

orgasmic state arises one moves into an experience of complete timelessness. Five minutes can feel like five hours, and vice versa. The minimum time for lovemaking should be about forty-five minutes to an hour, and of course two to three hours is even better. Once in a while, take a whole day in bed, making love again and again and again.

In general, people think about sex more than they actually have it. When they eventually get around to it, it's over in a few short minutes. Many a woman perceives herself as frigid because she cannot open up so quickly to a man (and because some man has told her she is so). This is not frigidity. This is a natural reluctance to enter the sex act the way it is commonly done these days—as just another task in a busy day, without adequate preparation. If given sufficient time, women *love* to make love—especially when warmed up to a full-body *yes*.

In foreplay, much depends too on the intention and awareness of the *giver* of the touch or the kisser of the breasts, lips, and nipples. The intention prowling behind the scene can be to excite and make horny and lustful. The opposite intention would be to love, to innocently say a sweet hello, to awaken from slumber. The role of foreplay is to energetically raise the octave in woman; however, when a man's intentions are loving, raising the woman's sexual temperature is *not* always an absolute necessity. You might embrace and caress for hours, or you might just "plug in" with soft penetration as explained in chapter 8. When lovers take the serene approach to sex and the man offers the famous "cool hand" to his woman, she will start to really turn on, perhaps even to her own surprise. As the woman melts into her female positive pole at the breasts, the man can focus on his own positive pole, in the perineum, central to the pelvic floor, rather than in the head of the penis itself. The energy then rises upward by itself. You do not have to concern yourself with the ascending energy: it happens without you. Your focus is in retaining the energy, not letting it leak out. A leaking pool has to be sealed before it can fill up. Both of you can relax, floating in that filling pool. Stay with it. Don't be tempted to pursue some avenues of excitement that send you racing off to the end.

Make a Date to Make Love

When you notice that there is a shortage of intimacy in your life, when daily commitments get in the way of your love life, when lovemaking ceases to flow spontaneously, then you need to intentionally make a date with your partner. Make special appointments to meet and dedicate your time entirely to making love—just like you make an appointment to meet a friend for dinner, or go to a party or to a business meeting.

This may sound a bit unromantic but it works extremely well. Each person comes prepared to make love, and it ceases to be an accidental happening. In time your lovemaking feels similar to two instruments tuning to one another, to create a beautiful piece of music. Bodies are indeed like musical instruments in that orgasmic states are created through fine-tuning and sensitivity. Mastering a musical instrument requires tremendous dedication and practice; in the same way, it requires lots of practice in making love to create ecstatic experiences until one gets the real hang of it. A musical maestro has to practice daily; if he doesn't he soon notices it, and within a few days his audience notices it. The more you make love, the finer your experiences become.

Tantric "quickies" are very much the order of the day when there is not adequate time to arrange a love meeting. Or, when it is late at night and you're a bit tired, plugging in for ten or fifteen minutes with soft penetration before sleep is a wonderful way to end the day. It transforms the rest of your day when you plug in before going to work in the morning. The beauty of the tantric approach to sex is that you don't need heaps of energy to make love; neither do you have to feel horny or sexually charged—you don't go that long without making love. Instead, you begin to have sex as a matter of course, just as you have dinner and breakfast. Love is essential food. There is no need to wait around for lust to overtake you. Many women begin to feel the failure of lust in their lives as they get older and think that their sexuality is failing them. They don't yet recognize that excitement cannot last forever and that coolness and relaxation can take its place. It's pointless to long for or look for the former signs of the strong, fierce sexuality you experienced when you were younger. You do not even

have to really "feel like" making love; if you go ahead and open yourself and your body to love, in so doing you will receive endless love.

More Women Sharing Their Experiences

"Something new occurred in making love. It happened to me twice in the last weeks. When we were together, with very little and slow movements, orgasm came, and it felt completely different from the orgasm that I knew before. I ask myself if it is vaginal orgasm and if it is the orgasm that comes by itself when the body likes to orgasm? It was very soft, nonexciting, quiet. Afterward I felt filled up with new energy."

"Lovemaking has started happening, really in the sense of generating love. Also, my pleasure and my physical sensations are very strong. I am aware of this border between voluptuous space and sexuality—any small 'breaking of the rules' immediately brings a different space, and changes the union experienced before."

"I was totally in my mind and thinking during lovemaking in the afternoon. I felt that my husband was moving too slowly because I was wishing for the old release, but after a while my usual approach did not work—my husband tried it but suddenly I realized that I did not want it.

Then I told him my feelings, that I did not want to continue looking for an orgasm, and told him that I wanted to now go inside, so I closed my eyes and did so. All this time we were in penetration. When I came back we looked in each other's eyes and for a few minutes he slowly, slowly moved his penis inside me. I had an explosion of energy, in the vagina first and then very soon after that in the head. It was another dimension of energy. I think it was an orgasm, but not of a sexual quality—it was one from another world. I cried intensely and then I was laughing. At first my husband was confused and then we were totally together."

"We decided to sit in silence for a few minutes after making love, and that was great—the energy turned in again and I felt very silent and centered."

"My *aha!* of the day was when I realized that 'presence' in itself brings a feeling of total well-being, even ecstasy, even though 'nothing' happened, even though there was tension and an intense burning in my vagina, even though my partner was freaked out. So nothing was perfect. Still, I experienced such a feeling of being present. The eye contact, the breathing, the awareness of my vagina, of the birds outside, of the river. Everything became perfect with my acceptance."

"In my relationship we've both always wanted to move somewhere else with our lovemaking, but we didn't know how. There's a part that's delighted and another part that is scared, but we both don't want to turn around and go back to the old. It is very beautiful and very fragile."

"The more I relax inside the more I encounter a sudden feeling of lovingness—it comes and goes and has nothing to do with personal/psychological stuff—it is not emotion. It has nothing to do with me."

"This is the first time I've touched that part of my body. . . . I can feel my pelvic floor, my ovaries, my uterus from the inside—there is so much more space."

"We are having a very good time. After meeting with you I started to understand lovemaking on a deeper level. There was much more relaxation and I was no longer waiting for 'ecstatic energy things.' I started to see making love as another form of meditation, relaxation, and regeneration, not as a means for having 'super sex.' Now we enjoy all kinds of sex as it is expressing itself right in the very moment."

"We are well and happily making love. Our lives are going in different directions in one way, as my work is so different from my partner's and I am away a lot. However, having our regular dates for lovemaking, which we give just as much priority as anything else, it doesn't seem to matter. It is a rhythm of being apart and being together that feels very good, and it is a great experience for me. My man tells me that it is great for him too. This being together in love makes such a lot of difference! It leaves so much

room for other things that we don't share without making us feel we are drifting apart.

"Lovemaking sometimes seems to me like it is about experiencing the full range of living life. It's the process of unlearning so much, of just being and experiencing whatever is happening at this very moment. It is so interesting to observe what happens when I am in my mind, entertaining concepts about how things should be or should not be versus when I am just fully present to whatever there is, loving every moment of it. Lovemaking like this is like a life school for me, and I am learning a lot by shifting my focus from 'shoulds' or 'should nots' to paths of fun and ecstasy. This has a strong effect on my work and on my whole life, which in return enhances the quality of our lovemaking. So it's just great."

"Even though in my mind I knew already that I did not have to please my man, I noticed that wanting to please still came up at times as a subtle pressure in my body. It showed itself in slight tension and a loss of energy sensations, and after some time even in not being interested in sex at all. This brought me into a deep insecurity and the feeling of being dysfunctional. For me it has been very important to have support from other women who have already been through these issues, which encouraged me to find my own truth—maybe it is even better to say 'to trust the truth of my body.' When I began to see the start of lovemaking as a soft, relaxed, and curious search for the entrance into a delicious and beautiful love garden instead of an effort to 'come into my energy,' things changed. It was no longer my responsibility to find my sexual energy to make my beloved happy. It became more like a journey together through a labyrinth, and the guide is my body. Both of us—my beloved and I—don't know where the entrance is today, because there is no recipe and it can be somewhere else every day, the way in can be new every time.

"Sometimes we find the way in, sometimes not. But if not, it is no longer my 'fault' for not being sexual enough. There is mystery to finding the 'magic word' to open the door. And to find this entrance it becomes totally important to listen to every little sign the body gives—to feel whether any touch or movement or even any thought is opening me up or closing me

down and to dare to share this with my beloved, sometimes with words and sometimes with body language. It is beautiful if the man is able to surrender and let himself be taken by 'the hand' of the woman's body, so that the woman's body is allowed to be the guide for both. But if this is not possible for him, or if he is disappointed, I think it is important for the woman to go on trusting her own body and not to compromise. For me this way of lovemaking is still not easy all the time, but I definitely feel it is the right way for me."

The Role of Relaxation

Not to be underestimated, relaxation is pivotal in woman's searching for satisfying orgasm. It is the real experience of sensuality as consciousness begins filtering through the body. The energy usually *ex*pressed turns inward and becomes *im*pressed. It sinks into the body, into oneness with the senses. Touch, sound, breath, eyes, hair, silky skin—all of these speak to us when we are relaxed enough to listen.

When a woman relaxes into herself, the adventure for a man is as momentous. A man needs only a couple of experiences to confirm how naturally the male energy responds to the presence of a complementary passivity—the sheer delight to be found in being welcomed, received, absorbed, and expanded through woman. Mistakenly, man has helped to make woman more male through his insistence on excitement. Yet ironically, man's sex obsession is a search for this very dynamic experience where his energy simply moves through him, drawn by an equal and opposite force—and both are fulfilled.

If you are single and without a regular partner with whom to make love, experimenting is more difficult—but not impossible. While you are making love, even if it is the first time with a new partner, just try a key practice. It might be bringing awareness to your positive pole, or slowing down. Or you may like to look into his eyes. How does he respond? It is very interesting to see what happens! If you continue to meet again to make love it is good if you can explain to the person that you are interested in experimenting with making love. Tell him a bit about how you feel and

what you would like to experience. Again, it does help if you are on the same wavelength. Sometimes it simply doesn't work to talk about it—perhaps you don't even speak a common language, in which case just try relaxing into sex, experimenting on your own. Notice what works. Notice what happens. Keep bringing in awareness.

Tantric Inspiration

Many people would like to relax, but they cannot relax. Relaxation is like a flowering: you cannot force it. You have to understand the whole phenomenon—why you are active so much, why so much occupation with activity, why you are obsessed with it.

Remember two words: One is "action" and the other is "activity." Action is not activity, activity is not action. Their natures are diametrically opposite. Action is when the situation demands it, you act, you respond. Activity is when the situation doesn't matter, it is not a response; you are so restless within that the situation is just an excuse to be active.

Action comes out of a silent mind—it is the most beautiful thing in the world. Activity comes out of a restless mind—it is the ugliest. Action is when it has relevance, activity is irrelevant. Action is moment to moment, spontaneous. Activity is loaded with the past. It is not a response to the present moment, rather, it is pouring your restlessness, which you have been carrying from the past into the present. Action is creative. Activity is very destructive, it destroys you and it destroys others. . . .

Remember, activity is goal oriented, action is not. Action is an overflowing of energy; action is in this moment, a response, unprepared, unrehearsed. The whole existence meets you, confronts you, and a response simply comes. The birds are singing and suddenly you start singing—it is not activity. Suddenly it happens. Suddenly you find it is happening, that you have started humming—this is action.

OSHO, TRANSCRIBED TEACHINGS,
TANTRA: THE SUPREME UNDERSTANDING

Awareness and Sensitivity Exercise
Activating the Microcosmic Orbit

Give yourself half an hour or more for this exploration. You can do this exercise sitting upright in a chair with a straight spine and both feet on the floor.

Close your eyes and tune in to two energy channels, or meridians: one running up the back of the body and the other down the front of the body. The channel at the back begins at the perineum, between the anus and the vagina, and runs up the sacrum and low back, up the spine, over the top of the head, to the roof of the mouth. The channel at the front runs from the tongue down the throat, heart, solar plexus, and navel, to the perineum. When these two main channels are open, the energy will circle automatically in a loop that Mantak Chia calls the *microcosmic orbit*.[2]

The tongue is the bridge that connects the yang male energy channel along the back to the yin female energy channel along the front. Place the tongue on the soft palate at a point toward the rear of the mouth cavity, about one and a half inches behind the teeth. It is a slight stretch for the tongue. (Closer toward the teeth is okay too, if the suggested tongue position is not comfortable.) By completing this route you get the yin and yang harmonizing, enabling you to increase the energy flow and vitality throughout your body. The direction of energy flow can also be reversed—moving up the front and down the back.

To awaken the energy at individual points along the way, use your inner vision. Attempt to sink your mind into your body, to the point you wish to activate, and soon you will feel warmth or energy or chi beginning to flow there. Each person will experience this energy activation differently; just stay attuned to your sensations in the body. The best place to start the circle is by focusing deep into the navel, and from there flow downward to a point just above the pubic bone (a point corresponding to the ovaries), then to the perineum, the coccyx, the lower back (on the same level as the navel), the mid back (on the same level as the solar plexus), behind the back of the neck just where it joins the head, the crown of the head, the point between the eyebrows, the tongue/palate, the heart, the solar plexus, and returning finally to the navel. Concentrate on the energy points and circling the energy; it is not necessary to focus on the breathing.

When you are finished, always complete the circle at your navel center and store energy there. To store energy, place your right fist on your navel and concentrate your attention there. Rotate your fist counterclockwise thirty-six times in an increasingly large circle, then reverse the direction, rotating clockwise twenty-four times while shrinking the circle back to the navel. Allow a little smile at the lip corners during the whole exercise, and notice the feelings of harmony and love. Rest for five to ten minutes after finishing.

After you get the feeling of this circle, you may hook up with it any time you are making love, to great effect. It is especially nice in yab yum, where you are in a sitting position and in line with Earth's gravitational field.

Awareness and Sensitivity Exercise
The Solar Plexus and the Third Eye

While you are making love—or any time, as a matter of fact—it is possible to intensify the focus on the solar plexus area by looking down to the point of your nose, which will give the sensation of the eyes crossing. Holding this eye position for a few moments enables you to sense into the solar plexus very deeply.

To help activate the third eye, between the eyebrows, almost close the eyelids and then start flickering them up and down very quickly *while at the same time* looking upward, directing your eyes toward the center of your forehead. Again there will be the sensation of the eyes crossing. Gradually look back as far as you can without strain. After a few attempts at this you will begin to get the sensation of something locking or converging in the area between the eyebrows. Close your eyes and continue to hold awareness at the third eye—the sensations at this energy point will be greatly intensified. You may only be able to do this for a few short seconds at first, but that is a good start.

Try these two practices on your own first before trying them during lovemaking. You can actually do them in sequence, looking down to the solar plexus, then looking up to the third eye a few minutes later, then down again and up again three or four times.

Circling energy through the microcosmic orbit, or lifting the lip corners into an inner smile, or simply placing the tongue on the soft palate, or connecting with the solar plexus or the third eye—the stimulation of all or any of these energy phenomena even just for a few seconds will have an impact on the sexual experience, and can be utilized at will during lovemaking.

Partner Exchange Exercise
Let Lovemaking Come by Itself

Before you move into love, sit silently together for fifteen minutes holding each other's hands crosswise. Sit in darkness or very dim light and feel each other. Get in tune with each other by breathing together: when your man exhales, you exhale; when he inhales, you inhale. Within a few minutes you will get into it. Breathe as if you are one organism—not two bodies but one. And look into each other's eyes with soft vision.

After fifteen minutes, take time to enjoy each other and play with each other's bodies. Don't move into love unless the moment arises by itself—not that you make love but suddenly you find yourself making love. Wait for this—do not force it. Go to sleep—there's no need to make love. Wait for the moment to arise even if you wait two or three days. It will come, and when it does love will go very deep. It will be a silent, oceanic feeling. Love is something that has to be engaged in like a meditation. It is something that has to be cherished, tasted very slowly so it suffuses deeply into your being. It becomes such a possessing experience—as if you are there no more. It is not that you are making love—you *are* love. Love becomes a bigger energy around you; it goes beyond you both.

10
Mastering Love and Overcoming Emotions

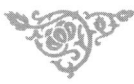

What is love? Love is the fragrance, the radiance of knowing oneself, of being oneself. . . . Love is overflowing joy. Love is when you have seen who you are; and then there is nothing left except to share your being with others. Love is when you have seen that you are not separate from existence. Love is when you have felt an organic orgasmic unity with all that is. Love is not a relationship. Love is a state of being. It has nothing to do with anybody else. One is not in love, one is *love. And of course when one* is *love, one* is *in love—but that is an outcome, a by-product, that is not the source. The source is that one is love.*

OSHO, TRANSCRIBED TEACHINGS, THE GUEST

As we now know, tantra sees human energy in terms of polarity: feminine energy as "being" and masculine energy as "doing." Within woman, the inner masculine is active, logical, and result-oriented; while in man the inner feminine is receptive, intuitive, and process-oriented. Tantra takes a step further to say that the highest spiritual polarity in existence is love and meditation, that woman embodies love and man embodies meditation. This implies that woman's inner man is meditative and man's inner woman is

loving. To be whole human beings, operating with wisdom, passion, authenticity, and spontaneity, we need to master both energies: masculine and feminine, meditation and love. Woman gets more meditative the more she loves and man gets more loving the more he meditates. In more precise sexual language, to love in woman means to welcome the penis in and surrender to its power. And to meditate in man means to merge with and become utterly present in his penis, inside woman, in stillness.

Distinguishing between Emotions and Feelings

Yet for too many of us, deep personal and societal wounding through sex prevents us from balancing our energies in a way that serves us. We repress the memories of our hurts, suppress our real feelings and energies, and then unconsciously begin to control or manipulate others or fail to channel our energies in a wise or creative direction. As we change the way we make love, we initiate an alchemical process of awakening the inner opposite polarity within, which in time enables us to use both energies powerfully and productively. This, in turn, helps us to dissolve the emotional patterns that have caused us pain in the past and to create the life and love we deeply desire in the present.

To create the life of sustained loving harmony that so many women desire, an important step to take is to keep emotion out of love. As Osho says, "love is a state of being," and "one is not *in* love, one *is* love . . . it has nothing to do with anybody else." With the new input about harnessing polarity and female orgasmic potential, you might be able to conceive of a day (or at least a few hours at a time, a few days of the week) of *being* love as a state that is sustained and not associated with the highs and lows of relationships. But these highs, and the painful and difficult lows filled with emotions, where love becomes scrambled up with irreconcilable feelings and fears: what is all this about? Despair or resignation can set in when a couple can see no way out of the cycle of conflicts.

Regaining female power is dependent upon knowing the difference between feelings and emotions, and knowing that "love has to be separated from this category of emotions." (See the tantric inspiration at the end of

this chapter.) The crucial understanding here is that emotion comes from the *past*, while love and true feelings arise in the *present*. When too much past stuff gets dragged into everyday life, love is quick to wane. Love has its tendrils in the delicacy of the now. That doesn't mean that you should think of emotion as some kind of demon. Emotion itself is fine; what is important is that you are *aware* that you are emotional, that you know what is happening when it is happening. This understanding changes everything.

Symptoms of Emotion

Until now we have had no frame of reference to understand what is truly going on in the split second when emotions surface, the instant when, out of the blue, the love boat begins to rock dangerously. What we need is self-awareness. The immediate physical symptoms of emotion can be described variously as "suddenly feeling paralyzed," or as if "a wall suddenly comes down," or as a moment when it is impossible look the other in the eyes, or having the awkward sensation of feeling disconnected from everything, utterly separate, lonely, totally misunderstood, physically collapsed. Often we find ourselves full of vengefulness and wanting to hurt back. We start blaming our partner for the situation, using the accusing words "You never . . ." or "You always. . . ." Or, alternatively, a jumble of feelings tumble around inside that are impossible to find words for. When one of these types of "emotional attacks" takes place, we must recognize that emotion is in play. It takes some practice to recognize emotion, but after a while it does become obvious.

This inner acknowledgment immediately puts things more into perspective. Emotion is, in reality, the resurfacing of an accumulation of old feelings, repressed feelings, feelings that had to be swallowed, that we did not dare to show or express *at the time* when the feeling was actually taking place—in a previous present, during some unhappy incident many years ago. This is why so often emotional reactions are quite disproportionate to the slight comment or mild action that triggers the emotion. The trigger itself does not usually warrant the huge upset that follows in its wake. What is really happening is that old, unexpressed feelings begin

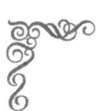

to resonate and bubble up inside and create confusion. When you acknowledge these old feelings for what they are and work their negative effects out of your system, emotional reactions will begin to cease. In a few years your partner can say precisely the same words to you, and nothing happens—the comment slips by you like water off a duck's back.

Using Love to Overcome Fears Created by Lack of Love

As women we carry many emotions, which means we are loaded with layers of unexpressed feelings. The source of unhappiness is most usually due to a lack of love, perhaps to abusive and hurtful sexual experiences of the past, where there was a total absence of respect and love. Even if a woman has not been intentionally abused, the current style of aggressive, insensitive sex can be acknowledged by a woman's body as a subtle form of abuse. This implies that basically all of us are emotional about the lack of love, not only in the past but perhaps even now. Deep fears are instilled by the unloving treatment that negatively affects a woman's capacity to love and be loved. Fear demands the need for protection and defense, so it is with good survival reasoning that woman protects herself from man.

However, to heal the existing situation and bring it back into balance (within us and between us) there is only one option open—if lack of love instilled fear, love is the direct method to dissolve the fear and thereby end the patterns of emotionality. A woman must trust her nature and allow herself to be loved by a man and open up to him (provided he is willing to be conscious in the tantric way), which means dropping the defenses, games, and emotions that form our personality but have nothing to do with the vulnerable sensitivity of our true selves.

The truth is, from our earliest years we have been developing feelings of being separate, of being wrong, of being unworthy, of not being good enough. We, who were manifested on earth as an expression of unhindered energy, become separate from ourselves, from each other, and from the whole of existence. As we cut off from our pure energy we also cut off from our *love source,* and gradually a false self develops around us as fear replaces

security and joy. The fear is due to imprints made by an absence of love in the immediate surroundings (family and parents), and the fear provokes a child into acting differently in order to try to get approval (or disapproval, through rebellion, where at least some attention is gained) in order to gain the love so necessary for survival. And so our parents begin to write the script for us, for who we are and how we should behave, and we gradually lose our authenticity.

Emotionality is an unconscious, automatic reaction to a situation or circumstance, like when a switch is flicked off and light turns to dark. It can even be a learned habit: some women learned to be emotional as young girls by mimicking their mother's behavior. As the years go by, we as women begin to define ourselves according to our emotions, our little and big ups and downs, thinking this is who we really are. It is as if we are in a movie and the situation is not actually real. Only the past makes it real. (If we were to wake up one morning without our memory, with no past, what then?) But in spirit and essence we are all love, and to keep love alive love has to be separated from the backlog of stored emotions we are not so aware of. As we begin to release these old feelings consciously (whenever we notice they arise) they cease to hold our energy down.

The Solar Plexus and Emotion

In addition to the emotional alarm signals, like suddenly feeling paralyzed or disconnected, you can learn to recognize states of emotionality in the solar plexus. Consider this area as a sensor for recognizing emotion, because this is where emotions will gather and create a lot of discomfort. Emotions try to seek discharge in various ways—through irritation, complaining, nagging, passing on your frustration to the children. When you develop awareness of the solar plexus, the moment someone says something that strikes an uncomfortable chord in you, you will notice something going on there telling you that you are emotional, that something unresolved is being triggered. For woman it is good to have the solar plexus free of tensions to allow for unobstructed flow of sexual energy between the breasts and the vagina.

Many women will feel nauseous when first relaxing into lovemaking, but this is nothing to be concerned about. It is a sure sign of the surfacing of old feelings asking for release. Nausea is a by-product of the sexual energy expanding and pushing the restricting emotions out of the body. An ancient tantric technique is to drink a large amount of salt water and put a finger down the throat to open the solar plexus and keep it open. Even the vomit reflex alone, without any discharge, works wonders in releasing tensions of the solar plexus. There is an immediate feeling of expansion, as if something toxic has left you.

Verbalize Emotion, Separate, and Physically Move the Body

The very moment that you recognize that you are emotional, through the solar plexus or in whatever other way you recognize it, the first step is to inwardly acknowledge that you are emotional. The second step is to say it out loud to your partner. "I am emotional." This verbalization instantly brings a touch of relaxation, because at least now your partner knows that *you* know that *you* are emotional, which takes him out of the picture and no longer makes him responsible for your unhappiness. It is a difficult step to take, to admit you are emotional by actually saying so, because the ego will be fighting like crazy trying to blame the other. But in reality, until you take yourself back to yourself and acknowledge the past, your love life will remain a series of good times followed by bad times.

In such circumstances, having said the words "I am emotional now" to your partner as gracefully as possible, physically leave the room, adding the words "I need some time to myself and will return soon." Close the door gently and go outside or to another room in the house and take some time alone. (Do not drive off and feign that you are abandoning the relationship in that moment.) This is not switch-off time, but the time to switch on and release or get in touch with these old feelings residing in your system. In fact, when emotions get activated they move through a layer of connective tissue in the body called fascia. This explains why sometimes at the onset of an emotional attack you will feel that onset in your body very clearly, almost as

if a substance with density is swirling through the body. (Indeed, fascia does weave dimensionally through the body and from head to toe about five times, connecting the superficial layers with the deepest physical layers.)

Now, to get rid of these emotions you need to help them out of the body where they are stored. It is essential to physically move your body so that the old feelings can be burned up. Be active in some way: hit a pillow, bang on a drum, jog, chop wood; if you are able to have a good scream that also helps, but that depends on your neighbors and your level of privacy. Gibberish nonsense talk also works to release emotions. Have a little catharsis—be crazy for a while! Whatever you do, be active. This is not always the easiest choice because emotions leave us feeling collapsed and exhausted and more like curling up in bed to nurse them. The surprising fact is that when you return to your partner after physical release you are likely to experience that the sense of separation/disconnection is reduced, that you can make eye contact, that the wall between you is crumbling. If this is not the case, then another bout of body movement is called for, until the wall has crumbled to the ground.

This sounds almost too simple, but it works. And it certainly wins hands down over the alternative option of dragging the emotions around for a few days, heavyhearted and miserable, wondering what has become of love until eventually, sleepless nights later, one side breaks down into tears, gives up the fight, and starts to express the feelings lurking behind the emotions. You have experienced this yourself many times, I'm sure: the very instant one side gives up and starts to express inner feelings the fight is over. We pick up the remaining threads of love and start again.

A woman friend who uses body catharsis through chaotic movement as a meditation has shared this with me:

> I continue to marvel at how cathartic movement frees a lot of my psychological holding, a certain mental rigidity that collects and periodically builds up through the activities of my day-to-day life. As a result of movement catharsis, I find I have more patience and focus in dealing with all aspects of my life. In addition, I find that cathartic movement is especially complementary to my yoga practice. I love practicing yoga, but there is something serious and rigid about it that wild dancing movement seems

to free up and balance. Catharsis is a dredging-up process. Many people don't really want to look very deeply into what exists below the surface of the ego. I have found that the work of catharsis creates more softness, sensitivity, and receptivity within me, while at the same time creating dynamic and healthy boundaries. When some barriers and armoring are broken down and released, softer aspects within myself are contacted. At the same time, some weaker part of myself receives acceptance and become more vital and powerful.

The question may come up as to why is it necessary to separate physically to deal with emotions. One of the telltale traits of emotion is that it enjoys discussion and argument, each one trying to convince the other why *he* or *she* is right. Emotion is full of ego. If you do stay in each other's presence when emotionally activated, it is really best if you can say "I feel . . ." and *only* talk about yourself. This is the most direct way to step out of emotion: to talk about what you are feeling at a deeper level, to express and release your hidden feelings. Bring the congestion of emotions from the solar plexus—where it is likely to have formed a knot—up to the heart, and get into your inner feelings for real. Do not make your partner responsible for creating unhappiness in you. Reach behind the emotion and find what is truly happening inside of you, the old hurts buried away that have nothing to do with this individual in front of you. He has only been a trigger for the cache of unexpressed feelings within.

Even if perhaps this person *is* in some way responsible for some of the hurts you carry from the past, the fact that you did not express your deeper feelings at that time, and repressed them instead, is really the issue in the present. If feelings had been authentically released at the time, they would not keep bubbling up inside of you. At least you would have felt a great deal better for having expressed the feelings, even if a particular issue remains unresolved between you. Through expression you cease to drag emotions around with you that accumulate year by year. Instead you keep yourself free from the past, straight and up to date.

Emotions are really toxins (which is what you feel swirling around in the fascia) that will poison the atmosphere, striking deadly blows at the

person we most love, the one closest to us. This is a big problem—we unconsciously put all our unresolved feelings onto the person we most love, and thereby contaminate the love. We say the most awful things to our partner in an attempt to unburden ourselves of our emotions. Emotional statements stick like glue in the mind, and turn around in the thoughts endlessly, long after the fight is over. Did he *really* mean that? Am I really like *that*? And then *the mind will create more emotions from thinking over the past too much*. In truth, love cannot withstand too much emotion; it is like a delicate and fragile flower that requires awareness to keep it flourishing. Love will slowly slip through our fingers when we let emotion have the upper hand.

Conventional Sex Creates Emotionality

Another source of emotionality lies hidden in conventional sex. When energy moves downward, as it does in conventional sex with its conventional discharge, tension and anxiety are by-products.[1] This is why arguments and dissatisfactions easily follow. Sexual tensions eventually create an overcharge in woman, a subtle false-positive charge, and these accumulating tensions have to be discharged in some fashion. More often than not this happens through some kind of fighting, and often the tensions show up in premenstrual syndromes. When emotions are in the air they easily spawn excitement, which gives rise to the famous fucking-after-a-fight syndrome, a strategy commonly used to heal a rift between lovers. In reality, trying to patch up things like this is a vicious cycle, because through that same fuck women acquire more charge, which can flare up into emotion at any moment. This explains why, even in the absence of an argument, after a so-called good fuck a fight can start so easily.

Because of our emotional patterns, as women we can tend to get a bit high on emotions and begin to believe that this intensity is a part of love, that a good throwing around of china is an expression of our love. I have heard Barry Long say in a public gathering that all anger is, in reality, the result of sexual frustration. This certainly gives food for thought—and if you look at all the wars around us, and how little satisfying sex is being

enjoyed on Earth, it appears that he speaks the truth. Women have difficulties and frustrations with conventional orgasm, so they are quite likely to have anger about this lurking within. Many women feel deep rage toward men for their abusive behavior, a rage that extends beyond the personal to the collective level.

Expressing Feelings in the Here and Now

In addition to (a) attempting to keep the past in the past by recognizing when emotion steps in, and (b) experimenting with relaxing into sex to avoid adding emotions to the store you already have, the art now becomes one of (c) staying in touch with your feelings, beginning to *feel what you are feeling*. To keep love fresh and free of emotion, it is essential to express feelings *as* they arise! Do not hang on to your feelings for an instant, unless you are in a hopelessly inappropriate situation. Move with the rising feeling and don't let your mind talk you out of it. Allow the tears to flow, the laughter to erupt, the roar to express itself, jump up and down, *do* something fast! Above all, do not repress feelings and in so doing form fresh emotions, which happens very quickly. Equally as quickly, any sadness, pain, anger, or frustration, if *fully* lived *as it is happening,* will have a life span of about eight seconds or so in intensity, after which it is all over.

When you practice consciously expressing anger there are a few hard and fast rules that come with it, and these are not to be broken under *any* circumstances. If you feel anger, do *not* direct it onto your partner, even if on the surface your emotions are convincing you that he is at fault. Do not touch him or do anything physically to hurt him—do not even face him. Turn to face in the opposite direction, showing him your back; then let a deep roar emerge from your belly.

The first time I allowed my anger to flow it was an unforgettable experience. In the very instant that I felt the rising anger for being blamed for something I did not do, I contacted a deep, roaring sound in my belly, that was so powerful it shot me up into the air to virtually touch the ceiling (which was higher than most ceilings are). By the time gravity pulled me back to terra firma a second or two later, it was all over. I felt no anger, no emotion, no resentment—nothing. I stepped back into the moment without hesitation, ready and willing to continue communicating.

When anger arises, welcome it knowing that it is an old tension existing within you and it can be transformed. By expressing it for yourself you are released from its restrictive grip. Contacting feelings is a cleansing experience—energy that was locked suddenly becomes available. When you express a feeling or transform an emotion you feel lighter, expanded and fresh, connected to your partner, open and soft, clear and radiant, even loving. Emotions bring the experience of quite opposite qualities: darkness and gloom, despair and collapse. The whole range of positive experiences is what shows up when you share your feelings.

Woman Needs to Make Love for Her Continuing Health

Just as tension is the by-product of energy moving downward (as in conventional sex), silence is the outcome of energy moving upward (as in tantric sex or meditation).[2] Relaxing into sex brings you into a state of being that is quite apart from the whole range of emotions. Through relaxing and reaching the orgasmic state, we reach a rare peace and fulfillment, a state in which our energy is regenerated and we become filled with love, not only for the beloved but for any person around us. As energy moves upward through the centers (chakras) it cleanses them, purifies them, and makes them dynamic and alive.

However, at present women suffer extreme menstrual syndromes with hormonal ups and downs and lack of self-value alongside fears of aging, menopausal anxieties, and disappointment and often disinterest in sex. At a certain point sex is considered by many women to be too much hard work with very little reward, and for this reason they give it up. I heard a research statistic mentioned by a U.S. television show host recently revealing that 45 percent of happily married couples did not have sex in the last six months!

For men, too, the situation is dire. Until given the chance to enjoy the flowering of sex through direct experience, man cannot imagine it. And since excitement and ejaculation are the only tricks he knows, he is not giving much thought to trying something different. These tricks, however,

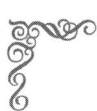

are only superficially satisfying, while in the depths a bubbling sexual pool remains untapped. A man's inability to channel his real life force leads to frustration, aggression, anger, restlessness, obsessive fantasizing about sex—in sex and out of sex—and all manner of sexual perversions. When the tantric energy circulates freely through him he feels himself, finally, as more of a man. At the end of a workshop recently I overheard a man saying to Raja, my partner, "This is the first time in my life of fifty-four years that I have been given any insights or guidance on what it means to be a man." And that was not the first time I've heard this.

When a woman knows it is possible to use her sexual energy rightfully, allowing it to circulate throughout the body orgasmically, her sense of self changes and she *wants* to make love. Sex becomes less to do with the other or with getting something and becomes more a way of valuing and loving oneself, of being with oneself. With insight into her body mechanisms she is able to direct her sexual energy and so be more in command of her life. The process of the body getting older and perhaps less attractive becomes of no real concern, in the sense that she knows how to attract the male principle when a man is in her presence, how to draw and drink from him, through understanding the deeper layers of sexual energy. It has nothing to do with how she looks or how old she is. She bypasses the superficiality of sex and steps directly into the female element, which is passive, relaxed, receptive, sweet, serene, open. Such an ambience in itself stimulates man to respond to woman in a way quite different from how he usually responds.

Perhaps only a woman can really and truly break the cycle of unconsciousness in sex. When sex is balanced and in accord with her female design, a woman has some leverage, some authority in sex, and a new confidence in herself. Her man will be in wonder and even a bit awestruck to learn how the same elements—the penis and the vagina—can produce two such vastly different experiences.

The Emotion of Jealousy

Jealousy is perhaps the most debilitating and excruciating of emotions, more frequently experienced by women than by men. Jealousy is con-

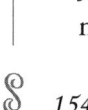

cerned with possessing and controlling another person; it is not an expression of love for that person. Jealousy has its roots in comparison, and we are taught to compare ourselves in all kinds of ways, particularly in the sexual sphere. Easily and instantly we can have overwhelming feelings of inadequacy and feel threatened by another woman giving or receiving attentions from the man we love. In the conventional picture, a new and fresh pretty, tilted face represents a bit of excitement to a man, excitement being his main stimulus for sex at present. However, when a woman steps away from excitement as the basis of the sexual experience, she finds a real rootedness in her deeper self; then she is not so easily knocked off center.

Comparison is a useless activity because each individual is unique and incomparable, and once this understanding settles in you, it is possible for jealousy to disappear. Sex certainly creates jealousy, but jealousy is a secondary thing. So it is not a question of how to drop jealousy. Jealousy cannot easily be dropped while we are trapped in conventional sex. The question therefore is how to transform sex into love. And in this love, jealousy disappears.

> *Don't repress it, express it. Sit in your room, close the doors, bring your jealousy into focus. Watch it, see it, let it take as strong a flame as possible. Let it become a strong flame, burn into it and see what it is. And don't from the very beginning say that this is ugly, because that very idea that this is ugly will repress the jealousy, will not allow it total expression. No opinions. Just try to see the existential effect of what jealousy is, the existential fact. No interpretations, no ideologies. Just let the jealousy be there. Look into it, look deeply into it and so do with anger, so do with sadness, hatred, possessiveness. And by and by you will see that just by seeing through things you start getting a transcendental feeling that you are just a witness; the identity is broken. The identity is broken only when you encounter something within you.*
>
> OSHO, TRANSCRIBED TEACHINGS,
> *TAO: THE PATHLESS PATH*

Divesting Interest in Peak Orgasm and Ejaculation

We know that many a man is obsessed with producing a peak orgasm for a woman because it validates him as a lover. And we understand that this attitude has grave consequences, for both men and women—that peak orgasms leave a residue of tension that become a source of emotions in woman (and man), and that, in trying to produce excitement and orgasm in woman, man easily ejaculates, which is against a woman's long-term interests.

But some women are equally identified with their lover's ejaculation. They say quite clearly that, for them, their man's orgasm is an essential part of the sexual act. A woman of this persuasion feels that in the very moment of releasing his semen he gives himself utterly to her, he shares something of his essence that he can do with no one else. In reality, each ejaculation is an enormous disempowerment of man, for it represents an incalculable amount of energy in sperm life—approximately two hundred *million* to five hundred *million* sperms, or potential human beings, per ejaculation. Huge amounts of creativity are lost by the male species through habitual and uncontrollable ejaculation! Ejaculation has become the norm, and woman can easily get into supporting man in this.

Yet with her capacity to influence the sex act by discovering the source of her orgasm in her breasts, any woman can begin reconfiguring her sexual reality to guarantee a life of love and a love free of emotion. The fragrance of a woman settled in her essence exerts an attractive force on man that alters the whole nature of the sexual act—it is a dimensional shift.

The stakes are enormous. Until a woman approaches sexuality in a truly feminine manner it is difficult or impossible for a man to change. Until man can manage to satisfy one woman utterly and completely, he will never feel himself to be a true man, in spite of any other achievements and successes. The need for man to feel himself as masculine, for woman to feel herself as feminine, and for both to have orgasmic experiences through each other is a burning need for humanity today. Without this spiritual sexual expression the human race will slowly die from starvation and become extinct through a dire shortage of love.

The Division between Sex and Heart's Love

Perhaps most women have at times (if not all the time) experienced a drastic and dramatic split between the experience of sex and the feelings of love. Sex can so easily feel dirty and animal and uncaring while love is something sweet and pure and beautiful. A majority of women have had countless experiences of loveless sex, and as a result many women choose a sexless life, at the same time attempting to love a man very dearly. Or instead, they choose to be alone.

But this solution of abandoning sex because it is not deeply moving comes at some cost to woman herself. As mentioned, lack of love and loving in woman results in all kinds of ill health, psychological disturbances, and emotional problems. For a woman, sex itself is not a dire need while love is an absolute need, and always remains one to the end of her life. The effort lies in bringing these two seemingly conflicting worlds into synchronicity. The route to that state is to connect sex with the heart (and love) *through* sex, not by avoiding it. Sex with any level of awareness creates love naturally, as a by-product; it follows simply and sweetly. Awareness is alchemical. Combining these two poles in her own body—sex and love, the earthly and the otherworldly—is the optimum for health and continued happiness for women.

Many women report that sometimes the heart feels like it is being touched internally, penetrated and opened by the penis, particularly when the penetration is deep and prolonged as suggested in chapter 6. When physical love reaches to this level of exchange through polarity, love is generated as a tangible reality between a man and a woman. In being so profoundly touched, woman connects with her love and in overflow showers love on man, thereby completing the circuit of love and joy. Remember this again and again: *any* level of awareness in sex will create love—it is the awareness itself that transforms sex into love. To repeat a common phrase: it is not what we do but how we do it. Woman is love, this is the quintessence of her very soul; thus, to her love is as essential as food. She requires the opportunity to relax into her feminine nature and receive the contentment and regeneration of orgasmic experiences to sustain her life. The

sincerity and willingness of a man is clearly a contributing factor to woman's orgasmic experiences, but the responsibility—even for this—lies in woman's hands. Through sex woman can regain her original power as female.

One Woman's Journey

I am fortunate to be able to include here a written report by a woman from Switzerland, now a good friend, whom I first met during a "Making Love" retreat several years ago. She and her partner have been experimenting very sincerely with tantra since then. Recently I slipped her an email asking her to write, if she wished, a few lines to quickly encapsulate her experience. Instead of the two or three lines I expected she sent a comprehensive and sincere assessment of her transformation, and I am grateful to her for doing so. Her experience can be an encouragement and inspiration to every woman.

> The most amazing development in our sexuality and lovemaking is this: The plugging in (the "tantric quickie"), which we do at least twice a day when we are together [they live together half of the week] is somehow healing deep wounds in our bodies *and* souls without our conscious effort or contribution. Fully beyond our heads (quite unusual for us), the bodies are doing this healing all by themselves! I enjoy sex much more, am always ready to make love provided there is enough time, and the pressure to perform is gone, as well as the fear of being hurt again. S. now knows his penis can come into my vagina anytime, which makes it less desirable somehow. But also, his urgent physical "baby needs" are finally fulfilled. He really seems to finally get what he needed most throughout his life with the plugging in!
>
> So when we are exhausted from working too much, we now peacefully plug in and go to sleep instead of the earlier dramas of having to have an exciting sex act at any cost because if we didn't have sex every day, something wasn't normal in the relationship (thus spending two or more difficult hours trying to achieve something, under performance pressure, with fancy underwear and toys, etc., instead of sleeping, which

was what our bodies really needed . . .). When we wake up at night, we either plug in again or make love. The first one to awaken in the morning asks the other one to plug in once more.

This has made us into peaceful human beings—no more fighting in the office, which we did daily before we learned from you. And if we do fight, we know that we are not taking enough time for love and have skipped our weekly appointments for making love. This skipping unfortunately still happens quite often. We are so performance-driven and responsible for our company, with twelve employees, and our garden, that we have difficulties with making time for love a top priority. (Interestingly, when we do just that and go away for a full week to a "Making Love" workshop, orders come in like crazy—this has happened two times now!) S. is getting what he needs to a point where I feel he really wants me as his partner, and has stopped wondering if there is anyone better out there. I feel the same way, especially when life with him is not stressful. Then it's all that I have ever dreamed of; we come into love deeper and deeper! We're even talking about getting married.

The other great help was your teaching about the difference between emotions and feelings. We are still both working hard at the "daring to express our feelings" part. I still sometimes don't dare to express them in order to minimize stress when it is already here. But then my resentments toward the stress come out in other ways, in aggressions—so I don't serve the whole if I don't say what I feel! My head knows that, but the little girl inside is still afraid to lose the love she needs so badly.

I'm working on that. It was amazing how few times we had to go jogging or screaming or cleaning before we recognized being emotional quickly enough to stop the fighting. Only a total of about five times—but we are used to recognizing patterns amongst the two of us, which was also very helpful. My breasts are still very sensitive and accept touch only when it happens in a fully loving way. They want S.'s or my own hands to go away immediately again when they feel manipulated. This is a tough one. It would take several sessions of loving touch to more easily welcome touch at my breasts—I better start planning for them!

In our third time of attending your "Making Love" workshop I had a beautiful release inside. A great pain came up in my vagina or uterus shortly before my period. I usually never have that. When I got up at night to go to the toilet and came back, it had gotten so bad I woke up S. and asked him to plug in to make it better. We started talking about the pain, and at some point I said "I carry this pain with pride." S. asked "For whom?" and I instantly replied "For my father, of course." S. said, "But your father doesn't see you, is not interested in you, and thinks you're crazy anyway!" All of which is true. I realized the little girl in me still does everything she can to win her father's love, because she wasn't able to reach him with her great love for him when she was little. So I took my pillow (standing for the little girl) into my arms and finally cried about this. The tears and mourning washed away my core belief that love doesn't have a chance (because it didn't have one back then). This belief had led to my subtle dismantling of love whenever it showed itself, with a little criticism here and some aggression there—I seem to have done that in order not to reexperience the disappointment of not reaching somebody with my love, which was so overwhelmingly big when I was a child and had left me so very lonely. After the crying and recognizing what it was telling me, the pain in my belly slowly went away. I'm very careful now to give love a real chance, especially with S. and my children. . . .

Women Sharing Experiences

"Another 'aha!' realization that keeps coming to me is never to take anything of my partner's response as personal *and* not to exclude anything. It reminds me of the well-used phrase 'Tantra does not exclude anything.' I also had to let go very early in the process of this idea and identification that I am a very fucked up and wounded woman. To disengage from the emotional, over and over, is a delight."

"I connected with my own rejection wound. I've been in it for days—in pain and panic and not able to see my way. It's like a rewinding. Right now I'm back to ages seven to eleven, realizing how much this little flower has been abused. I feel compassion for myself, my partner, all the unconsciousness. . . . From this wound I have rejected others, especially men. Everything has been about projection. I cried for hours."

"The wounds seem all to be in the heart—all about receiving love and giving love. When a lot of rejection is there, there is a closing to receiving love and a disbelief that my love has value to a man."

"Today I really connected with the eyes as a key. Keeping eye contact kept us both present and lifted me right out of the emotions and past movies, and I found that I can trust my intuition about how to move into this space. Also, opening my eyes with the focus being 'in' and not 'out' helps me to stay connected almost as much as if I have my eyes closed."

"I had major energy release happening during the lovemaking; it was electrical. The non-movement brought up all my 'no' to penetration, 'no' to man."

"After six or seven days I felt so much energy building up inside. We had an exquisite meeting where I felt all the boundaries in my vagina melt away, which made my man's erection very strong. We were very blissful, present for a long time. After that for three days everything went the other way, my Christian judgments coming in full force—bad sleep, feeling restless and prudish, all kind of things came up for me. Our sexual meetings have gone to a deeper level it seems. The mind freaks out, reacts; the vagina has become more and more tense to a point that the whole pelvic floor is in contraction. This morning it was impossible to make love. We talked through our genitals—abuse was strong on both sides—both from outside. I have three rapes in my history as well as my personal abuse of my genitals by fucking when I didn't feel like it. It is still tight everywhere, but strangely enough, by sharing our tightness, lying very close together, I still feel very connected to my partner and loving and friendly."

"I got the impression I never learned so much about real love as I did in this week. I was always looking for this feeling and hoping I would meet it one day. Yes, I came near to it but in a different way in certain moments in meditations in the awareness training I've done over the past ten years. But in my daily life with my husband I had many returning moments of sadness. Our relationship was really good and deep; we have been together for twenty-three years and I always had the impression we loved each other, were there for each other, cared about the other, went through difficult times together, enjoyed life together, had good conventional sex, all was so good, and—there was a big and—I many times felt a big sadness deep in me. I had this 'idea' of love that I felt was covered over on a very deep level. In all these years I carried big doubts within myself. Doubts about whether I really loved my man compared to the love I had as an 'idea.' Then I doubted whether that love could exist on our Earth-level of existence. I carried all these questions in me. During the week I started to get closer to real love. I could not imagine that my love for my man could get so strong and fine at the same time. We spent such wonderful hours, we shared so many things, I was crying sometimes just because I was so happy to get closer to this deep love. I am so thankful for this big gift!"

Tantric Inspiration

This has been my observation: It is difficult for people to love, but there is one thing that is even more difficult than to love, and that is to receive love. To love is difficult, but to receive love is almost impossible. Why? Because to love is in a way simple, and one can do it because it is not against the ego. When you love somebody you are giving something, and the ego feels enhanced. You have the upper hand, you are the giver, and the other is at the receiving end. You feel very good; your ego feels enhanced, puffed up. But when you receive love, you can't have the upper hand. Receiving, your ego feels hurt. Receiving love is more difficult than giving love. And one has to learn both—to give and receive.

And to receive is going to transform you more than giving can do, because in receiving love your ego starts disappearing.

OSHO, TRANSCRIBED TEACHINGS,
I SAY UNTO YOU, (VOL. 1)

Question on Emotions

[This passage begins with a personal question by a female disciple to Osho.]

> Beloved Master,
>
> So often a feeling that I can't describe fills my heart and my whole being. During the other morning's discourse it felt like overwhelming love for you and the whole. But now I realize that the same feeling or a very, very similar feeling also comes up in fear, anguish, throbbing pain, helplessness, and frustration. I am trembling and confused. Beloved Master, can you say something?

Osho answers:

There is certainly something very similar in very different emotions: the overwhelmingness. It may be love, it may be hate, it may be anger—it can be anything. If it is too much then it gives you a sense of being overwhelmed by something. Even pain and suffering can create the same experience, but overwhelmingness has no value in itself. It simply shows you are an emotional being.

This is typically the indication of an emotional personality. When it is anger, it is all anger. And when it is love, it is all love. It almost becomes drunk with the emotion, blind. And whatever action comes out of it is wrong. Even if it is overwhelming love, the action that will come out of it is not going to be right.

Reduced to its base, whenever you are overwhelmed by any emotion you lose all reason, you lose all sensitivity, you lose your heart in it. It becomes almost like a dark cloud in which you are lost. Then whatever you do is going to be wrong.

Love is not to be a part of your emotions. Ordinarily that's what people think and experience, but anything overwhelming is very unstable. It comes like a wind and passes by, leaving you behind, empty, shattered, in sadness and in sorrow.

According to those who know man's whole being—his mind, his heart, and his being—love has to be an expression of your being, not an emotion. Emotion is very fragile, very changing. One moment it seems that is all. Another moment you are simply empty.

So the first thing to do is take love out of this crowd of overwhelming emotions. Love is not overwhelming. On the contrary, love is a tremendous insight, clarity, sensitivity, awareness. But that kind of love rarely exists, because very few people ever reach to their being.

OSHO, TRANSCRIBED TEACHINGS,
OM SHANTIH SHANTIH SHANTIH

Awareness and Sensitivity Exercise
Self-Massage of the Solar Plexus

If you find the solar plexus congested or uncomfortable at any time, it is very important to dissolve the tensions that have collected there; otherwise you may discharge them in other ways. Massage is helpful for increasing awareness of the area.

Lie on your back with your arms at your sides, in an aligned position as suggested in previous exercises, with about twenty to thirty minutes to yourself. Take a few deep breaths into the belly and solar plexus area. Then make your fingertips into a pointy tool by placing them back to back, with fingernails touching. Bring your hands to the solar plexus area and very lightly place this tool on the skin about half way between the arch of your rib cage and your navel. Rest here for a few moments using hardly any pressure—like a butterfly alighting on a flower—and soon you will begin to feel the heartbeat pulsing in the solar plexus. If you feel no pulse after several minutes, increase the pressure slightly. Keep your attention on your fingertips and feel the pulsing of the heart.

After a few minutes pull the fingers away from the heartbeat but don't lose contact with the skin. It is a fraction of a movement, just a hairbreadth. Take two or three nice deep breaths through the solar plexus into the belly, and then deepen your contact again to return your fingertips to the pulse of the heartbeat. Continue this process of feeling the pulse and then giving the pulse space by pulling away for as long as you are comfortable with the exercise. When you have finished, pull away from the solar plexus extremely slowly. Place one hand on top of the other over the solar plexus, keeping your eyes closed and resting for a few minutes.

Awareness and Sensitivity Exercise
Cathartic Exercise for Repressed Emotions

It is an excellent idea to create the space to intentionally contact unexpressed anger. Whenever you feel that you cannot get below the stomach, that you are not reaching into your belly, when you feel somehow superficial, you can walk and pant like a dog. You will need three things: a half hour of privacy; a room with the door closed; and, ideally, the liberty to make some sound without arousing the curiosity of your neighbors. This kind of anger is usually embedded deep in the body, which makes it difficult to work with directly. However, indirectly something can be done with anger so as to release accumulated frustrations.

Simply pretend that you are a dog by letting your tongue stick out and hang down. Walk around on the floor on all fours (hands and knees) and take fast panting breaths through your mouth. As you do this, the passage down the throat to the belly will open. Pant for thirty minutes and soon anger will flow easily and beautifully. Let your whole body become involved in it. You can even bark and growl at your reflection in the mirror.

If anger is a constant stumbling block for you, I suggest you do this panting exercise daily for a period of about three weeks. Once anger is released, you will have the feeling of body energies awakened very deeply and you will feel an inner freedom—you will no longer be in bondage to unexpressed feelings held in the body.

11
Woman as Lover During Menstruation, Fertility, Pregnancy, Motherhood, and Menopause

$\mathcal{A}$ woman, simply by virtue of being a woman with the capacity to bear children, is subject to the influence of hormones that affect her life and her sexual expression in powerful ways, and these must not be underestimated. A whole class of these effects is produced by the very knowledge that, for much of her life, sex for a woman is inextricably linked with the possibility of pregnancy. It starts with menstruation at puberty, and from then onward in many cases an unadulterated fear of accidentally getting pregnant lies between a woman and her full immersion into sex. Deep-seated fear can be a great hindrance to the experience of sex as something natural and beautiful.

The Contraception Issue

Many women, particularly in their teenage years, are bound to have had experiences of an excruciating longing to have sex and a simultaneously profound *no* to it. Usually in these circumstances the contraception issue has not been addressed or acted upon. This inner conflict of yes/no creates great tension in a woman and affects her ability to genuinely open up, to herself and to a man. And even if she does open up, she is likely to retain a subtle *no* of underlying resistance, when so much is at stake. If a woman is compelled to set out with a basic unwillingness to open up and relax, this contraction does not help the expansion of female energy. Tensions about pregnancy will influence and affect a woman's presence, her pleasure, and her entire perception of sex.

Fertility awareness becomes essential if a woman really wants to let go into lovemaking. Without it, the riskiness of the situation, the resistance to it and the wanting of it, can serve to intensify the excitement to a point that she will willy-nilly thrust herself into the experience, throwing all caution to the wind. It starts out with a no, and yet the woman is slowly getting excited, still saying no but enjoying the sexual feelings. At a certain point the excitement reaches a peak with the overwhelming desire for penetration, and the *no* rapidly flips on its head into a *yes*, and this is certainly not the moment to halt the proceedings to insert a diaphragm or roll on a condom. Thrusting oneself into sex like this is to enter the act with an already high level of excitement, with less awareness, and usually with the desire for orgasm—all of which pretty much guarantees ejaculation. Which of course makes the risks of pregnancy even higher.

For all of these reasons it is really essential that a woman, especially when young, take complete responsibility for contraception and not leave it up to the man. A woman does herself a great service if she takes precautions against unwanted pregnancy: much energy is liberated into the sexual experience. A woman who has had the joy of a vasectomized man entering her life will know what an incredible relief it is not to even *think* about contraception. Not ever! Making love becomes so joyful and easy—just an unconditional *yes* away.

Often women in workshops will ask the question, "What about making love during menstruation—is it good or bad?" Basically, to make love at this time is perfectly fine; it is a super-safe time relative to the fertility cycle and can even ease menstrual symptoms such pain or irritability. It really depends on the personal choice and preferences of the two people involved. There are no general rules to be made and each woman has to find her own way with her partner in this.

When Sex and Fertility Make Friends

Keeping track of a woman's fertility cycle is the most helpful way to avoid or invite pregnancy. Perhaps the best tool for this is the Sympto-Thermal Method. Having a working knowledge of this method empowers women, in that they remain in closer contact to the cycles of their bodies and puts them in a position to have greater control over contraception. Nature gives us subtle signs telling us when a woman is fertile: ovulation is accompanied by a temperature rise (sympto-thermal), which indicates the passing of an egg being released from the ovaries to travel down the fallopian tubes to the womb. At the same time, there are changes in the cervical fluid. In the Sympto-Thermal Method, the temperature rise is always interpreted in correlation to cervical fluid observation, and together these reveal ovarian activity. This method is taught by two major world organizations: a Catholic organization called the Natural Family Planning (NFP) Institute and the non-religious-affiliated Fertility Awareness Method (FAM) schools. Instructions in the Sympto-Thermal Method can be obtained from these organizations and others all over the world. Some women manage to learn the method on their own just by reading a competent book, but it is recommended that they discuss their charts at least once with a Sympto-Thermal counselor and, importantly, that they fully include their partners.

It is commonly understood that having sex but refraining from ejaculation is not a sufficiently safe form of contraception. Accordingly, the Sympto-Thermal Method, the so-called "natural contraception" method, is not considered sufficiently safe by its antagonists. Instead, the multi-billion-dollar hormone industry, and thus, most gynecologists and other

doctors, discourage women from getting involved with their own fertility cycles. Advocates of the natural approach insist that the Sympto-Thermal Method is the best-kept secret around, and the underlying reason is monetary: consumption of expensive pills to forget about body cycles is preferred, and so there is precious little promotion of self awareness and how to better take care of ourselves.

For women who do wish to know more about this method, I have included a detailed introduction in the appendix at the back of the book. Although you should not consider this account complete, I have included all the contact information you will need on how to learn more.

Choosing to Have a Child

When a woman feels ready to have a child and truly wishes for one, it is very much advantageous to all concerned to *consciously* conceive that child, to ensure that the pregnancy results from a planned ejaculation to coincide with ovulation, not an accidental ejaculation. A couple should build a special ritual around such a conception experience, creating a temple for making love, providing a sacred space into which to invite a new being into life. A child entering the world is easily able to sense welcome or a lack of welcome; she feels how she has been longed for or accommodated by the new parents, whether they have changed joyfully or adjusted reluctantly to fit her into their usually already busy lives. Feelings of being unwelcome will be in force in this new being in spite of all of the loving attentions that may subsequently be poured on her. A child who has truly been invited into the world displays a completely different psychology and life force.

One basic way in which a baby can sense the lack of welcome on planet Earth is through a lack of breast-feeding. Many mothers today do not have the time or the patience to devote themselves to breast-feeding, and further, some women fear they will ruin their breasts by breast-feeding and thereby decrease their sexual attractiveness. Breast milk contains all the vital ingredients essential for developing a healthy immune system in a child, so breast-feeding is basic to human life. Yet today not many women

breast-feed their children for more than a few weeks. Much less common is breast-feeding for twelve to eighteen months.

Sex during Pregnancy

Pregnancy, planned or not, raises the question of how to proceed with a sexual life for the following nine months. As the pregnancy advances many women become reluctant to engage in sex, becoming concerned that in some way the baby will be hurt through sex, and this concern increases as the pregnancy progresses. This is perhaps the first time that a woman becomes conscious of the aggressive, unloving quality of the conventional sexual exchange. Feeling a need to protect her unborn child, she begins to turn away from sexual overtures by her man. This withdrawal often creates tensions within the relationship; by the time the baby arrives, not much sex has been had at all in the preceding months.

With the conscious and loving tantric approach to sex, and soft penetration with the possibility of erection in the vagina as described in chapter 8, sex is easy to engage in. It is such a completely organic approach that a woman will feel in herself that absolutely no harm can come to the fetus. On the contrary, women in my workshops who have attended in the seventh to the ninth month of pregnancy all report a positive response from the fetus. Tantric sex creates more space for the baby, because the belly relaxes. The movement of the fetus increases, and in some cases tantric lovemaking has even stimulated the act of the fetus turning to the head-down position important for birth. The life force generated during sex radiates through the whole body, with beneficial outcome for both mother and child. It can act as a preparation for birth. In addition, this lovemaking nourishes the loving bond between man and woman, which is the foundation of parenthood.

Sex after Birth and while Breast-feeding

After the birth of a child, a woman's reluctance to engage in sex tends to increase. Some of this disinclination can be an outcome of the birth experience itself and the intensely physical process a woman goes through. If it was a difficult birth, with tears and stitches at the entrance of the vagina

for instance, a woman will feel naturally unwilling to open up to sex. A tantric friend of mine reported that she had two completely opposite experiences giving birth: the first was very hard and very long and the second took only six hours. Though the second birth was intense, it was a natural birth and was a very empowering experience. After the birth of her first child she noticed she could not even entertain the *thought* of getting interested "down there"—it seemed that feeling sexual was simply light years away. My friend required five months of healing before she felt physically available to make love with her husband. When she finally agreed, she experienced the soft penetration and presence of the penis inside her as a tremendously healing experience. Many tears and tensions were able to flow out of her system. In contrast, with her second child she resumed lovemaking (tantric style, as she had done up to the birth) shortly after the birth and continues to make love regularly (one to four times a week), along with breast-feeding and caring for her two children.

In the case of cesarean birth there is often pain and discomfort associated with the surgery and healing of the wound, as well as a general sensation of being cut off from the pelvic basin—the genitals and pelvic floor. With vaginal birth, many women are given an episiotomy—a cut from the vaginal entrance into the perineum—as a routine procedure that is done with the intention of preventing the possibility of any tearing during birth. In these cases penetration is associated with pain in the vagina. So it follows that if birth has occurred without surgical invasion or difficulties, the mother is more likely to be open to sexual exchange. Her body is relatively intact and carrying no traumas that need time to heal in the body and the psyche.

Apparent Loss of Libido after Birth

As a creative expression of the female element, giving birth is a profoundly transforming process for a woman. For some women the birth process can be an orgasmic experience. Birth energetically expands a woman's system and thereby increases her overall receptivity and sensitivity. As a consequence of giving birth a woman feels more feminine, more connected to her innate female nature.

So it is quite understandable that, in these new circumstances, a new

mother is not as interested in sex as she was before the birth—in sex of the conventional kind, at any rate, in which her delicate feminine senses are transgressed. The conscious, tantric approach to sex poses no problems for a woman because it does not involve the machinations and strenuousness demanded by convention. Perhaps the commonly experienced loss of libido after childbirth is due to nothing other than resistance to the conventional approach to sex—not a resistance to sex itself. For a woman as mother, it is important to move into the spiritual expression of sex, which requires raising that same energy that produced the child. This will bring her, as woman, more love, vitality, and wisdom. Sex is a powerful way of indirectly nourishing a child.

At present in the field of medicine the loss of libido is attributed to prolactin, a hormone that is secreted after giving birth and is absolutely necessary for breast-feeding. Prolactin is a physiological requirement of the body, because without it the breast milk is unable flow. Prolactin works as a relaxant for the breasts, and naturally calms and relaxes the mother in preparation for breast-feeding. Incidentally, prolactin is also used in psychiatry for its calming effects. Knowing the role of prolactin in milk production, a woman can feel more relaxed about the calm state of her libido. It is an internal body process, so to feel tired or lacking energy while breast-feeding a child is perfectly normal. As well, breast-feeding represents a huge commitment, as an adequate schedule is about six or seven times a day for at least four to six months. So when a woman does not feel attracted to the rigors of normal sex, it may be unrealistic to call it a loss of libido!

Breast-Feeding Enhances Lovemaking

In the tantric picture, to be relaxed is actually considered a great advantage, and a woman will be naturally more open and receptive while she is breast-feeding—a gift! (Soft penetration is quite feasible during breast-feeding itself.) It is possible also to support the flow from the breasts by connecting with the inner energy circle flowing from the breasts to the vagina and back again to the breasts. A tantric friend of mine who breast-feeds with awareness of the breasts as the positive downward-radiating pole says she finds the experience very nourishing; it even gives her a certain sexual

fulfillment by virtue of completing her inner circle. She says that the circular connection, the tuning in to her body, creates a calm, peaceful atmosphere around her, which gives the baby a sense of security, and this in turn helps the baby relax into drinking. By making the experience a nourishing one for herself, a woman can avoid exhaustion or irritability, extreme sensitivity in the nipples, and feeling empty and drained of reserves after feeding.

Remember, breast-feeding prevents ovulation, so as long as a woman is breast-feeding she is protected by natural contraception.* You can add this to the advantages of breast-feeding. It is really the perfect period of time for making love. You can be almost certain that during this time there will be no ovulation, which gives you time to get back in sync with your partner. A woman can be infertile for about eighteen months if she breast-feeds for this length of time; however, after six months she should seek more information from a fertility counselor.

The World Health Organization recommends a minimum of one year of breast-feeding, which makes it difficult or impossible for a new mother to work away from the home. In Sweden, mothers are paid by the government for one year to assist them financially in order to encourage breast-feeding, in recognition of the vital importance of mother's milk to the building of a child's immune system and future health.

All in all, sex after giving birth can be a great healing force, and women are encouraged not to abandon being a lover when becoming a mother. In the tantric context one starts to view life very differently, to see that a conscious approach in sex can be a unifying force, as things that are normally held apart (sex and parenthood) are brought together in harmony. You can engage in unassertive tantric sex in the vicinity of babies because it is a loving and natural happening—unlike conventional sex, which is more animalistic and places adults in an embarrassing situation when children happen in on them.

---

*The contraceptive protection is about 95 percent as long as a woman is breast-feeding her baby at least six times a day; not more than six hours pass between feedings; and the baby is consuming no other liquids in addition to the breast milk. If these rules are not followed, ovulation could occur.

Sex and Parenthood

Over and above the actual birth experience and its impact on a woman's sexual willingness, birth marks the significant transition from woman to mother. It is an experience of great energy expansion; with it a woman's energy changes and becomes more feminine, receptive, and loving. The qualities of motherhood are instilled through the birth process. A total shift in consciousness occurs—love wells up from an inner source and flowers into an utter devotion to the well-being of this fragile new life. Woman becomes 100 percent present to the needs of her child. A natural absorption with the child makes her less accessible to man, and it may become impossible to tear herself away from tending to the baby to notice the needs of her partner. From a woman's perspective it can seem an insurmountable effort at this time to open up to making love and to her man himself.

However, the love between a couple really needs to be nourished. Lavishing attentions on the child and excluding the man leads to the possibility of the man feeling unwanted, getting restless, and seeking "entertainment" elsewhere. It is well documented that, when a man is continually refused sex by his woman-turned-mother in the early years of parenthood, his eyes will start to roam. When sex is not available at home, inevitably he will find alternative sources. Thus it happens frequently that a man will move on permanently to greener pastures, leaving a woman stranded, babe and all.

Given the innate male-female polarities, sex is more essential for the male; it is not as optional as it is for women. As passive pole, women do not really appreciate this important difference between the sexes. I remember a twenty-year-old mother recently telling me, with innocent girlish surprise on her face, that she had *no* idea that sex was so important to a man. This sharing followed a spate of arguments with her man over the issue of availability for sex, which had some frightening emotional touches to it.

Well, the simple truth is that sex is extremely important for a man. A mother must find a balance between the two, and understand that love between man and woman will sustain the love for the child and the harmony in the home.

A new mother is often overconcerned about a child's physical needs and comfort, smothering the baby with attention instead of attending to the ambience surrounding the baby. As *mother* a woman has responsibility to her child and as *woman* she has responsibility to her man, the father of her child—an almost equal responsibility, if she wants her child to grow up in the ambience of love rather than conflict. And this is not to mention the responsibility of woman to *herself* to obtain nourishment and love and tenderness and so avoid the buildup of emotions. The love field that bonds and surrounds the parents is as vital a food to a young child as is the breast milk of the mother. Children are extremely sensitive to this; they draw on the nourishment love provides, and where there is an absence of harmony and lack of love there is a shrinking (due to fear) in the core of the child's energy system. They become tense and wary, possibly restless and demanding, even if well fed and properly taken care of. If this unlovingness continues and the years accumulate, the children will grow up to be overly emotional and afraid and not as filled with love as they might otherwise have been.

Parents are not aware of this when they fight in front of their children. When a sensitive new life is engulfed by tensions and arguments, a defensive, contracting fear sets in and a child easily grows up learning to express herself with an emotional personality; thus problems in life and relating begin. Parents need to keep all evidence of their fights away from their children. They need to take responsibility for their states of emotionality, following the steps suggested in chapter 10, to prevent the toxic vibrations of emotionality from having an influence on a child. Children are exceptionally sensitive to the atmosphere between the parents for as long as they are living at home, which can be for seventeen years or more. Many parents have said that when they started to make love more often, after participating in my workshop, it had a positive impact on the children. The children became less demanding and more content in themselves, and the usual squabbles between the children diminished dramatically. Parents concern themselves with informing and educating their children in any number of ways, yet they often overlook the basic requirement of love in a family, the very glue that keeps a family together. Parents who make love and live a loving life as a consequence give the best possible preparation and education to their children.

Sex during and after Menopause

The final cycle through which all women pass, whether they have had a child or not, is menopause—the ceasing of monthly menstrual bleeding. Many women hold menstruation dear, as it represents their womanhood. Thus many a woman begins to dread menopause because it appears as a threat to her femininity and attractiveness.

But this is true only when you look through conventional eyes. If a woman makes an attempt to step away from conditioned sex (with luck, early in her life, though it really is never too late to start), she receives a profound understanding of femininity and the real nature of sexual attraction. She knows it has nothing to do with outer appearance but with an ageless and powerful force residing within her. This brings a confidence and clarity way beyond the limiting concerns of the physical aging process. In fact, as you embrace tantric sex more and more, you feel better and better about yourself and getting older holds no great anxiety. Of course, the body itself may manifest a few telling signs, but the spirit remains ever young. A woman who learns the art of tantra empowers herself to make love until the end of her days, if this is her wish, without need to give it up with menopause and then old age.

Many women report that penetration becomes extremely painful during menopause, and I have met women in workshops in a relationship crisis because of this. Some have been unable to have sex for several years because of this uncomfortable symptom. Adding to this problem can be a lack of lubrication often experienced during this phase of hormonal change. Conventional sex becomes impossible for many women during menopause. However, tantra offers us the possibility of soft penetration, from which an erection is able to grow, and women who have tried this say there is absolutely no pain. Suddenly new doors open through which lovemaking can enter again in all its glory.

In my experience of working with women in menopause I can report that a conscious approach in sex is of great benefit. Women who have commenced with a tantric approach during menopause say they very definitely notice a relaxation of many of the menopausal symptoms. Hot flashes, for

example, flow down to the ground as if a channel has been opened. Some of the emotional difficulties are also relieved. Unfortunately there is not enough research being done in this area; however, a body of evidence is bound to emerge as more and more women begin to embrace tantric principles.

Menopause marks the time of a great rise in creativity for a woman—now free from the bondage of her hormonal aspect (the biological expression of sex)—and she naturally moves into a more serene state of equilibrium. The difficult ups and downs that can come with menstruation are left behind. No monthly bleeding to deal with is a great liberation and not something to be feared as some kind of intrinsic loss. Instead, the continuum of love and lovemaking can now go on undisturbed by the monthly onset of ovulation and menstruation. And most of all, it is very liberating to no longer have to worry about birth control.

Tantric Inspiration

And this is my observation—that if grownups are a little more meditative, children imbibe the spirit very easily. They are so sensitive. They learn whatsoever is there in the atmosphere; they learn the vibe of it. They never bother about what you say. What you are—they always respect that. And they have a very deep perceptivity, a clarity, an intuitiveness. You may be smiling but they will immediately know that it is false, because your eyes will be saying something else—and more than that your whole body will be saying something else—that you are angry, that you are just pretending, that it is just a policy.

They may not be able to formulate it in so many words, but they immediately feel it. So never be untrue with children because they will immediately know it. And once a child comes to know that his parents are untrue, his whole trust is lost. That is his first trust in life, his very base, and if that is lost he will become a skeptic. Then he cannot trust anybody. He cannot trust life, he cannot trust God, because those things are very far away things. Even the father deceived, even the mother deceived; even they were not reliable, so what to say of anything else now?

Once a child learns . . . and every child is going to learn; it is impossible to deceive a child. There is no method discovered up to now on how to deceive a child. He simply knows where you are, who you are. It is intuitive, it has nothing to do with his intellect. In fact the more intellectual he will become, the more he will lose this intuitiveness, and he will not be able to see things as they are. Right now a child is immediate. He simply looks through and through. He looks at you and you are transparent. So never be deceptive.

Love him and allow him to be a little meditative and much is possible.

OSHO, TRANSCRIBED TEACHINGS,
THE PASSION FOR THE IMPOSSIBLE

Tantric Meditation
Radiating Love

It is advantageous to take some time to practice love on your own. Sit upright in a comfortable position, alone in your room for about thirty minutes. Close your eyes and bring your awareness to your heart/breasts, and feel yourself to be loving. Radiate love from your heart and imagine that you fill the whole room with your expanding love energy. Soon you will feel yourself vibrating with a new frequency. If you feel yourself swaying, as if you are a wave in the great ocean of love, allow it. Let your whole room be filled with love. Intentionally create vibrations of love energy around you, and you may start to feel that something around your body is changing. It can feel like a warmth rising around your body, like a deep orgasm. You will feel yourself becoming more alive. If you feel moved to dance or sing to express your love, allow it. Through meditating on love you are likely to experience that you are the source of love, and not—as you have always thought—that love comes from somebody else. When you are able to connect to the love within yourself, it is a preparation for transforming your lover into a person with the right receptivity for you.

12
Tantric Orgasm and Same-Sex Partners

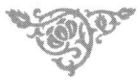

This letter came to me in e-mail form during the final days of completing this manuscript.

> I happened upon your Web site while doing some investigation on tantric sex. I think you have an excellent Web site and especially found the excerpts from the book to be interesting and informative. However, I have a question related to tantric sex and everything I have read about it so far.
>
> First, let me give you a bit of background. I have been in a relationship with a man for over fourteen years. We stopped having sex several years ago—not by my choice, but by his. He is not interested in sex and nothing I have done to try and change the situation has helped. He refuses to see a counselor or go to any workshops, and simply accepts the "fact" that he has a low sex drive. Even when we were having sex, it was infrequent and not very satisfactory, despite my attempts to try different techniques to get him interested. He assures me that his lack of drive has nothing to do with his love for me and I know he does not seek other partners.

TANTRIC ORGASM AND SAME-SEX PARTNERS

A few years ago, I ended up—out of desperation—having an affair with another woman. It was not something I sought out necessarily, though I was vulnerable and had at times in my life felt attractions to women. What I discovered through this affair was that, for me, sex with a woman was much more pleasurable than I had ever experienced with a man. The reason was that it was not "goal oriented" sex and had more to do with sensual pleasure. Often, my female partner and I never had orgasms, but would make love for hours. Of course, I recognize that I could just as easily have had a female partner who had bought into the idea of sex being all about the orgasm. I think this is how we are socialized in Western cultures and therefore even lesbians buy into this view.

When I began reading about tantric sex, it brought to mind my affair and my feelings about lesbian sex. It seemed to me that two women are more likely to naturally practice a more tantric style of sex, because we are more sensual (and I know we could argue that this, too, is related to the way women are socialized). However, I noticed that there is very little written about homosexual sex as it pertains to tantric practices. It seems most of the reputable tantric Web sites are extremely heterosexually oriented. My attempts to find anything on tantric sex for lesbians lead me mostly to pornographic Web sites or to workshops for lesbians with nothing written on the topic. And, although I remain in my chaste, heterosexual relationship, I identify myself as bisexual and would like to see more balance. Is there a reason that most of the books are for heterosexuals? Is it related somehow to the spiritual origins of tantric practices that perhaps don't allow for homosexual love? I am just curious—and I'm not sure you have the answers, but I am sure there are many gay and lesbian people out there wondering the same thing.

This is only one of several messages that I have received over the last few years asking me the same question: what about tantra and homosexuals? It is sometimes also asked during my heterosexual couple workshops, because most people have a homosexual sibling or friend. While I cannot say I have confirmed answers, I do have insights into how tantric principles can be applied between bodies of the same sex. My own tantric exploration has been within the heterosexual sphere, although every hug I share with a person is a tantric moment, be it a man or woman.

For many of us, exploring sexuality with a same-sex partner is part of a progression of natural sexual development. Human sexuality makes its first appearance in an auto-erotic way, in the exploration of the pleasures of one's own genitals in early childhood. This will usually change within a few years into a curiosity about the genitals of others of the same sex (homosexuality). There can also be a simultaneous interest in the genitals of the opposite sex, hence the ubiquitous "doctors and nurses" games that children create intentionally to explore each other's genitals. The actual attraction to the opposite sex (heterosexuality) for the purposes of sexual intercourse comes as a later, third, phase.

Society frowns upon and discourages innocent sexual interaction between children in their search to know themselves. Part of this is because it often happens between siblings, due to their proximity to each other, and the fear is that it will foster incestuous relationships. When we as children are discovered while attempting to fulfil our sexual curiosity, we get punished, made to feel we have done something wrong, made to feel guilty about the pleasure we have elicited from our genitals. If we manage to get away with it undiscovered, we nevertheless feel guilty for having done something secretly and therefore wrongly. Through fear of sex and lack of understanding of true sexuality, the sexual/life energy becomes repressed in each of us.

For some people, exploration with the same sex can extend into teenage years through the forced separation of the sexes, as in unisex boarding schools. Monasteries or other institutions that hold men and women apart will automatically encourage sexual exploration with the same sex. As the basic life force, sex is a drive that demands expression. What matters is whom you choose—or who is available—to consummate this expression with.

For survival we are designed to reproduce, which makes heterosexuality the next step in human sexual expression. (There *is* a fourth stage, at which an exceptional individual fully transcends sex through having embraced its elements deeply and then lives in twenty-four-hour ecstasy.)

Many people in later years, especially women, will opt totally out of sex because it fails to satisfy. (For some men this is a less easy choice, hence the many perverse ways some men release their sexual frustrations.) Women easily become autosexual again, or they become asexual, avoiding their own genitals completely. Some women deliberately choose a same-sex partner or find themselves emerging with an attraction to their same sex. A couple of lesbian women have told me that they felt they were born lesbian and were never really interested in males at any time. In fact, they were attracted to other girls before they even knew what sexual attraction was. There can be many reasons for abstention, just as there can be for the homosexual option.

But as I see the situation at present, for countless generations now we have been without positive reflection of man's and woman's sexual potential and the love that is so created. This lack of example is due to the very misunderstanding of sex itself, the theme of earlier chapters. As things stand, in the absence of guidance or insight into sexual expression, it can be easier to avoid the challenge presented by the unknown opposite sex (a complex challenge, given the level of sexual misunderstanding). Instead one can choose either to abstain from sexual contact completely, or to stay with the same sex because that sex is known and understood, since it is also a part of oneself.

Awareness of Present Moment, Relaxation, Sensitivity

If I were to simply divide the tantric approach in half, there would be a) the essential aspect of the so-called present moment, and b) the essential aspect of bodies existing as equal and opposite forces. As far as the first aspect goes, any two people, homosexual or heterosexual, can be increasingly more present to each other, more in and down in the body and aware of themselves, and thus more sensitive to their partners, their children, their parents. The more physically close we are, as in the case of lovers, the greater the opportunity to practice awareness and create the present between us. For same-sex partners, as with heterosexuals, the tantric principles apply all the way.

Tantra tells us to be aware of what we do and how we do it, to unhook slowly from excitement and drift toward relaxation, to practice being here and now and not so pinpointed on a goal. The implication is that for *all* lovers the effort is toward *not* using the genitals solely for climax purposes. The attempt is still to retain the energy so that it can spread through the body and empower the body, and to avoid the repeated discharge of life energy. It continues to mean that love should be a meditation rather than an activity.

For any two people, eye contact—using receptive soft vision as described in chapter 2—will profoundly intensify the meeting, as will relaxing into orgasm, as discussed in detail in chapter 9. Slowing down in any or all movements will enhance the experience tremendously. Consciously breathing will expand your body energies beautifully. Kissing deeply with the lips adds intimacy and intensity. Any awareness, and the challenge that comes with it, creates a bond, a sense of a unifying force encompassing greater intimacy and love. This happens because awareness transforms sex into love. And love is what we are all longing to receive and to give. Presence, silence, stillness, the essence of meditation and relaxation can be developed as a heart-opening link between any two people. Even a person alone will benefit from more inner awareness, more stillness and relaxation, meditation, less focus on the goal in any daily activities, less doing and more being in the here and now, enjoying the moment.

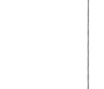

Opposite Polarities and Genital Correspondence

Many of the guidelines listed above can be used with equal effect by both heterosexual lovers and homosexual lovers. However, most of the guidelines for sexual intercourse pertain to heterosexuals and will therefore not apply. Nevertheless, the information can be of value in reconceiving how one goes about genital intercourse, and why. Heterosexual guidelines do not apply because of the sameness of the genitals in same-sex partners: the genitals do not correspond with each other and fit one into the other. The genitals are equal but they are not opposite; instead of a hand in a glove there is a glove and a glove, or a hand and a hand.

Tantra is based on the union of male and female aspects as equal and

opposite forces. Without the sexual organs corresponding there exists little possibility, as I see it, for the subtle exchange of organic sexual energies—where the penis in response to the vagina awakens the inner streamings in the bodies, the connection itself acting like a jump-start to a different dimension of the inner world. This opposition, attraction, and electromagnetic interplay inherent to the penis and the vagina cannot function in the same way for homosexual couples. This is a disadvantage because the gay or lesbian couple is not able to just hang out and let the current run, as a heterosexual couple can do.

With women couples, for example, where the overall polarity is feminine, there will be a meeting of two receptive genitals, negative with negative (vagina-vagina) and positive with positive (heart/breasts-heart/breasts) instead of vice versa, positive to negative, which completes the circuit. The absence of the tantric aspect of genital correspondence in homosexual sex requires a complete re-viewing of the genitals and how to use them in applying tantric principles to create higher states. The first shift is already mentioned in the previous section: a stepping away from stimulation and excitement to discover ways of containing the sexual energy and so inviting it to rise upward, not discharging it.

The same challenges of moving away from one's sexual conditioning apply to homosexuals as to heterosexuals. Perhaps it might be more difficult, especially for gay men, to find a passive, more feminine way of being with each other's genitals, instead of constantly seeking intensity of sensation. The problem with excessive stimulation is that it makes the genitals insensitive; they begin to lose their capacity to feel, and slowly nothing turns you on any more, the old tricks don't seem to work. Then there is a need and desire for more and more stimulation, which in some cases can leave a person feeling quite numb to himself. The inner sensitivities have been blasted with an overdose of sensation. Sensitivity arises with awareness, so when we use our bodies insensitively to satisfy our sexual minds, we are closing ourselves down to our inner treasures. The guideline for any couple interested in tantra, homosexual or heterosexual, is always to seek sensitivity rather than sensation. Sensation dulls while sensitivity awakens inner sources of delight and pleasure.

The Auto-Ecstatic Individual

Having stated clearly the genital need of equal and opposite forces as essential to tantra, I remind you now that our basic inner set-up is bisexual. This is indeed the very foundation of tantra. Each one of us contains male and female poles, which makes each individual essentially auto-ecstatic. It seems rather obvious, then, that there has always been and will always be a variety of sexual expressions among human beings. In the homosexual connection, the inherent potential of the sexual situation is limited, first because reproduction is not possible, and second because of the lack of alignment in polarity. But I am certain that the ultimate potential of the individual is not affected, because ultimately the source of orgasmic states lies within each person; it is an inner celebration of the male and female elements. So it becomes more a question of how we get there, how we awaken our inner ecstatic potential. In homosexuality and heterosexuality the routes are similar and at the same time diverse.

On my way to deliver the completed manuscript of this book to the publisher, I fortunately and unexpectedly met a friend who then sent me the following report about her experiences with sex.

A woman shares her experience: "My entire life I have been bisexual. Sex used to be frustrating with both the sexes. This temporary fit of ecstasy left me almost always feeling empty afterward. So I was insatiable, a true nymphomaniac. Then many years ago I participated in a group with Diana—we called it 'The Tantra Experiment.' It changed my view and experience of sex completely. Here I was practicing how to *not* run with my hormones and lust, learning to relax into sex. Nothing really tantric was happening yet, but mysteriously it was the most fulfilling sex I had ever had. After that I was only interested in tantric lovemaking, which at that point only happened with men. When a woman crossed my path I would have a short fling, but I did not want to go back to what I called 'doing' sex.

"Everything changed when I met my female partner four years ago. To my great astonishment, the famous 'circle of energy' happened without genital penetration. A kiss or an embrace was enough to set off the silent implosion. My mind was like scrambled eggs. I could not comprehend it. It

shattered a lot of beliefs and ideas I had about male and female. After all, the male and female reside in every human being; it seemed that we both have integrated these polarities and can rest in the silence of being and heart. This is a total energetic penetration! Sometimes one of us is more in the 'male,' outgoing energy and the circling goes in one direction. Sometimes it goes in two directions at the same time. At times it is full on and at times not. One thing is that we cannot 'do' it. Maybe there are ways to direct the energy that we are not aware of yet. In my experience, the difference between tantra with the opposite sex and tantra with a same-sex partner is that with the opposite sex the genital penetration almost always allows for the circle of energy to happen, or at least more easily. At the same time, right now I am menopausal and there is not always enough sexual energy available to allow for the tantric orgasm. The ecstatic melting then happens purely in the heart."

The Focus of Sexual Exchange for Women

As far as women go, a tantric approach means shifting away from an over-focused clitoral approach that encourages excitement and toward a style in which the breasts are loved and understood as the focal point of the female energy system. As explained in chapter 5, breasts are the source of the energy in a woman's deepest orgasm; an orgasmic state can be experienced just through deeply loving the breasts. (A woman can lavish love on her own breasts as well, to arouse herself into an expanded state.) The energy of the breasts accumulates and spreads downward, resonating in the vagina. For this there is no necessity of penetration by a penis.

Instead of going for excitement and orgasm, a lover should treat the clitoris more gently and passively, so as to create a flow of energy backward into the vagina. In fact, she should treat the vagina itself gently. Any phallic substitutes will naturally lack the electromagnetic intelligence possessed by the penis in relation to the vagina. In particular, there is perhaps less perception and sensitivity in the upper vaginal region, which is significant in deep penetration by the penis for the accessing of ecstatic energies in women. A lifeless, phallic-shaped object cannot meaningfully communicate with the receptive feminine pole; however, mechanical vibrations

emanating from them can do something to awaken the more subtle energies. Fingers certainly have much more sensitivity than a vibrator but only when offered with a delicate, loving, conscious touch. There are beneficial therapeutic massage techniques that can help to release tensions that are held in the vagina and obscure its polarity. (These require personal instruction and are therefore beyond the scope of this book.) However, fingers will naturally lack the perception, finesse, and catalytic effect of the "magnetic" penis head (chapter 6). If simulating vaginal penetration, the guideline would be to do so in a fashion that steers away from friction and excessive building of excitement (resulting in more tensions). Move toward relaxation and the sustained presence of the finger(s) (short nails!) as the receptive partner absorbs, while primarily focusing on the heart and breasts. The receptive partner may feel a circling downward to the vagina that returns upward to the heart via the inner "magnetic rod." Or she can positively direct the imagination toward the inner circle of energy: breasts-vagina-breasts. In this way it is possible for a woman to experience an ecstatic state without necessarily involving a clitoral orgasm and an undue discharge of energy, just as in the case of a heterosexual woman, who may have the additional help of the penis in the vagina to open the inner channels.

Homosexual Love and the Feminist Movement

For many feminists today, the clitoris has become a symbol of woman's sexual freedom because through it woman is able to reclaim her long lost orgasm. This movement is certainly well motivated but perhaps a little misled in that what has emerged is an intensified focus on the clitoris, with a corresponding abandonment of the vagina and the receptive pole of feminine energy. The clitoris, through a buildup of excitement, is used as a "positive pole" for discharge, not as a link back into the vagina to connect with the receptive energies. With the focus on the clitoris also comes talk of multiple orgasms (which are indeed possible, and will always be a temptation); however, these are based primarily on excitement, with its consequences of tension and emotionality.

Because at present we see this major identification with the clitoris as

TANTRIC ORGASM AND SAME-SEX PARTNERS

the center of female sexuality, some feminists may view the relative de-emphasizing of the clitoris in the tantric picture as a step backward for the feminist movement, and for women in general. It is also quite possible that women who are unfamiliar with (or inexperienced in) the intrinsic power of yielding or giving way through a more absorbent and receptive approach will strongly react to my tantric suggestions on the feminist level. They may feel a resistance to giving up the male approach, which they have used in freeing themselves sexually. However, with understanding of the connection between peak orgasm and distressing states of emotionality (see chapter 10), women may see that they need to explore themselves on a different level when together as lovers.

In tantric exploration, women should avoid the temptation to go for the so-called male approach because basically it is an imitation of man, who is at this time completely unconscious in his sexual expression and by no means a reflection of the qualities of true masculine force. Trying to be like a man only makes a woman hard and tough and inaccessible. To begin with, a woman should go for being feminine and as a consequence, her *real* inner man will awaken. Naturally within any two people (heterosexual or homosexual) a certain kind of polarity can develop—one may shift to become the more responsible, worldly, doing type (positive) while the other becomes the more encompassing, loving, being type (negative)—but in sexual love with one another, women should not really attempt to copy men. Rather, two women can find the feminine way to make love by reconfiguring the essential elements.

Recently I spoke with a good friend who has many gay and lesbian couples as close friends. She told me that this is what she observes: the gay couples tend toward being more womanlike while the lesbian couples tend to being more manlike. *Both* of the partners in each couple tend toward the equal and opposite that is lacking in their couple. This can be understood as a balancing of polarities, which for sure it is in a certain sense; but unfortunately, I repeat, for a woman to be like a man is not to her ultimate advantage.

Where homosexuals are at an automatic disadvantage is in not being able to "hang out" with genitals united and let sex happen by itself, the way

190

that heterosexual couples can. The tantric union of male and female elements produces the current of sexual (life) energy, providing an ongoing focus for awareness and a source of great pleasure. It is possible to sustain hours of penetration without doing much at all. The correspondence of the genitals encourages a "being" approach—in fact, sex presents the perfect circumstances for meditation.

In contrast, the homosexual lack of correspondence leads to a more "doing" approach, which easily turns to excitement and peak orgasm. Nevertheless the thrust should always be toward "being" even while a certain amount of "doing" may be required, and of course all kinds of doing can be radically modified by using awareness, as suggested earlier in the chapter. It is likely that female homosexuals, when they drop the orgasm-oriented style of sex, tend toward a meditative type of sexual expression more easily than male homosexuals, simply by virtue of their overall negative polarity.

I sent this chapter to a friend of mine who has had sexual experiences with both men and women, asking for her comments. I am most grateful to her for her response, which follows.

A woman shares her experience: "So, I read your chapter and I'll tell you a little of what my experience has been. Having known the tantric way with men, it has always been a conflict for me to be with women, knowing that the advantages of opposite polarity are not possible. However, for many other reasons, I keep finding myself drawn to relationships with women over and over again.

"I'm still in the search of what can or can't be done with a woman, and I'm trying to understand a little bit more what happens energetically when I am with a woman. I think it would take a lot more experience than what I have to give really conclusive answers, but I have had some experiences (one was very strong) that might give a little direction as to where to begin.

"Whether I was with a man or a woman, I had never liked being penetrated by anything other than a penis (fingers, vibrators, etc). When I had sex with a woman, I was limited to caressing, touching, and oral sex, which always led to orgasm because the clitoris was always involved.

"Then, with a female partner, I decided to try penetration with a finger with the specific intention of not seeking excitement and orgasm. I asked her to gently penetrate me and not move inside—a simulation of silent penetration with a penis. I could feel the two pulses, my vagina's and her finger's. It was delicious to just feel the pulsation there with no movement or stimulation. After a little while the pulses started synchronizing and it was a pretty delicious experience, with no need of excitement or orgasm at all. We did it several times and I started noticing a mini, mini, mini similarity to sensations I've had with men, very subtle energy flowing throughout the body.

"Then came the issue of still having memories in my body of having been raped as a child. As I had mentioned to you when you were in the process of writing about sexual abuse and its effects, the problem for most women in this situation is that while the polarity created by a gentle penetration by the penis is a great way to cleanse those memories from the vagina, most woman in severe trauma will not get to that point. Often they fear intimacy or they can't attract men or they have turned to relationships with women or, as a means of repeating the pattern, they end up attracting the wrong men who certainly can't be very meditative about sex. For myself, once the memory was there it was simply impossible, for several of the above reasons, to get myself into such a healing situation with a man.

"Back to the silent penetration exercise with my female partner: Once again I asked her to penetrate me gently with a finger and to not move. When the pulses started synchronizing, I asked her to start applying a very soft pressure in different directions, first up, staying there for a while with both of us in silence. And sure enough, a lot of energy started moving. Then she applied pressure on the diagonal, then to the right, and so forth—slight pressure with the whole finger. Most of the time I experienced a very silent cleansing, just feeling and breathing, while a couple of times there was a little more, crying and strong emotions coming to the surface. It was pretty unbelievable to be dealing with my past trauma it in this way.

"After we did this several times, the energy in my vagina was clearly more open and the penetration without movement became more and more pleasant. Once, I *did* have an experience that could be compared to a tantric one with a man. How that happened without the opposing polarity of the penis and vagina, god knows. It just did. It was certainly not as intense or as obvious as my experiences with men, but then again, I haven't delved into this that much.

"Clearly the first aspect of tantra, as you mention in the chapter, is the first opening for gay couples. About the second aspect and the polarity issue, the above is the only thing I can share for the moment. Maybe this approach could open a door for lesbian women. I really can't say for sure."

I have heard it suggested that in homosexual couples, the polarity of one partner can energetically shift into its opposite, so that same-sex couples will begin to internally balance each other on a polarity level. This implies that in one lesbian partner the negative vagina would shift to a positive phenomenon, and the breasts to a passive one. I am inclined to doubt this, especially in view of the fact that when a woman has a breast or her cervix removed, the magnetic phenomenon present in the physical tissues continues to exist on an energetic level.

In saying this I am aware that there is very little research done on homosexual experience, and research could perhaps prove me quite wrong. A friend recently told me that a lesbian she knows, who has been interested only in women from the beginning of her sexual life, feels that she has an "etheric penis." Perhaps something of this nature is possible without an actual change occurring in the body energy. Certainly, if she is talking about an "inner penis," which is the experience of a constantly alive magnetic rod, then I can relate to this feeling. With the current emphasis in sex being toward excitement, not toward meditation, we will need a major shift in consciousness for a reliable body of material on homosexual tantric experience to emerge in order to give substance to its practice.

Because this is a book for women, I am not saying much about gay men; however, the many principles of tantra will of course apply to them, in the sense that the energy is encouraged to stream inward and upward toward the heart (positive to negative) instead of being discharged from the positive. And not unlike the dildo/penis replacement, I do feel it is unlikely that the highly erotic zone of the anus can successfully replace the electromagnetic cavity of the vagina. (This applies also to the case of heterosexuals who take part in anal sex, although the female internal connection via the anus may perhaps be different from that of the male). It is likely that the anal approach is seldom slow and easy—that is, tantric style—but instead reflects the conventional style of going for stimulation, excitement, and ejaculation. Until the anus is not used for stimulation and eroticism, we will not know whether there is some internal, magical, electromagnetic connection to be made there.

Tantric Spiritual Background Is Heterosexual

From its origin tantra has been oriented toward heterosexuality. The subject of our study here, the so-called left hand path of tantra, uses the sexual current on a physical level for an outer union (man and woman), which leads to an inner union, which results in states of meditative ecstasy.*

In India we find a multitude of temples that are now thousands of years old (the most famous ones being in Khajuraho) containing statues of man and woman in sexual union. Usually these stone partners are maintaining some acrobatic position in which, when viewed conventionally, one cannot imagine how they achieve any kind of sex at all. But with the advantage of tantric eyes, knowing that the penetration of the vagina can be sustained for hours and produce endless delight, one sees that these statues do represent reality, positions and all! The remarkable thing about many of these statues is that you can actually see the ecstasy alive in their faces and you feel it radiating as you look at them. The people who built those temples in ancient times, especially the sculptors of the statues, were not artisans but artists, living the very experience they were creating in stone. Their personal inner experience was embodied in stone; their ecstasy is still palpable thousands of years later.

---

*The right hand path is the school of the Buddhist tantric meditation practices in which sexual energy is employed on a symbolic level; the practitioner uses visualization to stimulate the inner union.

The emphasis on heterosexuality in these spiritual practices is not due to a sexual prejudice but exists because tantric experiences arise with ease between the opposite forces of male and female. Tantric sex is the most direct and natural route to awaken the inner opposite force within oneself, the outer opposite being used to reach the inner opposite. Woman can use man to awaken her inner man. Without the genital correspondence, which in and of itself creates intense ecstatic moments, a sustained, meditative state of union for hours at a time becomes more difficult. But for sure it is not out of the question. To really explore the tantric frame as a homosexual requires deconditioning the stimulation-as-sexuality attitude and rediscovering sensitivity as a door to bliss—the same tasks required of heterosexuals.

Masturbation and Self-Love

On the question of masturbation, or self-love, once again the tantric principle applies: anything done with awareness cannot be wrong or unnatural. It is not what you do but how you do it. As always, experiment with loving yourself in a way that does not depend exclusively on excitement but on expansion of energy through relaxation. Retain the energy in your body without automatically discharging it. While masturbating, avoid unnecessary contractions in the body or in the vagina, and don't be too demanding of the clitoris. If you have an orgasm, don't force it—relax into it, take it all very slowly. The masturbation that includes more and more intense stimulation to the clitoris or vagina can slowly deaden the very sensitivity that is sought, in the end leaving not much pleasure at all.

Include the breasts in your experience. Make them the focus, make the shift away from the clitoris as you discover the new doorway to sexual expression. Stroke, caress, and expand the energy through your own body or your partner's. A woman alone, or on her own, can enhance her femininity by meditating on the breasts as suggested at the end of chapter 5. Lesbian women can use this practice to support the awakening of the orgasmic energy in the body, doing it as a separate practice or as part of foreplay. Then, during lovemaking, massage your own breasts and also show your partner how to touch your breasts. Even though with two

women together there will be more knowing about how breasts feel while being touched, it is a beneficial practice to be guided by the one you love. In the same way, explore the clitoris and the surrounding area, sharing and discovering what kind of touch supports the sensations and sensitivity in your body and what distracts from your more subtle inner feelings and delicate sensations.

Applying Tantric Principles to Same-Sex Relationships

Quite a few years ago in Mexico City I had the opportunity to work with a group of nine gay couples who were all HIV positive. I was given the concluding day with them as the grand finale of a six-month-long intensive healing program that included meditation and natural therapies, which had assisted their physical and psychological conditions tremendously. I was invited for the final wrap-up because the therapist wished for the men to be left with a positive impression about sex. Most of them had really disastrous sexual backgrounds and exceptionally negative imprints about sex, as well as a sexually transmitted disease to top it off. In these painful and challenging circumstances it was not easy for them to view sex with any feelings of contentment or joy.

As at that point I had never imagined applying tantra to homosexual couples, I at first balked at the invitation from my friend, the therapist. After some thought, I told her that I would present the aspect of tantra that pertains to inner awareness and creating the present moment. I would not, however, be willing to explain the picture of the innate polarities and how the male-female interaction is conceived by nature. But my friend was insistent—I was to give the complete picture—and I reluctantly agreed, not really seeing the point of it.

The morning was a beautiful experience. Leading the male couples through a structure that brought them into the present moment with each other, I saw before my eyes a profound transformation that turned out to be a great teaching for me: a conscious, sensitive merging into each other; relaxing into the now of the body; melting into tender, powerful

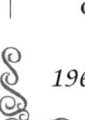

hugs. Silence and sincerity and love filled the air. It was so touching that at times I had tears in my eyes, as did many of the men themselves.

At the end of the morning one man shared the wish that he had found this space, or known how to find it, with his lover years earlier. It would have made all the difference; and now it was late for it, given the knowledge that he was nearing the end of his life.

After a break for lunch, we resumed in the afternoon with a discussion of the male-female polarities, the interaction of the penis and vagina, the breasts, and erection. The information was received with much interest and I felt and saw no resistance at all among the men. We finished with a meditation imagining the energy circles in our own bodies, then had tearful, loving farewells before going our separate ways.

This impressive experience gave me the authority to say that *all* couples, regardless of gender, definitely have positive, inspiring experiences when they use tantric principles during intimacy. Every couple can benefit from being more aware and relaxed when making love, and all human bodies have both positive and negative polarities within them. As more homosexual couples experiment with tantra, I look forward to their feedback on how they have put these ideas into practice to engender successful and loving relationships.

Tantric Inspiration

Man has to transcend sex, whatsoever kind of sex it is, because unless you go beyond your biology you will never know your soul. Meanwhile—before you go beyond—it is your freedom to be whatsoever you want to be.

Don't make a problem out of it. Nothing has to be done about it. I don't tackle individual problems. My whole approach is that there are millions of diseases and only one cure and that cure is meditation.

You meditate—homosexual, heterosexual, bisexual... You meditate. Become more still and more silent. Create inner emptiness. Become more transparent. And then things will start changing. You will be able to see what you are doing to yourself. And if it is right you will go on doing it with more joy, with more totality, with more intensity, with more passion. And if it is wrong it will simply drop, just like dead leaves falling from a tree. So I cannot suggest any specific method because to me all the problems are arising because we have become minds and we have forgotten that deep down there is a space within us which can be called no-mind. Entering that space, no-mind, will give you perspective, vision, clarity.

Meditate. Sit silently watching your thoughts—homosexual, heterosexual, whatsoever they are, it doesn't matter. You watch, you become the witness. Slowly, slowly a distance will be created between you and your thoughts. And one day suddenly—the realization that you are not your mind. And that day a revolution has happened within you. After that day you will never be the same again. A transcendence will have happened.

OSHO, TRANSCRIBED TEACHINGS,
THE BOOK OF THE BOOKS, VOLUME 9

Tantric Meditation
The Golden Flower

Do this meditation early in the morning or when you are going to sleep at night.

Lie down comfortably in your bed, on your back, with about half an hour to yourself. Relax for a few minutes with your eyes closed. When you breathe in, begin to visualize great light entering from your head into your body, as if a sun has just risen close to your head—golden light pouring into your head, as if you are hollow and golden light is pouring in at the top and going deeper and deeper, all the way down and out through your toes. As you breathe out, visualize darkness entering through your toes, a great dark river entering through your toes, traveling all the way up and out through your head.

Do slow, deep breathing so you can visualize this. Go very slowly. Breathing in, let golden light come into you through the top of your head; it is here that the Golden Flower opens. The golden light will cleanse your whole body and will fill it with creativity. This is male energy. When you exhale, you let darkness, the deepest darkness you can conceive, like a dark night, come from your toes upward like a river, and out through your head. This is feminine energy. It soothes you and makes you receptive. It calms you and gives you rest. Then inhale again and let the golden light enter in. Keep breathing in this manner for about twenty minutes and then relax after that for another ten minutes.

You can do this early in the morning, when you just start to wake and are still wavering between sleep and waking. Right there, start the process of breathing in the light and breathing out darkness for twenty minutes. If you do the meditation at night and you fall asleep doing it, the impact will remain in the subconscious and will go on working. After a three-month period you will begin to notice that the energy that was constantly building up and concentrating itself in the sex center is no longer gathering there. The energy is going upward; the energy begins rising by itself.

Conclusion
Embracing Our True Feminine Power

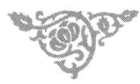

*W*ith the unmasking of woman's true role in sex and the profound implications of true femininity, it is possible that you will find contradictory feelings arising simultaneously—an uplifting sense of inspiration or empowerment along with the heaviness of feeling overwhelmed and intimidated by new input, daunted and unsure about how to proceed, how to alter the way of making love *in reality*. Rather than getting bogged down in all the pros and cons, simply take immediate action by starting to refocus on the body right away. Even this very second, while sitting and reading, relax the jaw and shoulders, the belly. Enjoy two or three nice deep breaths as the pleasure of a physical letting go spreads through you. Or rest with your awareness in the breasts and nipples for the next few minutes, sensing them from within, radiating warmth outward. Close the eyes and enjoy feeling rooted in your body; it is the link to your being, a natural bridge to the endless source of love residing within you.

Shifting awareness from mind to body, as you have just done and as you

CONCLUSION: EMBRACING OUR TRUE FEMININE POWER

are encouraged to do by the tantric meditations offered at the end of each chapter, will gradually have an impact on your body. As sensitivity increases, subtle yet powerful shifts will be detectable in your energy system. Shifts of awareness back and down into the body can be done at will at any time. In place of being caught up in the endless circling train of thoughts, begin directing attention inward, merging internally with any pleasant sensations present in your body. The next time you embrace your lover or make love, make similar shifts of awareness, from the outer to the inner. Start out innocently; be childlike, stepping to the side of the known sexual you, and sink into your body. This instantly creates a more relaxed unhurried "tantric" state of being, without the pressure of big goals and expectations clouding the simple reality of two human bodies together. Take small experimental steps each time you make love or hug (porously) or kiss (lingeringly). While hugging, caressing, kissing become merged with the experience of *how* you are doing it, so that the whole experience evolves in graceful slow motion, choreographed by inner awareness. Experiment with some of the guidelines given in the earlier chapters, then attempt others, then begin putting together various combinations according to what your experience reveals to you.

You will find it advantageous to play with reducing excitement, thereby reducing the urges for conventional orgasm, and losing the creative potential of lovemaking. Introducing awareness allows you to move into the encounter in a sensual catlike way, connected to what is happening as it is happening. Let it be a mobilization of all your senses. Intensify your awareness of your vagina; consciously transform its quality into a receptive channel, instilling it with an absorbent, drinking quality, which is enticing, alluring, inviting, available, and welcoming to the male force. Also bring the breasts into awareness and see what impact this has on your responses. What deepens your yes; what reduces your yes? What expands your body energy; what causes a shrinking? What heightens sensitivity; what deadens sensitivity? Pursue any avenues that interest to you in particular. For instance, if the clitoris is a place you emphasize, experiment with including it in a more relaxed undemanding way or leaving it out or leaving it to later. The inner attitude should be investigative, rather than

being an attitude of impatient expectation or demand for immediate results. Instead, cultivate an attitude of observation, standing back and challenging routine patterns, then witness what happens. As an outcome, you will gradually establish the truth in yourself. It is a challenge to confront oneself in this way, let me not lull you into thinking it necessarily effortless. Of course it takes an effort to break away from the past but it is the effort of being aware, not the effort of doing. In time it becomes less and less effort to remain rooted in the body; one is simply present with joy.

In the process of bringing awareness to habitual, unconscious sexual habits a gradual inner transformation takes place. You will emerge with new eyes, new values, new insights, indeed you will view and experience all of life from another perspective. Reinventing yourself as a woman or arriving at your femininity anew will be the result of a slow, steady pursuit. By following an inner inquiry you embrace the willingness to reveal a deeper layer of yourself to yourself. Osho encourages us in this way:

And this merger [sex] should not become unconscious, otherwise you miss the point. Then it is a beautiful sex act, but not transformation. It is beautiful, nothing is wrong in it, but it is not transformation. And if it is unconscious then you will always be moving in a rut. Again and again you will want to have this experience. The experience is beautiful as far as it goes, but it will become a routine. And each time you have it, again more desire is created. The more you have it, the more you desire it, and you move in a vicious circle. You don't grow, you just rotate.

Rotation is bad, because then growth is not happening. Then energy is simply wasted. Even if the experience is good, the energy is wasted, because much more was possible. And it was just at the corner, just a turn, and much more was possible. With the same energy the divine could have been achieved. With the same energy the ultimate ecstasy is possible, and you are wasting that energy in momentary experiences. And by and by those experiences will become boring, because repeated again and again, everything becomes a boring thing. When the newness is lost, boredom is created.

If you remain alert you will see: first, changes of energy in the body, second, dropping of the thoughts from the mind; and third, dropping of

CONCLUSION: EMBRACING OUR TRUE FEMININE POWER

the ego from the heart. And when this third thing has happened, your energy, that sex energy has become meditative energy.[1]

Doubts can easily surface and dampen our creative and courageous responses to the truth. Mind, with its many voices, will begin with excuses to put us off taking action now, encouraging us into postponement. Doubts are triggered by our fear of the unknown, a fear of standing naked, stripped of our stylized skills and strategies, and a deep fear that our control will be lost. However, witnessing instills a new control, the control of the witnessing self, the control that arises through awareness. This type of control is so natural that you never ever feel that you are controlling. In reality, through understanding and experiencing the feminine body from a new perspective, woman will not be devalued or depreciated in any way. In fact this new awareness is a tremendous empowerment.

When we (man and woman) learn to understand one another's psychology and physiology, we can embrace our biology and our spirituality as one. With a multidimensional quality to it, sex has a far deeper significance than the production of children. It is also fun; it is play; it is prayer; it is meditation; it is a merging into oneness, into love; it is true spirituality.

For many a man (as he knows himself now), sex is not a spiritual phenomenon but only a physiological release, more in the direction of an emotional release of pent up tensions and feelings. For women sex is always, to large extent, a spiritual phenomenon, which is why women easily feel offended in sex. Unless love happens as part of a greater spiritual experience she has trouble opening up to it. Participation in loveless sex is the precise reason that so many millions of women have completely forgotten what orgasm means. Women have become sexually repressed due to man's nonunderstanding of the difference between the sexes. But it is not man's fault, personally; he too is a by-product of the social, sexual misunderstanding in force today.

The tragedy of this repression of woman and her sexual power is that whenever man's and woman's real nature is not allowed to go according to its inner needs it turns sour, becomes poisoned, crippled, or paralyzed; it can even become perverted. If woman is corrupted by man, man himself

CONCLUSION: EMBRACING OUR TRUE FEMININE POWER

cannot remain natural either. After all, the woman gives birth to the man. If woman, as mother, does not express her sexuality naturally, her children will not learn a natural expression either. Woman certainly needs a great liberation but not through imitation of man, not through being equal to man by being exactly like him. Instead, woman's true liberation will come through being an authentic and opposite force to man.

It is an undeniably painful reality that today millions of women on Earth continue to be dominated by male sexual unconsciousness, subjected to all kinds of inhumanity, humiliation, and aggression, suffering untold emotional and physical pain as part of daily living. For these unfortunate women the fine tuning of "feminine energy," is the remotest of their concerns because, tragically, reality is dominated by the sheer struggle for survival. As women from a more privileged sector of society (which we are if holding this book in our hands) we can join our hearts in the silence of prayer, willing days of peace, love and balance to manifest on Earth. Any change in the global sexual situation cannot be dependant on a mass solution. It needs to emerge from individual consciousnesses and spread outward into the collective consciousness in true homeopathic fashion. Each woman, through understanding herself more intimately, has the capacity and power to transform her living situation into one that is satisfying and nourishing to her, thereby passing higher values down the generational line.

Returning full circle to the introduction of the book, we, as women from the privileged sector of society, are in a position to be responsible to ourselves for creating love and not letting things run on lovelessly as they have for hundreds of years. Never underestimate our intrinsic power as female members of the species. Women are very powerful people, not in the muscular sense but as far as their resistance is concerned, their life energy is concerned, their sex energy is concerned, their tolerance is concerned. Woman's whole functioning is intrinsically graceful, insightful, loving, compassionate. Henceforth woman should not rely on permission or cooperation from man before taking experimental steps to find her true self through sex. Try things out, in and out of bed, independent of your partner and what he thinks or expects or wants. Observe what happens within yourself and

CONCLUSION: EMBRACING OUR TRUE FEMININE POWER

between yourself and your partner on an energy level. If your man is worth his salt his response will follow your lead, trusting and sensing the capacity for natural authority that all women have in sex when given the chance.

Since time immemorial women have been a collective force in healing, wisdom, and spiritual evolution but in this technological age we have become emotionally confused and have lost contact with our feminine truth. Feminine growth requires the willingness to feel anything and everything, including old and painful emotions, which often have less to do with the present than with the past. Recalling the difference between a feeling and an emotion is one of the most helpful keys in living a joyful, loving life. Remember, emotions themselves are not wrong but where we put the blame can be wrong, and damaging. Conquering states of emotionality, getting to the root of the emotions by expressing the feelings hiding behind them, and handling emotions in a conscious way is a powerful gift to creating inner balance. It is a step in maturity. Succumbing continually to upsurges of emotion keeps us in a childish frame to which the unfulfilled past keeps coming back in cycles, spilling over into the now in seismic upheavals.

Woman can begin to cut away from the myth that she is basically emotional, unstable, and given to bouts of moodiness. At the personality level, we as women have "learned" to be emotional, but emotion is not an aspect of woman's essential nature. The heart—at the center of our true being—knows only one language and that is the language of love. When searching and longing for love, it is very easy to lose oneself in the other, thereby unconsciously and accidentally giving up the power and grace of our feminine birthright. By opening consciously to man, inviting him in, while at the same time remaining true to our own feminine awareness, we transform sex between man and woman into love—a sublimely spiritual experience.

I leave you with these final words from Osho:

> Remember this: Tantra is a love effort towards existence. That is why so much of sex has been used by Tantra: because it is a love technique. It is not only love between man and woman; it is love between you and existence, and for the first time existence becomes meaningful to you through a woman. If you are a woman, then existence becomes for the first time meaningful to you through a man.[2]

Appendix
The Sympto-Thermal Method of Fertility Awareness

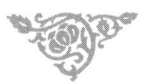

When a woman wishes to become intimate with her own fertility cycle, for contraception or for conception, possibly her best bet is to learn the Sympto-Thermal Method.* The brief introduction contained here should familiarize you with the method, but please do not consider it as definitive. It explains the basics of how the method works, but space doesn't permit a thorough explanation of all the possible exceptions to the rule that should be considered if you want to use the method for truly reliable birth control. If you would like to give the Sympto-Thermal method a serious try, please consult the Web site mentioned below for further guidance.

Instructions in this method are available worldwide. The SymptoTherm Foundation in Switzerland offers addresses and contact information for

---

*Contributors to the Sympto-Thermal Method information contained herein are R. Harri Wettstein, Ph.D., M.B.A., M.A., Director of Bioself SA, Geneva, Switzerland and secretary of the SymptoTherm Foundation, Morges, Switzerland; and Christine Bourgeois, president of the SymptoTherm Foundation.

APPENDIX: THE SYMPTO-THERMAL METHOD OF FERTILITY AWARENESS

the main organizations that teach this method on its Web site: www.symptotherm.ch. Each organization has its own competent network of counselors. For beginners, the SymptoTherm Foundation recommends the Bioself fertility indicator (www.bioself.com) as an educational tool, together with a good textbook about the method.

The Sympto-Thermal Method was developed by Catholic researchers in the early 1950s. The term was coined by Professor Josef Rötzer, an Austrian doctor who was one of its pioneers. Many universities are still conducting clinical and scientific research on this method, but its present form of practice has about twenty years of solid experience and statistical data testifying to its safety.

The original motive for the development of this practice was to find a "natural" alternative to so-called artificial contraception (which is prohibited by the Vatican) in order to enable Catholic couples to enjoy sex during infertile days, at times when pregnancy was not advised or desired. Paradoxically, the Fertility Awareness Method (FAM) schools and other secular organizations are indebted to the Catholic Natural Family Planning Institute, with which they do not agree on the issue of condom use. Thus, strict Natural Family Planning use of the method always implies periods of abstinence, whereas FAM has nothing against protected sex during the fertile phase. But FAM also recognizes that the use of a contraceptive device (condom, cervical cap, diaphragm) during fertile parts of the cycle diminishes contraceptive safety, and suggests that a contraceptive be used in conjunction with the Sympto-Thermal Method to prevent any failure.

The word *sympto-thermal,* as it relates to ovulation, means that there is (a) a temperature rise, indicating the passing of an egg (ovulation). This rise is always interpreted in relation to (b) observation of the cervical fluid, which also reveals ovarian activity. Other observations, such as breast tenderness and intermenstrual pain (e.g., a few sharp shooting pains associated with ovulation), can also help a woman attune to her cycle and become aware of when she is fertile and when she is not. The Sympto-Thermal Method always uses two signs—body temperature and vaginal secretions—and then "cross checks" them against each other.

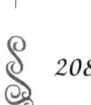

APPENDIX: THE SYMPTO-THERMAL METHOD OF FERTILITY AWARENESS

How the Sympto-Thermal Cross-Check Works

A woman's monthly cycle, starting with the first day of her menstrual period as day one, will continue with some six infertile days and then enter into the fertile phase until after ovulation. Ovulation will occur near the middle of the cycle, but there is considerable variation in the exact timing of ovulation from one woman to another. With careful observation, over time a woman can become familiar with the pattern of her cycle and know when to expect ovulation each month. To be safe, she must consider herself fertile for several days preceding and following ovulation. However, by observing her waking body temperature and her cervical mucus, a woman can confirm ovulation and know when she has entered the second, absolutely infertile phase of her cycle.

Determining the Peak Day

To determine the beginning of the postovulation infertile phase, a woman first must learn to spot the *peak day:* this is *the day of her most fertile cervical fluid.* The most fertile fluid, or mucus, looks and feels like clear, slippery, uncooked egg whites. It is very elastic and can be stretched into a long string between finger and thumb without breaking—in contrast to the sticky, opaque infertile mucus that breaks immediately when thumb and forefinger are pulled apart. Once a woman has observed fertile mucus, she can pinpoint her peak day of fertility by noting the first day that the mucus quality changes drastically and begins to dry out—that is, the peak day can only be identified for sure by mucus changes the day after. That last day of slippery mucus should be considered the peak day.

    A woman must observe the quality of her cervical fluid until she can identify it precisely. It might take her several cycles to really become familiar with her own peak symptoms. Each month she will record her peak day in her personal calendar or note it in the special chart provided in the manual. Her peak day may be the ovulation day. This is especially probable if she has on that day what some 10 percent of all women can feel—a few spasms of penetrating ache in the belly. This ache occurs on the side of the abdomen where the ovulating ovary lies.

According to scientific studies done by ultrasound tests with women who do not feel this kind of ache, there remains a 10 to 20 percent chance that ovulation occurs up to three days before or three days after the peak day. The minimal fertility window must take account of these six days of possible fertility. Because the egg lives for approximately eighteen hours after ovulation, and because sperm cells can survive for up to five or six days in the cervical crypts and folds, the fertility window generally extends to a minimum of eight days. Irregular cycles require extra vigilance.

Once the woman has spotted her peak day and noted it in her personal calendar or her cycle chart, she counts *until the evening of the third day* to fix the most probable end of her fertility. For example, let's say Wednesday is the peak day. She counts Thursday as the first day (it is also the day of her peak-day verification) and Friday as the second. She may expect infertility to begin the evening of the third day—Saturday evening in this example. How can she be absolutely sure about this forecast? By using the second sign, the temperature, as verification on Saturday morning.

Confirming Ovulation with Temperature

When practicing the sympto-thermal method a woman learns to observe her waking body temperature as a cross-check to her cervical mucus observations of fertility. To get an accurate reading of her waking temperature, she should take her temperature right after she wakes up in the morning. (It's okay go to the bathroom before taking the temperature or even to make tantric love *while* taking it, but excessive activity should be avoided before getting a reading.) For the first (estrogen-dominated) part of her cycle, a woman's waking body temperature will be slightly lower than her temperature after ovulation. Once ovulation has occurred, the waking temperature will rise slightly, due to a higher proportion of the hormone progesterone in the woman's body. So a woman can confirm the occurrence of ovulation by noticing when her waking temperature goes up. When a woman has observed three elevated waking temperatures—at least 0.2°C higher—following at least *six* of the lower temperatures, she will know that she has entered the infertile phase of her cycle and that she will remain infertile until her next menstruation, when her new cycle begins.

APPENDIX: THE SYMPTO-THERMAL METHOD OF FERTILITY AWARENESS

Only an adequate temperature rise can certify that the ovulation process is completely finished and that the absolutely infertile (progesterone) phase of the cycle has been established. (Such minute changes in temperature can be read only by special thermometers known as basal body temperature thermometers. The Bioself indicator [see page 208 for contact information for the Director of the Bioself company] is a most convenient and reliable tool for measuring temperature changes relative to the ovulation cycle.)

Exceptions

Occasionally the third high temperature may occur one or two days before the peak-day forecast would suggest (Thursday or Friday rather than Saturday, in our example here); in other words, the temperature rises before the peak day. (The Bioself indicator shows green too early.) It is then the viscosity of the cervical fluid that indicates Saturday evening as the beginning of the infertile phase. This cross-check determines the end of fertility fixed by the peak plus three days. This exception is very rare.

The following exception is more common. It is not risky, but it does extend the the fertile phase.

Let's continue with the same example. This time, the temperature does not rise immediately after the peak day, so that, on Saturday morning, the third high temperature is still not there. (The Bioself indicator shows red.) On Sunday morning, however, the fourth day after peak, the third high temperature is confirmed (the Bioself indicator shows green); thus, the absolute infertile days start Sunday evening, the fourth day after peak day.

The principle of cross-checking at work in these two exceptions, as everywhere, is this: *You always have to respect the fertility sign that comes last.*

What if the Bioself indicator still does not show green on Sunday or Monday morning? This means that ovulation *did not occur* and that the woman can expect another ovulation development with a *second peak day*. A woman can have two or more peak days especially when under stress. It is always the *last* peak that begins the count to the second, postovulatory phase. However, if the last peak day is not followed by the temperature rise before the next bleeding, the woman has had an anovulatory cycle.

In such situations, the woman fortunately can apply a general rule:

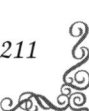

From the fourth evening after the peak day, whatever happens to the temperature curve (the Bioself indicator will continuously show red), the woman can consider herself as *relatively* infertile, as she is in the beginning of her cycle. The couple can safely have unprotected sex in the evening of every dry day while the woman daily keeps an eye on any potential new ovulation activity, indicated by the start of cervical fluid secretion. If the cycle remains anovulatory until the next bleeding, the woman might have an ovulation hidden by this bleeding. Only the temperature rise can confirm or refute this supposition.

Is Cross-Checking Always Needed?

Cross checking is only needed to screen out the exceptions noted earlier in this section. Once the woman really masters all fertility signs, according to her experience and her needs (provided her cycles remain strictly within the same pattern), she may concentrate on a single-sign approach: only the cervical fluid observation or only the temperature observation. But in doing this she may diminish the contraceptive safety provided by the cross-checking.

This, in a nutshell, is all a woman needs to know if she wants her sexuality to make friends with her fertility. The Sympto-Thermal Method also works during breast-feeding and perimenopause; it has its place in all types of cycles, during all gynecological ages. Using the Bioself indicator is the easiest way to learn and to manage this method.

Notes

Owing to the existence of a number of earlier editions of Osho's books, the author has provided the relevant chapter number instead of the page number for Osho references. The most recent publication details have been used.

Author's Introductory Note
1. Osho, *The Tantra Experience* (Pune, India: Rebel Publishing House, 1998) and Rufus C. Camphausen, *The Yoni: Sacred Symbol of Female Creative Power* (Rochester. Vt.: Inner Traditions, 1996).

Chapter 2
1. See Osho's *Fly without Wings, Walk without Feet and Think without Mind* (Full Circle Publishing, Ltd., 2000), chapter 5, question 3.
2. Mantak Chia, *Awaken Healing Energy through the Tao* (Santa Fe, N.M.: Aurora Press, 1983).

Chapter 4
1. Osho, *The Book of Secrets,* (New York: St. Martin's Press, 1998), chapter 34.
2. Julian Whitaker, M.D., and Brenda Adderly, *The Pain Relief Breakthrough* (New York: Plume, 1999).
3. Tantric *sutra* (or highly condensed telegraphic instruction) of the ancient tantric master Lord Shiva, elaborated upon in Osho's *The Book of Secrets,* chapter 71, sutra 98. *The Book of Secrets* explains Shiva's 112 tantric sutras. It was origianlly delivered as a series of talks, so Osho also answers questions from his audience about the sutras and about their experiences in meditation.

Chapter 5
1. Osho, *The Book of the Secrets,* chapter 68, question 4.
2. Ibid., chapter 67, sutra 95.

NOTES

Chapter 7
1. Natalie Angier, *Woman: An Intimate Geography* (New York: Virago, 1999), 57–81. Includes an interesting chapter on the clitoris.
2. For a remarkable description of the twenty-two different parts of the intricately formed female genitalia, see Rufus C. Camphausen, *The Yoni: Sacred Symbol of Female Creative Power*, 96–103.
3. Nik Douglas and Penny Slinger, *Sexual Secrets: The Alchemy of Ecstasy*, 20th Anniversary Edition (Rochester, Vt.: Destiny Books, 2000), 148.
4. Another Shiva sutra included in Osho's *The Book of Secrets*, chapter 75, sutra 103.

Chapter 8
1. Another Shiva sutra included in Osho's *The Book of Secrets*, chapter 47, sutra 70.

Chapter 9
1. Osho, *My Way: The Way of the White Clouds* (Pune, India: Rebel Publishing House, 1995), chapter 6, question 1.
2. Mantak Chia, *Awakening Healing Energy through the Tao*, 32.

Chapter 10
1. Osho, *The Supreme Doctrine* (Pune, India: Rebel Publishing House, 1997), chapter 5, question 3.
2. Ibid.

Conclusion
1. Osho, *My Way: The Way of the White Clouds*, chapter 6, question 1.
2. Osho, *The Book of Secrets*, chapter 43.

Recommended Books and Resources

Books and Resources by Osho
The Book of Secrets. New York: St. Martin's Press, 1998.
My Way: the Way of the White Clouds. Pune, India: Rebel Publishing House, 1995.
Sex Matters: From Sex to Superconsciousness. New York: St. Martin's Press, 2003.
The Tantra Experience. Pune, India: Rebel Publishing House, 1998.
Tantra: The Supreme Understanding. Pune, India: Rebel Publishing House, 1998.
Tantric Transformation. Pune, India: Rebel Publishing House, 1998.
(For more information about Osho, visit www.osho.com, a comprehensive Web site in different languages featuring Osho's meditations, books, tapes, and selections from his talks)

Audiotapes and Books by Barry Long
Love Brings All to Life Audio Tapes
Making Love 1 & 2 Audio Tapes
Raising Children in Love Justice and Truth. London: Barry Long Books, 1998.
Stillness is the Way. London: Barry Long Books, 1989.
(Barry Long resource materials are available from: BCM. Box 876, London WC1N 3XX U.K: info@barrylong.org; www.barrylong.org; Valeo Resources, 2820 Sunlight Drive, Clinton, WA 98236, U.S.A. blf@whidbey.net)

Books on Sexuality
Angier, Natalie. *Woman: An Intimate Geography.* New York: Virago, 1999.
Camphausen, Rufus C. *The Yoni: Sacred Symbol of Female Creative Power.* Rochester, Vt.: Inner Traditions, 1996.

RECOMMENDED BOOKS AND RESOURCES

Chan, Jolan. *The Tao of Love and Sex: The Ancient Chinese Way to Ecstasy.* Hounslow, U.K.: Wildwood House, 1977.

Chia, Mantak. *Awaken Healing Energy through the Tao,* Santa Fe, N.M.: Aurora Press, 1983.

Chia, Mantak, and Maneewan Chia. *Healing Love through the Tao: Cultivating Female Sexual Energy.* New York: Healing Tao Books, 1986.

Douglas, Nik and Penny Slinger. *Sexual Secrets,* 20th Anniversary Edition. Rochester, Vt.: Destiny Books, 2000.

Richardson, Diana. *The Heart of Tantric Sex: A Unique Guide to Love and Sexual Fulfilment.* Arlesford, U.K.: 'O' Books 2002. (First published in 1999 as *The Love Keys: The Art of Ecstatic Sex.*) Translated into German, Spanish, Italian, French, Chinese. Excerpt and further information: www.love4couples.com. Available from oshoviha@oshoviha.org, www.oshoviha.org.

Books and Resources on the Sympto-Thermal Fertility Awareness Method

Fuller, Rose and Rev. J. Huneger. *A Couple's Guide to Fertility: The Complete Sympto-Thermal Method.* Portland, Oregon: Northwest Family Services, 1996. www.nwfs.org

Kippley, John F. and Sheila K. Kippley. *The Art of Natural Family Planning.* Cincinnati, Ohio: The Couple to Couple League International, 1997. See www.ccli.org

Weschler, Toni. *Taking Charge of Your Fertility: The Definitive Guide to Natural Birth Control, Pregnancy Achievement and Reproductive Health.* New York: Quill-HarperCollins, 1995. www.TCOYF.org

A new book is due out soon by the British Fertility Awareness Organisation. See www.fertilityuk.org for more information about its release.

If you would like to contact the sympto-thermal experts who contributed their expertise to the appendix, feel free to e-mail, phone, or fax them using the contact information provided below:

R. Harri Wettstein, PhD, MBA, MA, Director of Bioself SA, Geneva, Switzerland, www.bioself.com., and Secretary of SymptoTherm Foundation, Grand-Rue 41-CH-1110, Morges, Switzerland, e-mail info<@>symptotherm.ch, phone/fax +41 21 802 44 18, www.symptotherm.ch

Christine Bourgeois, President of SymptoTherm Foundation, 8 Sécheron, CH-1132 Lully, Switzerland, phone/fax +41 21 802 37 35, email c.bourgeois@swissonline.ch, symptotherm.ch, www.symptotherm.ch

"Making Love"
A Tantra Meditation Retreat for Couples

The author (also known as Puja) and her partner, Raja,
facilitate week-long meditation retreats and
guide couples into the art of tantra.

For further information and further communication:
www.love4couples.com
www.livinglove.com

TANTRIC SEX FOR LOVERS

A Complete Guide to Tantric Sex in an Illustrated 3-Volume Boxed Set

Renowned tantric sex teachers Diana and Michael Richardson present practices to help couples learn how to keep their sex life sustainable, fulfilling, and enjoyable for decades.

Includes *Tantric Orgasm for Women*, *Tantric Sex for Men*, and *Slow Sex*

In *Tantric Orgasm for Women* Diana explores Tantra from the female perspective, revealing how relaxation is the key to achieving deep orgasmic states. She looks at how receptive feminine energy influences the male-female exchange and the role of the clitoris, breasts, and vagina in achieving orgasm.

In *Tantric Sex for Men*, Diana and Michael show men how to move beyond goal-oriented sex and relax into sex as a meditative union. They include foreplay approaches, explore the benefits of deep sustained penetration, and explain how to perform soft penetration and avoid premature ejaculation.

Slow Sex is a step-by-step guide for committed couples to awaken the body's innate mechanism for ecstasy and pleasure and help create a deep and restoring love. With illustrations of various positions for eye contact, deep penetration, and soft penetration, Diana shows how the practice of slow sex can also provide a vehicle to achieve higher consciousness.

These three books enable committed couples to develop a personal tantric sex practice, enrich their relationship, and harness the power of sex to access extraordinary realms of sensitivity, sensuality, and higher consciousness.

DIANA RICHARDSON, a pioneer of the Slow Sex movement, is a disciple of tantric master Osho and a teacher of holistic massage and deep tissue rebalancing. She is the author of 8 books across her more than 35 years of involvement in holistic bodywork and tantric wisdom, including *Tantric Sex and Menopause*. **MICHAEL RICHARDSON** is a teacher of t'ai chi, practitioner of shiatsu, teacher of the Gurdjieff Sacred Dances, and a disciple of tantric master Osho. Together, Diana and Michael have been teaching the art of Tantra and guiding couples in the art of slow, conscious sex in their life-changing weeklong "Making Love Retreats" since 1995. They live in Switzerland.

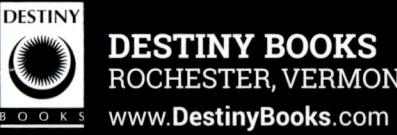

DESTINY BOOKS
ROCHESTER, VERMONT
www.DestinyBooks.com

ISBN 978-1-64411-956-3

55000

9 781644 119563